The Greenberg Rapid Review

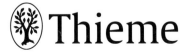

The Greenberg Rapid Review

A Companion to the 8th Edition

Leonard I. Kranzler, MD, JD, FACS, FAANS
Clinical Professor of Surgery (Neurosurgery)
University of Chicago
Chicago, Illinois

Jonathan G. Hobbs, MD
Resident Neurosurgeon
University of Chicago
Chicago, Illinois

Thieme
New York • Stuttgart • Delhi • Rio de Janeiro

Executive Editor: Timothy Y. Hiscock
Managing Editor: Judith Tomat
Director, Editorial Services: Mary Jo Casey
Production Editor: Naamah Schwartz
International Production Director: Andreas Schabert
Vice President, Editorial and E-Product Development: Vera Spillner
International Marketing Director: Fiona Henderson
International Sales Director: Louisa Turrell
Director of Sales, North America: Mike Roseman
Senior Vice President and Chief Operating Officer: Sarah Vanderbilt
President: Brian D. Scanlan

Library of Congress Cataloging-in-Publication Data

Names: Kranzler, Leonard I., author. | Hobbs, Jonathan G., author.
Title: The Greenberg rapid review: a companion to the 8th edition / Leonard I. Kranzler, MD, JD, RACS, FAANS,
    Clinical Professor of Surgery (Neurosurgery), University of Chicago, Chicago, Illinois, Jonathan G. Hobbs, MD,
    Resident Neurosurgeon, University of Chicago, Chicago, Illinois.
Description: New York : Thieme, [2017] | A companion to: Handbook of neurosurgery. 8th ed., c2017. |
    Includes bibliographical references and index. | Description based on print version record and CIP data
    provided by publisher; resource not viewed.
Identifiers: LCCN 2016037898 (print) | LCCN 2016035166 (ebook) | ISBN 9781626232075 |
    ISBN 9781626232068 (pbk.)
Subjects: LCSH: Nervous system–Surgery–Examinations, questions, etc.
Classification: LCC RD593 (print) | LCC RD593 .G677 2017 Suppl. (ebook) | DDC 617.4/80076–dc23
LC record available at https://lccn.loc.gov/2016037898

Thieme Medical Publishers, Inc.
333 Seventh Avenue, New York, NY 10001 USA
+1 800 782 3488, customerservice@thieme.com

Thieme Publishers Stuttgart
Rüdigerstrasse 14, 70469 Stuttgart, Germany
+49 [0]711 8931 421, customerservice@thieme.de

Thieme Publishers Delhi
A-12, Second Floor, Sector-2, Noida-201301
Uttar Pradesh, India
+91 120 45 566 00, customerservice@thieme.in

Thieme Publishers Rio de Janeiro, Thieme Publicações Ltda.
Edifício Rodolpho de Paoli, 25º andar
Av. Nilo Peçanha, 50 – Sala 2508,
Rio de Janeiro 20020-906 Brasil
+55 21 3172-2297 / +55 21 3172-1896

Cover design: Thieme Publishing Group
Typesetting by Friedhelm Hübner Electronic Publishing GmbH

Printed in The United States of America by Sheridan Press 5 4 3 2 1

ISBN 978-1-62623-206-8

Also available as an e-book:
eISBN 978-1-62623-207-5

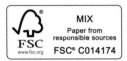

In appreciation for their example of scholarship, tradition, and love of family, this book is dedicated to the memory of:

Mr. Morris Kranzler
Mr. Louis Weinberg
Mr. Max Goldstein
Dr. K. Jeffery Kranzler
Mr. Charles Kranzler
Dr. Gershon Kranzler
Rabbi Alex Weisfogel
Mr. Nate Blum
Mr. Henry Kranzler
Mr. Harvey Goldstein
Mrs. Luiza Anghelo
Mr. Yerachmiel Kranzler
Mrs. Ruth Yudkofsky

Mr. Ben Teichner
Dr. David Kranzler
Mr. Alex Angheluta
Mr. Milton Saltzman
Mr. David Hurwitz
Mr. Kurt Loebenberg
Mr. Joseph Kranzler
Mr. Walter Rosenbush
Mr. Steve Rotter
Mr. Tobey Friedman
Mr. Python Anghelo
Mr. Arthur Kranzler

Mrs. Eva Teichner
Mrs. Ada Rotter
Mrs. Rina Rosenbush
Mrs. Dina Weinberg
Mrs. Chana Kranzler
Mrs. Rose Hurwitz
Mrs. Ruth Kranzler
Mrs. Helen Goldstein
Mrs. Betty Blum
Mrs. Rosalie Goldstein
Mrs. Eveline Kranzler
Mrs. Miriam Saltzman

In appreciation of my parents, Lillian (obm) and George Kranzler (obm).
And to my wife Uliana and children, Jenelle, Justin, and Jared.

Leonard I. Kranzler

No accomplishment would be possible without the unwavering and selfless love of my family, allowing me to pursue my aspirations and dreams without limits. They are the ones who made this possible. My friends and mentors who provide guidance, support, and an often needed voice of reason; I am grateful for all that you do. It is for my family, friends, and the countless others who are yet to be named, that I strive to be a better physician and most importantly, a better person. Thank you all.

Jonathan G. Hobbs

Below is a quote from Walden, a book that has provided inspiration, fostered self-reflection and a deeper understanding of what my family and friends mean to me, and how I want to approach life. It is my hope that these words will speak to you too, even in some minute way, that may give you hope and reason in those dark times we all face during our journey to become the person we want to be.

"I went to the woods because I wished to live deliberately, to front only the essential facts of life, and see if I could not learn what it had to teach, and not, when I came to die, discover that I had not lived. I did not wish to live what was not life, living is so dear; nor did I wish to practice resignation, unless it was quite necessary. I wanted to live deep and suck out all the marrow of life, to live so sturdily and Spartan-like as to put to rout all that was not life, to cut a broad swath and shave close, to drive life into a corner, and reduce it to its lowest terms."

— Henry David Thoreau, Walden: Or, Life in the Woods

Contents

Preface

This offering is a study and review aid. It is to be used in conjunction with *Handbook of Neurosurgery, Eighth Edition*, by Mark S. Greenberg. It permits the user, after reading a page, section, or chapter in Greenberg, to test retention of the details of that portion. Every question is directly referenced to Greenberg's text, where background information and context is readily available. An effort has been made to highlight the important facts in neurosurgical practice by posing questions to the reader that forces active involvement in the learning and review process.

The purpose of this textbook is to make clinicians aware of what they should expect to know using a rapid review format. It will help identify for readers what they already know as well as what is not known and provide a method by which an individual can verify the fact that has been learned. The reader can also have confidence that what has been highlighted as valuable has been identified by peers and by an editor who has been involved in neurosurgical education as coordinator of the Chicago Review Course in Neurological Surgery since 1974. Many questions were contributed by enrollees in the Chicago Review Course in Neurological Surgery as well as by young neurosurgeons and neurologists. In a nutshell, individuals at all levels of neurosurgical and neurological sophistication have contributed to this book.

It is expected that the reader will review the material multiple times until success in responding to the questions has been achieved. The question formats take advantage of the established ideas in learning theory:

- complex subjects broken into small bits
- fill-in-the-gap exercises in sentences and words
- progressive withdrawal of cues forcing the user to recall more and more of the details
- mnemonics or hints (some material has been arranged in "study charts" to aid mnemonic teaching techniques)
- Humor
- alternate arrangements of the material (the same facts presented in different formats)
- repetition

Moreover, this study guide is designed with answers appearing directly after the questions (we recommend that users cover the answers in the outer page margin) so that time is not wasted searching for correct answers at the back of the book. This format should further facilitate rapid review.

Please note that literature references and the index are present in the parent volume, *Handbook of Neurosurgery, Eighth Edition*.

Knowledge of this material demonstrated by correct responses to the questions can give confidence to the reader that much of the current scientific foundation of the specialty of neurosurgery has been mastered. This reassurance of a strong, up-to-date knowledge base should be helpful to the resident, the instructor, the neurosurgeon, and those who are planning to take written, oral, or recertification examinations.

Note to the Reader

Please call to our attention any mistakes that you identify. Please suggest any additional mnemonic devices that might help others in the field of neurosurgery. Be aware that medical knowledge is ever changing and that some items and opinions conveyed in these pages are controversial.

Leonard I. Kranzler
Jonathan G. Hobbs

Contact the authors at
KranzlerMD@gmail.com
jonathanhobbs@gmail.com

Acknowledgments

We acknowledge the cooperation and encouragement of Dr. Mark S. Greenberg. Our generation of neurosurgeons is fortunate that Dr. Greenberg has collated the literature of our field and presented it to us in such a concise, authoritative, well-balanced, and wise manner.

We also thank our contributors and the team of Thieme who helped us so much.

Special Acknowledgment

It has been a pleasure to work with and have the collective experience of our contributors. They have been insightful in their choice of questions, prompt and efficient, and fully cooperative. We thank each of you. For more details on the specific work of our contributors, please contact jonathanhobbs@gmail.com.

Uchenna Ajoku, MD
University of Port Harcourt Teaching Hospital
Port Harcourt, Nigeria

Jason L. Choi, MD
University of Chicago
Chicago, Illinois

Bhargav D. Desai, BS
University of Illinois-Chicago College of
Medicine
Chicago, Illinois

J. Palmer Greene, BA
University of Chicago Pritzker School of
Medicine
Chicago, Illinois

Dominic A. Harris, MD
University of New Mexico
Albuquerque, New Mexico

Jordan Lebovic, BA
Harvard Medical School
Boston, Massachusetts

Yimo Lin, MD
Oregon Health and Science University
Portland, Oregon

Raisa C. Martinez Martinez, MD
University of Chicago
Chicago, Illinois

Ryan A. McDermott, MD
University of Texas at San Antonio
San Antonio, Texas

Jose M. Morales, MD MSc
University of Chicago
Chicago, Illinois

Ramin A. Morshed, MD
University of California, San Francisco
San Francisco, California

Andrew W. Platt, MD, MBA
University of Chicago
Chicago, Illinois

Sean P. Polster, MD
University of Chicago
Chicago, Illinois

Sophia F. Shakur, MD
University of Chicago
Chicago, Illinois

Jacob S. Young, BS
University of Chicago Pritzker School of
Medicine
Chicago, Illinois

1

Gross Anatomy, Cranial, and Spinal

■ Cortical Surface Anatomy

1. Characterize the lateral cortical surface.   1.1.1

a. The pre-central sulcus is not_____.   complete

b. The middle frontal gyrus connects with   precentral, isthmus
the _____gyrus via a thin _____.

c. The central sulcus is separated from the   98%
sylvian fissure ___% of the time.

d. The tissue separating them is called the   subcentral gyrus
_____ _____.

e. The inferior and superior parietal lobules   intraparietal
are separated by the _____ sulcus.

f. The inferior parietal lobule is composed
of

   i.   the _____ _____   supramarginal gyrus (SMG)

   ii. and the_____ _____.   angular gyrus

g. The sylvian fissure

   i.   terminates in the_____,   SMG

   ii. which is the Brodmann area #___.   40

h. The superior temporal gyrus

   i.   terminates in the____,   AG

   ii. which is the Brodmann area #___.   39

**2. Complete the following regarding   1.1.1
surface anatomy:**

a. The middle frontal gyrus often connects   precentral gyrus
with the _____ _____.

b. The central sulcus joins the sylvian   2
fissure in only___%.

c. A sub-central sulcus is present in___% of   98
patients.

d. The sylvian fissure terminates in the   supramarginal gyrus
_____ _____.

e. The superior temporal sulcus is capped   angular gyrus
by the_____ _____.

3. **Matching. Match the following Brodmann cortical areas and their functional significance:**   1.1.2

Functional significance:
① primary motor cortex; ② Broca's area (motor speech); ③ Wernicke's area in the dominant hemisphere; ④ primary auditory area; ⑤ frontal eye fields; ⑥ primary somatosensory area; ⑦ premotor area; ⑧ primary visual cortex
Area: (a–h) below

a.	Area 3, 1, 2	⑥
b.	Area 41, 42	④
c.	Area 4	①
d.	Area 6	⑦
e.	Area 44	②
f.	Area 17	⑧
g.	Area 40, 39	③
h.	Area 8	⑤

4. **Complete the following regarding pars marginalis:**   1.1.3

a.	Is the terminal part of the _____ sulcus.	cingulate
b.	Is visible on axial view in___% of CTs and ___% of MRIs.	95%, 97%
c.	Is the_____ _____ of the middle paired grooves straddling the midline.	most prominent
d.	Extends into the hemispheres. On axial CT it is located just posterior to the widest_____ _____.	biparietal diameter
e.	It curves_____ in lower slices.	posteriorly
f.	It curves_____ in higher slices.	anteriorly

■ Central Sulcus on Axial Imaging

5. **Complete the following regarding central sulcus:**   1.2

a.	Is visible in almost___%.	95%
b.	Does it reach the midline?	no
c.	Terminates in the_____ _____.	paracentral lobule

■ Surface Anatomy of the Cranium

6. **True or False. The pterion is a region where each of the following bones comes together:**   1.3.1

a.	frontal	true
b.	sphenoid (greater wing)	true
c.	parietal	true
d.	temporal	true
e.	sphenoid (lesser wing)	false

7. **Matching. Match the bones/sutures that form the listed craniometric points.**   1.3.1
Bone/suture:
① lambdoid suture; ② occipitomastoid suture; ③ parietomastoid suture;
④ frontal; ⑤ parietal; ⑥ temporal;
⑦ greater wing sphenoid
Craniometric point:
a. asterion   ①, ②, ③
b. pterion   ④, ⑤, ⑥, ⑦

8. **True or False. The name of the junction of lambdoid, occipitomastoid, and parietomastoid sutures is**   1.3.1
a. pterion   false
b. asterion   true (Asterion is the junction of the lambdoid, occipitomastoid and parietomastoid suture.)
c. lambda   false
d. stephanion   false
e. glabella   false
f. opisthion   false

9. **The asterion junction overlies the**   1.3.1
a. ____sinus and the   transverse
b. ____sinus.   sigmoid

10. **Describe the visible landmarks of Taylor-Haughton lines.**   1.3.2
Bone/suture:
① Frankfurt plane (AKA: baseline);
② posterior ear line; ③ condylar line
a. perpendicular to the baseline through mastoid process   ②
b. perpendicular to the baseline through mandibular condyle   ③
c. inferior margin of orbit →upper margin of the external auditory meatus   ①

11. **The external landmark for the Sylvian fissure is a line from the lateral canthus to a spot three quarters of the way posterior along an arc running over the convexity in the midline from the _____ to the _____.**   nasion; inion   1.3.2

1

12. True or False. In relation to external landmarks the angular gyrus is   1.3.2

a. one finger's breadth above the zygomatic arch.   false

b. just above the pinna.   true (The angular gyrus is just above the pinna and important as part of Wernicke's area in the dominant hemisphere.)

c. a thumb's breadth behind the frontal process of the zygomatic bone.   false

d. at the junction of the lambdoid and sagittal suture.   false

13. True or False. The motor strip of the motor cortex lies   1.3.2

a. at the level of the coronal suture.   false

b. within 2 cm of the coronal suture.   false

c. 3 to 4 cm posterior to the coronal suture.   false

d. 4 to 5.4 cm posterior to the coronal suture.   true

e. 2 cm posterior to the mid-position of the nasion-inion arc.   true

f. 5 cm straight up from the external auditory meatus.   true

14. True or False. In the non-hydrocephalic adult the lateral ventricles lie   1.3.3

a. 2 to 3 cm below the outer skull surface.   false

b. 3 to 4 cm below the outer skull surface.   false

c. 4 to 5 cm below the outer skull surface.   true

d. 5 to 6 cm below the outer skull surface.   false

15. True or False. In the non-hydrocephalic adult the anterior horns extend   1.3.3

a. 1 to 2 cm anterior to the foramen of Monro.   false

b. 2.5 cm anterior to the foramen of Monro.   true

c. 3 to 4 cm anterior to the foramen of Monro.   false

16. True or False. The fastigium is located at   1.3.3

a. the midpoint of the Twining's line.   false

b. the floor of the fourth ventricle.   false

c. the apex of the fourth ventricle within the cerebellum.   true (The fastigium is the apex of the fourth ventricle in the cerebellum.)

d. 1 to 2 cm anterior to the coronal suture.   false

17. **List the surface landmarks of the following cervical levels:**   Table 1.4
    a. C3-4_____ _____   hyoid bone
    b. C4-5_____ _____   thyroid cartilage
    c. C5-6_____ _____   cricothyroid membrane
    d. C6-7_____ _____   cricoid cartilage

18. **Matching. Match the following surface landmarks and cervical levels:**   1.3.3

    Surface landmark:
    ① level of thyroid cartilage; ② cricoid cartilage; ③ angle of mandible; ④ cricothyroid membrane; ⑤ carotid tubercle; ⑥ 1 cm above thyroid cartilage (hyoid bone)
    Cervical level: (a-f) below
    a. C1-2   ③
    b. C3-4   ⑥
    c. C4-5   ①
    d. C5-6   ④
    e. C6   ⑤
    f. C6-7   ②

■ Cranial Foramina and their Contents

19. **Matching. Match the foramen with contents (choices may be used more than once).**   1.5.1
    Contents:
    ① nothing; ② middle meningeal artery; ③ VII facial; ④ V2; ⑤ V3; ⑥ V1; ⑦ IX, X, XI
    Foramen: (a-h) below
    a. superior orbital fissure   ⑥
    b. inferior orbital fissure   ④
    c. foramen lacerum   ①
    d. foramen rotundum   ④
    e. foramen ovale   ⑤
    f. foramen spinosum   ②
    g. stylomastoid foramen   ③
    h. jugular foramen   ⑦

20. **List the cranial nerves and the three branches of one found within the superior orbital fissure (SOF).**   1.5.1
    a. o_____   CN III oculomotor
    b. t_____   IV trochlear
    c. n_____   nasociliary nerve
    d. f_____   frontal nerve ophthalmic
                          division: all three branches
    e. l_____   lacrimal nerve
    f. a_____   VI abducens nerve

1

21. **List the other contents of the superior orbital fissure (SOF).**   1.5.1
a. s_____ o_____ v_____.   superior ophthalmic vein
b. r_____ m_____ a_____.   recurrent meningeal artery
c. which arises from the l____ artery.   lacrimal
d. o ____ b____ of the m____ m____   orbital branch of the middle
   a_____.   meningeal artery
e. s____ p____ of the ICA   sympathetic plexus of the ICA

22. **Another name for the transverse crest is _____ _____.**   crista falciformis   1.5.2

23. **Another name for the vertical crest is _____ _____.**   Bill's bar   1.5.2

24. **Draw and label the nerves in the right porus acusticus.**   1.5.2

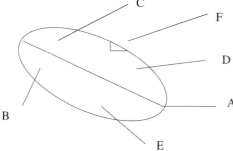

a. Bill's bar
b. Transverse crest crista falciformis
c. CN VII
d. SV—superior vestibular
e. CN VIII
f. IV—inferior vestibular

Fig. 1.1

25. **Label the diagram of the right internal auditory canal.**   1.5.2

a. Transverse crest
b. Acoustic portion of CN VIII
c. CN VII in facial canal
d. Superior vestibular nerve
e. Inferior vestibular nerve
f. Bill's bar—vertical crest

Fig. 1.2

26. **Matching. Match the nerves of the IAC**   1.5.2
    with the areas that they serve.
    Nerves:
    ① facial n.; ② nervus intermedius;
    ③ acoustic portion of VIII n.; ④ superior
    branch of vestibular n.; ⑤ inferior branch
    of vestibular n.
    Areas served: (a-h) below
    a. facial muscles   ①
    b. hair follicles   ②
    c. taste buds   ②
    d. hearing   ③
    e. utricle   ④
    f. superior semicircular canal   ④
    g. lateral semicircular canal   ④
    h. saccule   ⑤

■ Internal Capsule

27. **Most internal capsule lesions are**   thrombosis or hemorrhage   1.6.1
    caused by _____ or _____.

28. **Name the vascular supply for the**   1.6.2
    following components of the internal
    capsule:
    a. anterior limb   lateral striate branches of
                                  MCA
    b. posterior limb   lateral striate branches of
                                  MCA
    c. ventral posterior limb   anterior choroidal
    d. genu   direct branches of ICA
    e. optic radiations   anterior choroidal

29. **Name four thalamic peduncles and**   1.6.2
    where their radiations go.
    a. a____, f____ l____   anterior, frontal lobe
    b. s____, p____ g____   superior, postcentral gyrus
    c. p____, o____ & p____ a____ posterior, occipital & parietal
                                   areas
    d. i____, a____ a____   inferior, auditory area

1

30. **Draw the internal capsule and label which blood vessel serves which area.**
Hint: MIMA

1.6.2

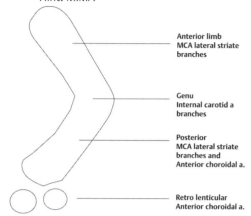

Anterior limb
MCA lateral striate branches

Genu
Internal carotid a branches

Posterior
MCA lateral striate branches and
Anterior choroidal a.

Retro lenticular
Anterior choroidal a.

Fig. 1.3

31. **Matching. Match the area in the internal capsule with its function.**

1.6.2

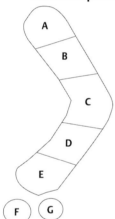

Fig. 1.4

Function: (a-d) below

a. Movement of face
b. Movement of foot
c. Vision
d. Hearing

C   genu
D   posterior limb
F   lateral geniculate
G   medial geniculate

■ Occipitoatlantoaxial-Complex Anatomy

32. **Matching. Match the ligaments of the occipito-atlantoaxial complex with the statements below.**
    Ligaments:
    ① apical; ② alar; ③ cruciate;
    ④ ascending portion; ⑤ descending portion; ⑥ transverse portion;
    ⑦ posterior longitudinal; ⑧ tectorial;
    ⑨ anterior longitudinal; ⑩ anterior atlanto-occipital
    Statements: (a-k) below   1.8

   a. Attaches the odontoid to the foramen magnum. ①
   b. Attaches the odontoid to the occipital condyle. ②
   c. Attaches the odontoid to the lateral mass of C1. ②
   d. Attaches C1 to the clivus and to C2. ③
   e. Attaches odontoid to clivus. ④
   f. Attaches C1 to C2. ⑤
   g. Traps the odontoid against the atlas. ⑥
   h. Extends cephalad to become the tectorial. ⑦
   i. Is the cephalad extension of the PLL. ⑧
   j. Extends cephalad to become the anterior atlanto-occipital. ⑨
   k. The cephalad extension of the anterior longitudinal ligament. ⑩

33. **The most important spinal ligaments in maintaining atlanto-occipital stability are the**   1.8
   a. _____ membrane and the   tectorial
   b. _____ ligaments.   alar

■ Spinal Cord Anatomy

34. **The dentate ligament**   1.9.1
   a. separates _____   dorsal
   b. from _____ roots in the spinal nerves.   ventral

35. **Which cranial nerve lies dorsal to the dentate ligament?**   CN XI spinal accessory   1.9.1

36. **How is the lateral spinothalamic tract (LST) somatotopically organized?**   Fig. 1.13
   a. Cervical is _____.   medial
   b. Sacral is _____.   lateral

37. **Which descending motor tract facilitates**   Table 1.7
   a. extensor tone?   vestibulospinal tract
   b. flexor tone?   rubrospinal tract

38. **The very large ascending tract closest to the dentate ligament is the _____ _____ _____.**

lateral spinothalamic tract (LST) (for pain and temperature from the opposite side of the body)

Table 1.9

39. **Matching. Match sensory function and anatomy.**
Sensory function:
① pain and temperature: body; ② fine touch, deep pressure and proprioception: body; ③ light (crude) touch: body
Anatomy: (a-i) below

1.9.2

a. Receptors
    i.   Free nerve ending — ①
    ii. Meissner's and Pacinian corpuscles — ②-③
b. First order neurons
    i.   Small — ①
    ii. Heavily myelinated — ②-③
    iii. Finely myelinated — ①
    iv. Large — ②
c. Soma in dorsal root ganglion — ①-②-③
d. Enter cord at
    i.   zone of Lissauer — ①
    ii. ipsilateral posterior columns — ②-③
e. Synapse in
    i.   Rexed layer II — ①
    ii. Rexed layer III and IV — ②
    iii. Rexed layer VI and VII — ③
f. Second order neurons
    i.   cross obliquely in anterior white commissure — ①-③
    ii. form the internal arcuate fibers — ②
g. and enter the
    i.   lateral spino-thalamic tract. — ①
    ii. medial lemniscus. — ②
    iii. anterior spinothalamic tract. — ③
h. Second order neurons synapse on the ventral posterior lateral nucleus of the thalamus. — ①-②-③
i. Third order neurons pass through IC to postcentral gyrus. — ①-②-③

40. **List the body area with the appropriate root.**

Fig. 1.14

a. Nipple, root: _____   T4
b. Umiblicus, root: _____   T10
c. Inguinal crease, root: _____   T12
d. Anterior thigh, root: _____   L2-L3
e. Posterior thigh, root: _____   S1
f. Lateral calf, root: _____   L5
g. Medial calf, root: _____   L4
h. Posterior calf, root: _____   S1
i. Big toe, root: _____   L5
j. Little toe, root: _____   S1

k. Sole of foot, root: _____   S1
l. Lateral shoulder, root: _____   C5
m. Lateral forearm, root: _____   C6
n. Thumb, root: _____   C6
o. Middle finger, root: _____   C7
p. Little finger, root: _____   C8
q. Medial forearm, root: _____   T1

**41. Complete the following regarding
upper extremity vs. trunk
dermatomes. Trunk sensory level is
reported at T3 on a trauma patient.**

Fig. 1.14

a. This is a little _____ the clavicle.   below
b. You must check the _____   arm
    dermatomes.
c. Dermatomes _____ to _____ are not   C5 to T2
    represented on the trunk.

2

Vascular Anatomy

■ Cerebral Vascular Territories

1. Cerebral vascular territories: Fig. 2.1
a. Anterior cerebral artery: frontal lobe and   caudate
   _____.
b. Posterior cerebral artery: occipital lobe   thalamus
   and _____.
c. Anterior choroidal artery: internal   optic tract
   capsule, medial globus pallidus, and
   _____ _____.
d. _____ _____ artery supplies   Middle cerebral
   the rest.

■ Cerebral Arterial Anatomy

2. Circle of Willis: 2.2.2
a. Intact in _____%.   18%
b. Hypoplasia of at least one of the   22-32%
   posterior communicating arteries occurs
   in ____ - ____%.
c. Absent or hypoplastic A1 occurs in   25%
   _____%.

3. Segments of the ICA: 2.2.3
a. Name the 7 segments of the ICA. (Hint:
   can **P**eter **l**augh **c**an **C**harlie **o**nly **c**lap)
   i.   c_____   cervical
   ii.   p_____   petrous
   iii. l_____   lacerum
   iv.   c_____   cavernous
   v.   c_____   clinoid
   vi.   o_____   ophthalmic
   vii. c_____   communicating

b. Now also name the main branches of   2.2.4
    each segment.
    i.   C1 c_____, no _____   cervical, branches
    ii. C2 p_____   petrous
    iii. C3 l_____   lacerum
    iv. C4 c_____   cavernous
         m_____ t_____   meningohypophyseal trunk
         a_____ m_____   anterior meningeal artery
         a_____
    v.   C5 c_____   clinoidal
    vi. C6 o_____   ophthalmic
         o_____ a_____   ophthalmic artery
         s_____ h_____ a_____   superior hypophyseal artery
         p_____ c_____ a_____   posterior communicating
                                                artery
         a_____ c_____ a_____   anterior choroidal artery
    vii. C7 c_____ a_____ divides   communicating artery
         into
         A_____   ACA
         M_____   MCA

4. **Name the branches of the**   2.2.4
    meningohypophyseal trunk:
    (Hint: dit)
    a. d_____ _____   dorsal meningeal
    b. i_____ _____   inferior hypophyseal
    c. t_____ _____   tentorial artery (artery of
                                                Bernasconi and Cassinari)

5. **Complete the following:**   2.2.4
    a. Occlusion of the i_____   inferior hypophyseal;
        h_____ artery results in _____ Sheehan's
        necrosis.
    b. This artery supplies the _____.   posterior lobe of pituitary
    c. It is a branch of the _____ artery. meningohypophyseal
    d. Occlusion usually occurs in _____ post-partum
        patients.

6. **Complete the following about the**   2.2.4
    ophthalmic artery:
    a. It arises from the _____ segment of 6th
        the ICA.
    b. _____% distal to cavernous   89%
        segment.
    c. _____% within cavernous segment.   8%
    d. Shape on lateral angiogram is   bayonet-like kink
        _____.

7. **Complete the following about the anterior choroidal artery:**   2.2.4

a. Name the 7 structures that it supplies. (Hint: gogoupl)

i.	g_____ p_____	globus pallidus
ii.	o_____ t_____	optic tract
iii.	g_____ of i_____ c_____	genu; internal capsule
iv.	o_____ r_____	optic radiations
v.	u_____	uncus
vi.	p_____ l_____ of i_____ c_____	posterior limb; internal capsule
vii.	l_____ g_____ b_____	lateral geniculate body

b. Occlusion may produce (Hint: 3Hs) _____, _____, and _____. hemiplegia, hemihypesthesia; homonymous hemianopsia

8. **Posterior communicating artery:**   2.2.4

a. _____ segment enters supracornual recess of the _____ _____ to supply _____ _____.   Plexal; temporal horn; choroid plexus

b. Origin is proximal to _____ _____ artery.   anterior choroidal

c. Larger than _____ _____ artery.   anterior choroidal

d. Anterior choroidal artery has hump, or _____ _____, where it passes through _____ _____ to enter the _____.   plexal point; choroidal fissure; ventricle

e. Travels between cranial nerves _____ and _____.   II, III

9. **Carotid siphon:**   2.2.4

a. Begins at the posterior bend of the _____ ICA and ends at the ICA _____.   cavernous; bifurcation

b. It includes 3 segments: ca_____, op_____, and co_____.   cavernous, ophthalmic; communicating

10. **External carotid artery:**   2.2.4

a. It lies _____ and _____ to the ICA.   anterior; lateral

b. Name its branches from proximal to distal. (Hint: salfopsmax)

i.	s_____ _____	superior thyroid
ii.	a_____ _____	ascending pharyngeal
iii.	l_____	lingual
iv.	f_____	facial
v.	o_____	occipital
vi.	p_____ _____	posterior auricular
vii.	s_____ _____	superficial temporal
viii.	i_____ m_____	internal maxillary

11. Recurrent artery of Heubner: 2.2.4
  a. Typically arises in area of _____   A1/2
     junction.
  b. Supplies h_____ of c_____,   head; caudate; putamen;
     p_____, and a_____   anterior internal capsule
     i_____ c_____.

12. Posterior circulation: 2.2.4
  a. _____% of patients have a   15-35%; fetal
     _____ circulation
  b. where PCA is supplied via _____   p-comm; vertebrobasilar
     instead of the _____ system.

13. Vertebral artery: 2.2.4
  a. The first segment enters the _____   sixth
     foramen transversarium.
  b. The second ascends _____ within   vertically
     the foramina transversaria.
  c. The second turns _____ as it exits   laterally
     the axis.
  d. The third curves _____ and   posteriorly; medially
     _____.
  e. The fourth pierces the _____.   dura
  f. Right and left vertebral arteries join at   lower pons; basilar
     the level of the l_____ p_____
     to form the _____ artery.
  g. Name its 6 branches. (Hint: **A** post**m**an
     puts **p**ostcards **a**way)
     i.   a_____ m_____   anterior meningeal
     ii. p_____ m_____   posterior meningeal
     iii. m_____   medullary
     iv. p_____ s_____   posterior spinal
     v.   p_____   PICA
     vi. a_____ s_____   anterior spinal

14. PICA: 2.2.4
  a. It arises _____ mm distal to the   10 mm
     point where the vertebral artery
     becomes intradural.
  b. Has an extradural origin in ____ - ____%.   5-8%
  c. Name the 5 segments.
     i.   a_____ m_____   anterior medullary
     ii. l_____ m_____   lateral medullary
     iii. t_____, contains _____   tonsillomedullary; caudal
          loop
     iv. t_____, contains _____   telovelotonsillary; cranial
          loop
     v.   c_____ s_____   cortical segments
  d. Name its 3 branches.
     i.   c_____   choroidal
     ii. t_____   tonsillohemispheric
     iii. i_____ v_____   inferior vermian

2

2

e.   The choroidal point on angiography is
     where the _____ artery enters the
     _____ _____ to supply the
     _____ _____.

choroidal;
4th ventricle;
choroid plexus

f.   The copular point on angiography is
     where the _____ _____ artery
     inflects _____.

inferior vermian;
inferiorly

15. **Posterior cerebral artery:**   2.2.4
  a.   Name the 3 segments.
       i.   P1 p_____
       ii.   P2 a_____
       iii. P3 q_____

peduncular
ambient
quadrigeminal

  b.   The medial posterior choroidal artery
       arises from the _____ or _____
       segment.

P1, P2

  c.   The lateral posterior choroidal artery
       arises from the _____ segment.

P2

  d.   Artery of Percheron is a _____
       anatomic variant where a _____
       trunk arises from _____ PCA to
       supply _____ paramedian thalami
       and rostral midbrain.

rare;
solitary;
one;
bilateral

16. **Persistent fetal anastomoses:**   2.2.4
  a.   There are _____ types.
  b.   They result from a failure to _____.
  c.   They include t_____, o_____,
       h_____, and p_____.
  d.   The most common type is _____.
  e.   The first type to involute is _____.

4
involute
trigeminal, otic, hypoglossal,
proatlantal
trigeminal
otic

■ Cerebral Venous Anatomy

17. **Cerebral venous anatomy:**   2.3.1
  a.   Dominance:
       i.   The _____ internal jugular vein
             is usually dominant.

right

       ii.   The _____ transverse sinus is
             usually dominant.

right

       iii. The _____ vertebral artery is
             usually dominant.

left

       iv.   The _____ vein of Labbé is
             usually dominant.

left

  b.   The main contributors to the vein of
       Galen are p_____ c_____ vein,
       b_____ vein of R_____, and
       i_____ c_____ vein.

precentral cerebellar;
basal vein of Rosenthal;
internal cerebral

  c.   The joining of the septal vein and
       thalamostriate vein with the internal
       cerebral vein forms an angiographic
       landmark called the v_____
       a_____ at the foramen of
       _____.

venous angle;
Monro

18. Cavernous sinus anatomy: 2.3.1

a. The cavernous sinus is a _____ of   plexus;
_____.   veins

b. Draw the right and left cavernous sinus
coronal view. On your drawing label the
following: 1. Oculomotor (III); 2.
Trochlear (IV); 3. Parkinson triangle; 4.
Ophthalmic (V1); 5. Maxillary (V2); 6.
Abducent (VI); 7. Carotid.

Fig. 2.1

c. Name 6 major contents of the cavernous   CN III, CN IV, CN V1, CN V2,
sinus.   CN VI, ICA

d. Cranial nerve _____ is the only   V2;
nerve of the cavernous sinus that doesn't   superior orbital fissure;
exit skull through _____ _____   foramen rotundum
_____; it exits through _____
_____.

e. Cranial nerve _____ is the only   VI;
nerve not attached to _____ dural   lateral
wall.

f. Parkinson triangle is bordered superiorly CN III and IV;
by _____ and _____ and   CN V1 and V2
inferiorly by _____ and _____.

■ Spinal Cord Vasculature

19. Spinal cord vasculature: 2.4

a. Supply of the cervical spinal cord comes   vertebral
from v_____ artery, d_____   deep cervical;
c_____ artery, and c_____   costocervical trunk
t_____.

b. Artery of _____ supplies spinal cord Adamkiewicz
from T8 to conus.

c. Artery of _____ is located on the   Adamkiewicz;
left in _____% and arises between   80%;
T9-L2 in _____%.   85%

d. _____ region is considered a   Midthoracic;
_____ zone and is thus more   watershed;
_____ to vascular insults.   susceptible

3

Neurophysiology and Regional Brain Syndromes

■ Neurophysiology

1. Answer the following concerning the blood-brain barrier (BBB):   3.1.1

a. What chemical opens the BBB?   Mannitol
b. What chemical closes the BBB?   Steroids
c. Which sites have no BBB? (Hint: pppcta)   Pituitary, pineal, preoptic recess, choroid plexus, tuber cinereum, area postrema
d. What pathology injures BBB? (Hint: histt)   Hepatic encephalopathy, infections, stroke, trauma, tumor

2. Complete the following statements about cerebral edema: 3.1.1

a. Cytotoxic
    i. occurs with h_____ i_____   head injury
    ii. occurs with h_____   hematoma
    iii. shape is c_____   circular
    iv. occurs with C_____   CVA
    v. BBB is c_____   closed
b. Vasogenic
    i. shape is _____   V-shaped (like fingers of white matter edema)
    ii. occurs with t_____   tumors
    iii. occurs with m_____   metastasis
    iv. treat with s_____   steroids
    v. with contrast it _____ and _____   enhances on CT and MR
    vi. BBB is o_____   open

3. Matching. Match the type of edema with the characteristics.   3.1.1
Type of edema: ① cytotoxic; ② vasogenic
Hint: cytotoxic—early letters of alphabet
vasogenic—later letters of alphabet
Characteristics: (a-l) below

a. BB disrupted   ②
b. BBB closed   ①
c. Head injury   ①

d. Tumor   ②
e. Enhances   ②
f. Does not enhance   ①
g. Not appropriate to use steroids   ①
h. Appropriate to use steroids   ②
i. Circular shape on MR   ①
j. V-shaped finger like extensions on MR   ②
k. Occurs with hematoma   ①
l. Occurs with CVA   ①

4. True or False. Cytotoxic edema has: 3.1.1
a. a disrupted BBB   false
b. expansion of the extracellular space   false
c. enhancement when contrast injected   false
d. no protein extravasation   true

5. Study Sheet.   3.1.1
a. Cytotoxic:
    i.   Closed BBB
    ii.   Head injury
    iii. Hematoma
    iv.   Circular shape
    v.   CVA
    vi.   Cells swell then shrink
b. Vasogenic:
    i.   Disrupted BBB
    ii.   Tumors
    iii. Metastasis
    iv.   Steroids
    v.   Protein extravasates
    vi.   Enhances on CT and MRI
    vii. Wide extracellular space
    viii. Stable cells

6. Fill in the blanks to complete the   3.1.2
    details of the Babinski reflex.
    (Hint: pcrstlpt)
a. lateral _____ stimulation   plantar
b. originates as a _____ _____   cutaneous reflex
c. and stimulates the _____   receptors
d. in the _____ dermatome   S1
e. that travel via the _____ _____   tibial nerve
f. to the spinal cord segments number   L4-S2; afferent
    _____ (_____ limb)
g. The efferent limb travels via the   peroneal
    _____ nerve
h. to the _____ _____   toe extensors

7. Summarize the Babinski sign.   3.1.2
a. receptor _____   S1 dermatome
b. afferent limb _____   tibial nerve
c. cord _____   L4-S2
d. efferent limb _____   peroneal nerve

3

3

8. **Fill in the blanks to complete the details of eliciting the plantar reflex.**   3.1.2
   a. Stimulate the _____ _____ surface   lateral plantar
   b. and the _____ _____   transverse arch
   c. in a _____ movement   single
   d. that lasts ____ - ___ seconds.   5 to 6
   e. Response consists of _____ of the _____ _____.   extension; great toe
   f. _____ of the small toes is   Fanning
   g. _____ clinically important.   not

9. **True or False. The Chaddock maneuver is described as**   3.1.2
   a. scratching the lateral foot   true
   b. pinching the Achilles tendon   false
   c. sliding knuckles down shin   false
   d. momentarily squeezing lower gastrocnemius   false

10. **Complete the following concerning Hoffman sign:**   3.1.2
    a. H (from Hoffman) is the _____ letter of the alphabet.   eighth
    b. If unilaterally present, Hoffman sign indicates a lesion above _____.   C8

11. **Complete the following concerning bladder physiology:**   3.1.3
    a. The primary coordinating center for bladder function is in the
       i. n_____ l_____ c_____   nucleus locus coeruleus
       ii. of the p_____.   pons
    b. This center coordinates
       i. b_____ c_____ (d_____)   bladder contraction (detrusor)
          with
       ii. s_____ r_____ (e_____ s_____).   sphincter relaxation (external sphincter)

12. **Voluntary cortical control**   3.1.3
    a. inhibits the p_____ c_____.   pontine center—nucleus locus coeruleus
    b. It originates in the
       i. a_____ f_____ l_____   anteromedial frontal lobes
       ii. and g_____ of the c_____ c_____ and   genu of the corpus callosum
    c. travels via the p_____ t_____   pyramidal tract
    d. to inhibit
       i. c_____ of the   contraction
       ii. d_____ and contraction   detrusor
       iii. of the e_____ s_____.   external sphincter

13. **Immaturity, infarct, or cortical lesions cause**   3.1.3
   a. inability to s_____   suppress
   b. the m_____ r_____   micturition reflex
   c. and result in i_____.   incontinence

14. **The efferents to the bladder**   3.1.3
   a. travel in the d_____ portion   dorsal
   b. of the l_____ c_____.   lateral columns

15. **Parasympathetic control**   3.1.3
   a. detrusor _____   contracts
   b. internal sphincter _____   relaxes
   c. travels via the p_____ s_____ nerves   pelvic splanchnic

16. **Somatic nerve**   3.1.3
   a. external sphincter _____   contracts
   b. maintains c_____   continence
   c. travels via p_____ nerve   pudendal

17. **Sympathetic nerve**   3.1.3
   a. provides bladder neck _____ and   closure
   b. travels via the i_____ h_____ plexus.   inferior hypogastric

18. **True or False. The detrusor muscle of the bladder contracts and the internal sphincter relaxes under**   3.1.3
   a. PNS stimulation   true (parasympathetic nervous system stimulation)
   b. somatic nerve stimulation   false
   c. sympathetic nervous system stimulation   false
   d. all of the above   false

19. **True or False. The following can cause detrusor hyperreflexia:**   3.1.3
   a. stroke   true
   b. spinal cord lesion (myelopathy)   true
   c. chronic bladder catheterization   false (Detrusor hyperreflexia can result from interruption of efferents anywhere from cortex to sacral cord.)
   d. multiple sclerosis   true
   e. Parkinson disease   true
   f. hydrocephalus   true
   g. dementia   true
   h. brain tumor   true

20. **True or False. Interruption of the efferents results in**   3.1.3
   a. atonic bladder   false—root lesion
   b. overflow incontinence   false—root lesion
   c. uncontrollable voiding   true
   d. reflex bladder emptying   true
   e. voiding triggered by critical volume   true

3

3

f. produced by myelopathy	true	
g. produced by head injury	true	
h. produced by certain drugs	false—detrusor areflexia	
i. produced by diabetes mellitus	false—automatic neuropathy	

21. **Loss of centrally mediated inhibition of the p_____ v_____ r_____ is mediated by supraspinal lesions.**
pontine voiding reflex
3.1.3

22. **The s_____ v_____ c_____ is located in the c_____ m_____, and results from lesions above the _____ spinal cord level, which correspond to _____ vertebral bodies.**
sacral voiding center;
conus medullaris;
S1;
T12/L1
3.1.3

23. **After acute suprasacral spinal cord injuries, there may be s_____ s_____, and as a result d_____ a_____.**
spinal shock;
detrusor areflexia
3.1.3

24. **When the spinal shock subsides, most develop _____ _____.**
detrusor hyperreflexia
3.1.3

25. **Match the injury to the etiology.**
Injury:
① suprasacral; ② infrasacral (below the S2 spinal cord level).
Etiologies: (a-d) below
    a. cauda equina
    b. conus medullaris injury
    c. transverse myelitis
    d. peripheral nerve injuries
②
①, ②
①
②
3.1.3

26. **Interruption of the p_____ r_____ a_____ may produce d_____ a_____.**
peripheral reflex arc;
detrusor areflexia
3.1.3

27. **Spinal stenosis urologic symptoms vary (detrusor hyperactivity or detrusor underactivity) and depend on the spinal level involved and the type of involvement depending on whether there is compression of the i_____ r_____ t_____ or m_____ involving the p_____ f_____.**
inhibitory reticulospinal tracts;
myelopathy;
posterior funiculus
3.1.3

28. **Cauda equina syndrome usually produces u_____ r_____, although o_____ i_____ may occur.**
urinary retention;
overflow incontinence
3.1.3

29. **P_____ n_____ usually produce impaired detrusor activity.**
peripheral neuropathies
3.1.3

30. N_____ d_____ patients have an areflexic bladder neck.

neurospinal dysraphism

3.1.3

31. True or False. Patients with multiple sclerosis develop voiding symptoms from demyelination primarily involving the

3.1.3

a. posterior and lateral columns of lumbar spinal cord.

false

b. lateral column of cervical spine.

false

c. posterior column of lumbar spine.

false

d. lateral column of lumbar spine.

false

e. posterior and lateral columns of cervical spinal cord.

true (posterior and lateral columns of cervical spinal cord)

32. True or False. Causes of urinary retention are

3.1.3

a. urethral stricture

true

b. prostatic enlargement

true

c. detrusor areflexia

true

d. herpes zoster

true

33. Evaluation of bladder function usually combines c_____ or v_____ with s_____ m_____.

cystometrogram; videourodynamics; sphincter myelography

3.1.3

34. Synthetic anticholinergics block p_____s _____ (m_____ a_____) without blocking skeletal neuromuscular or autonomic ganglia (n_____ j_____).

postganglionic synapses (muscarinic action); nicotinic junctions

3.1.3

35. The most widely prescribed anticholinergic for detrusor hyperreflexia is O_____, while T_____ is considered less effective.

Oxybutynin; Tolterodine

3.1.3

36. B_____ is indicated for post-op non-obstructive urinary retention and for neurogenic atony due to spinal cord injury or dysfunction.

Bethanecol

3.1.3

37. Following acute cauda equina decompression, patients may start T_____ to relieve urinary retention symptoms.

Tamsulosin

3.1.3

■ Regional Brain Syndromes

38. **Matching. Match region with deficit.**   3.2.1
Region:
① pre-frontal lobes; ② frontal lobe;
③ parietal lobe—dominant; ④ parietal—
non dominant; ⑤ occipital lobe;
⑥ cerebellum; ⑦ brain stem; ⑧ pineal;
⑨ olfactory groove
Deficit: (a-l) below

  a. apathy abulia   ②
  b. disorganized thoughts   ①
  c. contralateral neglect   ③ or ④
  d. language disorders   ③
  e. anosognosia   ④
  f. dressing apraxia   ④
  g. homonymous hemianopsia   ⑤
  h. truncal ataxia   ⑥
  i. ipsilateral ataxia   ⑥
  j. paralysis of upward gaze   ⑧
  k. poor planning   ①
  l. unilateral anosmia   ⑨

39. **Frontal eye fields for contra lateral**   3.2.1
gaze are

  a. located in the _____ frontal lobe.   posterior
  b. in Brodmann area _____.   8
  c. With a destructive lesion there, the   toward
     patient's eyes look _____ the lesion. (Hint: *destructive=toward*)
  d. With an irritative lesion there, the   away from
     patient's eyes look _____ _____ (Hint: *irritative=away*)
     the lesion.
  e. Usually the lesions are _____.   destructive

40. **True or False. Gerstmann syndrome**   3.2.1
includes

  a. agraphia without alexia   true
  b. left-right confusion   true
  c. digit agnosia   true
  d. tactile agnosia   false
  e. acalculia   true

41. **True or False. Gerstmann syndrome**   true   3.2.1
patients can read.

42. **True or False. Gerstmann syndrome**   false   3.2.1
patients can write.

43. **True or False. Cortical sensory**   3.2.2
syndrome includes:

  a. loss of position sense   true
  b. inability to localize tactile stimuli   true
  c. astereognosis   true
  d. loss of pain and temperature sense   false (Pain and temperature
                                  as well as vibration sense are
                                  preserved.)

44. True or False. Broca aphasia includes: 3.2.2

a. dysarthria — true

b. lesion is in area 44 — true

c. "apraxia" of motor sequencing — true

d. similar to conduction aphasia — false (Broca is a motor aphasia—faltering dysarthric speech. Conduction aphasia is fluent speech with paraphasias.)

45. True or False. Wernicke's aphasia includes: 3.2.2

a. fluent aphasia — true

b. lesion is in Brodmann areas 41 and 42 — false (The lesion is in Brodmann 39 and 40.)

c. speech devoid of meaning — true

d. normal intonation — true

46. Alexia without agraphia   3.2.2

a. means that the patient can _____ — write

b. but cannot _____. — read

c. Surprisingly, such patients can usually do what with numbers? — read and name them

d. Lesion is located in the _____ lobe. — parietooccipital

e. On which side? — dominant left

f. Serves to disconnect _____ _____ and — angular gyrus

g. _____ _____ — occipital lobe

h. also known as _____ _____ _____. — pure word blindness

i. This is contrasted with what syndrome? — Gerstmann's

j. Where patient can _____ — read

k. but can't _____ — write

l. also known as _____ _____ _____. — agraphia without alexia

47. Matching. Match the numbered syndromes with the lettered phrases.   3.2.2

Syndrome:
① Gerstmann; ② pure word blindness
Phase: (a-d) below

a. alexia without agraphia — ②

b. agraphia without alexia — ①

c. where patient can't read — ②

d. where patient can't write — ①

48. True or False. Regarding Foster-Kennedy syndrome: 3.2.3

a. usually from olfactory groove or medial third sphenoid wing tumor — true

b. contralateral anosmia — false (Ipsilateral not contralateral anosmia is part of the classic triad.)

c.	ipsilateral central scotoma	true
d.	contralateral papilledema	true
e.	contralateral optic atrophy	false (ipsilateral optic atrophy)
f.	usually from meningioma	true

49. True or False. Regarding Weber syndrome: 3.2.4

a. Weber syndrome includes CN III palsy with contralateral hemiparesis.   true

b. Weber syndrome includes CN VII palsy with contralateral hemiparesis.   false

c. Weber syndrome includes CN III palsy with ipsilateral hemiparesis.   false

d. Weber syndrome includes CN VI and VII palsy with contralateral hemiparesis.   false

e. Weber syndrome includes

i.	CN III palsy	true
ii.	contralateral hemiparesis	true
iii.	arm hyperkinesis	false
iv.	ataxia	false
v.	intention tremor	false

50. True or False. Benedict's syndrome is due to disruption of   3.2.4

a.	cerebral peduncle	true
b.	issuing fibers of CN III	true
c.	red nucleus	true

51. True or False. Millard-Gubler syndrome is due to disruption of   3.2.4

a.	nucleus of VII	true
b.	nucleus of VI	true
c.	corticospinal tract	true

52. True or False. Regarding Parinaud syndrome: 3.2.5

a. Parinaud's syndrome includes downgaze palsy.   false

b. Parinaud's syndrome includes lid retraction.   true

c. Parinaud's syndrome includes nystagmus retractorius.   false

d. When Parinaud's syndrome is combined with downgaze palsy it is known as the syndrome of the _____ _____.   Sylvian aqueduct

■ Jugular Foramen Syndromes

53. **True or False. Regarding jugular foramen syndromes:**   3.3.1
a. transverse sinus — false
b. CNIX, X, andXI — true
c. CN X, XI, and XII — false
d. sigmoid sinus — true
e. petrosal sinus — true
f. branches from the ascending pharyngeal artery — true
g. branches from the occipital artery — true

54. **Matching. Match the following numbered syndromes with the lettered lesions. Also indicate the nerves involved and the results of the lesion.**   3.3.2
Syndrome:
① Vernet's; ② Collet-Sicard; ③ Villaret's
Lesion: (a–c) below
a. Which jugular foramen syndrome is most likely due to an intracranial lesion? — ① involves CN, IX, X, XI taste, vocal cords and SCM (sternocleido mastoid muscle)
b. extracranial lesion? — ② above plus XII tongue
c. retropharyngeal lesion? — ③ above plus Horner

55. **True or False. A jugular foramen syndrome that spares CN IX is**   3.3.2
a. Vernet's — false
b. Collet-Sicard — false
c. Villaret's — false
d. Tapia — true (Tapia X, XII vocal cords and tongue)

4

Neuroanesthesia

■ General Information

1.	**Provide general information on neuroanesthesia.**	4.1
a.	Name the most potent cerebral vasodilator	CO_2
b.	Effect of hyperventilation on:	
	i. $PaCO_2$	reduces
	ii. CBV	decreases
	iii. CBF	decreases
	iv. Goal is end tidal CO_2 of ($ETCO_2$) ____ mmHg.	25-30 mm Hg
	v. Correlates with $PaCO_2$ of ___ - ___ mmHg.	30 to 35 mm Hg
c.	For every _____ degree Celsius change in temperature,	1
d.	there is a change in cerebral metabolic rate of oxygen by ____%.	7%
e.	Hyperglycemia can _____ ischemic deficits.	worsen
f.	Head of the bed elevation will have the	
	i. arterial blood flow	decrease
	ii. ICP	reduce
	iii. venous blood outflow	decrease

■ Drugs Used in Neuroanesthesia

2.	**Inhaled agents have the following effects on:**	4.2.1
a.	cerebral metabolism	reduce
b.	cerebral vessels	dilate
c.	cerebral blood volume	increase
d.	ICP	increase
e.	CO_2 reactivity	increase
3.	**What anesthetic drug may come out of solution and aggravate pneumocephalus?**	nitrous oxide 4.2.1

4. **To reduce the risk of tension pneumocephalus you would**   4.2.1
a. fill any space with _____   fluid
b. and turn off_____   agent
c. _____ minutes before closing the dura.   10

5. **Complete the following regarding barbiturates:**   4.2.2
a. They produce dose-dependent EEG _____   suppression
b. They cause peripheral vaso_____   dilatation
c. which may result in _____   hypotension
d. and _____ the CPP.   reduce

6. **Which barbiturate can decrease seizure threshold?**   methohexital   4.2.2

7. **True or False. Etomidate**   4.2.2
a. has analgesic properties.   false
b. can produce myoclonic activity.   true
c. can impair renal function.   true
d. may produce adrenal insufficiency.   true

8. **Ketamine is a _____ receptor antagonist.**   NMDA   4.2.2

9. **True or False. Morphine**   4.2.2
a. significantly crosses BBB   false
b. releases histamine which   true
c. produces hypotension   true
d. causes vasodilation   true
e. increases ICP   true
f. compromises CPP   true

10. **Characterize synthetic narcotics:**   4.2.2
a. Have the advantage that they don't   histamine release
    cause h_____ r_____.
b. An example is f_____.   fentanyl

11. **Benzodiazepines are _____agonists.**   GABA   4.2.3

12. **Dexmedetomidine (Precedex) is an _____ receptor agonist.**   alpha-2 adrenergic   4.2.3

13. **What is the only depolarizing paralytic agent?**   succinylcholine   4.2.4

■ Anesthetic Requirements for Intra-Operative Evoked Potential Monitoring

14. Answer the following questions concerning anesthesia requirements for evoked potential monitoring: 4.3
  a. What technique is preferred?   total IV anesthesia
  b. Second best is _____.   nitrous/narcotic
  c. Are muscle relaxants permitted?   yes

15. How should fentanyl be infused?   continuously, not intermittently   4.3

■ Malignant Hyperthermia

16. Regarding malignant hyperthermia: 4.4.1
  a. Due to block of _____ re-entry into sarcoplasmic reticulum.   calcium   4.4.2
  b. Earliest possible sign is _____ in end-tidal pCO_2.   increase
  c. Treatment with _____ IV is usually effective.   dantrolene   4.4.3
  d. In patients at risk _____ should be avoided.   succinylcholine   4.4.4

4

5

Sodium Homeostasis and Osmolality

■ Serum Osmolality and Sodium Concentration

1. A serum osmolality of _____ is associated with risk of renal failure.	> 320	Table 5.1

■ Hyponatremia

2. The diagnosis is hyponatremia if the serum sodium is less than _____ mEq/L.	135	5.2.1
3. Two common etiologies for hyponatremia are		5.2.1
a. S_____	SIADH	
b. C_____	CSW	
4. Minimal work-up for hyponatremia should include:		5.2.1
a. serum _____	[Na$^+$]	
b. serum _____	osmolality	
c. urine _____	osmolality	
d. assessment of _____	volume status	
e. urine_____	[Na$^+$]	
f. T_____	TSH	
5. The syndrome is SIADH		5.2.1
a. if the serum osmolality is less than _____ mOsm/L	275	
b. and the urine osmolality is more than _____ mOsm/L.	100	
6. Pseudohyponatremia occurs when _____ active solutes draw ____from the cells and _____the water fraction of plasma and produce artificially _____values.	osmotically; water; reduce; low sodium	5.2.1

7. Name osmotically active solutes that
   may cause pseudohyponatremia.   5.2.1
   a. g_____   glucose
   b. m_____   mannitol
   c. h_____   hyperlipidemia
   d. h_____   hyperproteinemia

8. Complete the equation to calculate   5.2.2
   serum osmolality
   Effective serum osmolality =   2.8

   $$\text{measured osmolality} - \frac{\text{[BUN](mg/dl)}}{\rule{1cm}{0.4pt}}$$

9. Matching. Match the symptoms with   5.2.3
   severity of hyponatremia.
   Hyponatremia:
   ① mild, < 130mEq/L; ② severe, <
   125mEq/L
   Symptoms: (a-i) below
   a. headache   ①
   b. cerebral edema   ②
   c. anorexia   ①
   d. nausea vomiting   ②
   e. muscle weakness   ①
   f. muscle twitching   ②
   g. seizures   ②
   h. respiratory arrest   ②
   i. difficulty concentrating   ①

10. SIADH is   5.2.5
    a. the release of _____   ADH
    b. without _____ stimuli   osmotic
    c. resulting in
       i.   _____natremia   hypo
       ii. _____volemia   hyper
       iii. with inappropriately _____ urine   high
            osmolality.

11. Complete the following regarding   5.2.5
    treatment of hyponatremia:
    a. Avoid _____ correction.   rapid
    b. Avoid _____ correction.   over
    c. Do not exceed _____mEq/L per hour.   1
    d. Do not exceed _____mEq/L per 24   8
       hours.
    e. Do not exceed _____mEq/L per 48   18
       hours.

12. **Matching. Diagnosis of SIADH depends on three diagnostic criteria. Match the laboratory value with the appropriate test.**   5.2.5

Hyponatremia:
① serum Na; ② serum K; ③ serum osmolality; ④ urinary osmolality; ⑤ urinary Na; ⑥ urinary K; ⑦ blood urea nitrogen (BUN) creatinine

a. low   ①, ③
b. high   ④, ⑤
c. normal   ⑥, ⑦

13. **Give the expected result for each test in the diagnosis of SIADH.**   5.2.5
a. serum Na _____   < 134 mEq/L
b. serum osmol_____   < 275 mOsm/L
c. urinary Na_____   > 18 mEq/L
d. urinary Na may be as high as _____   50-150mEq/L
e. serum BUN below _____   10
f. serum creatinine_____   normal

14. **Central pontine myelinolysis (CPM) is**   5.2.5
a. aka o_____ d_____ syndrome   osmotic demyelination
b. due to r_____ c_____ of hyponatremia   rapid correction
c. a disorder of p_____ w_____ m_____.   pontine white matter
d. Its symptoms are
   i.   f_____ q_____   flaccid quadriplegia
   ii. m_____ s_____ changes   mental status
   iii. c_____ n_____ abnormalities   cranial nerve
   iv. p_____ b_____ appearance   pseudobulbar

15. **Features common in patients who develop CPM are**   5.2.5
a. r_____ c_____   rapid correction
b. o_____ c_____   over correction
c. d_____ in _____ for more than _____ hours.   delay in diagnosis; 48
d. increase in Na by more than _____mEq/L within _____hours.   25; 48

16. **Treatment of SIADH includes:**   5.2.5
a. f_____ r_____   fluid restriction
b. s_____   salt

17. **Cerebral salt wasting (CSW) is**   5.2.6
a. r_____ loss of _____   renal; Na
b. as a result of i_____ disease   intracranial
c. producing _____natremia and a   hypo
d. _____ in extracellular fluid volume.   decrease

5

18. **List the expected patient laboratory result when comparing SIADH with CSW.**   Table 5.5
    a. Water: in SIADH _____, in CSW _____   SIADH: hypervolemic, CSW: hypovolemic
    b. Na (serum): in SIADH _____, in CSW _____   SIADH: low, CSW: low
    c. osmol (serum): in SIADH _____ , in CSW _____   SIADH: low, CSW: high
    d. osmol (urine): in SIADH _____, in CSW _____   SIADH: high, CSW: high
    e. Na (urine): in SIADH _____, in CSW _____   SIADH: high, CSW: high
    f. Hct: in SIADH _____, in CSW_____   SIADH: low, CSW: high

19. **What is the treatment of CSW?**   5.2.6
    a. Hydrate
        i.   with ___% _____saline   0.9% normal
        ii. at _____cc/hr.   100-125
    b. Use furosemide (yes or no?)   no
    c. Avoid _____ correction   rapid

■ Hypernatremia

20. **In neurosurgical patients hypernatremia is seen in**   5.3.1
    a. d_____ i_____   diabetes insipidus
    b. Define hypernatremia   Na > 150 mEq/L

21. **Characterize diabetes insipidus**   5.3.2
    a. Due to low level of _____.   ADH
    b. Urine output is < _____cc/hr.   200
    c. Specific gravity of urine is < _____.   1.005
    d. Serum osmolarity is normal or _____.   high
    e. Serum sodium is _____.   high

22. **In diabetes insipidus is the following low or high?**   5.3.2
    a. ADH is _____.   low
    b. Urine specific gravity is _____.   low
    c. Urine output is _____.   high
    d. Serum osmolality is _____.   high
    e. Serum sodium is _____.   high

23. **The etiology of diabetes insipidus can be**   5.3.2
    a. Neu_____   neurogenic
    b. Nep_____   nephrogenic

24. **Diagnosis of diabetes insipidus occurs when**   5.3.2
    a. urine output is above _____.   250cc/hr
    b. urine osmol is below _____.   200 mOsm/L
    c. specific gravity is below _____.   1.003
    d. adrenal function is _____.   normal

25. **Treatment of diabetes insipidus in**   drink;   5.3.2
    conscious ambulatory patient is to   thirsty
    instruct patient to d_____ only when
    _____.

26. **Treatment of diabetes insipidus in**   5.3.2
    comatose patient:
    a. IV fluid management with _____ at   D5 1/2NS + 20 mEq/L
       appropriate rate (75-100cc/hr).
    b. Replace _____ above base IV rate mL   urine output;
       for mL with _____.   1/2 NS
    c. If unable to keep up with fluid loss use
       i. v_____   vasopressin
       ii. d_____   desmopressin

5

6

General Neurocritical Care

■ Parenteral Agents for Hypertension

1. True or False. Nicardipine   6.1
a. is a calcium channel blocker.   true
b. does not raise ICP.   true
c. decreases heart rate.   false

2. Nitroglycerins can _____ ICP.   raise   6.1
a. It is a vaso_____   dilator
b. acts on v _____more than a____.   veins, arteries
c. which _____ LV filling pressures.   decrease

**3. Labetalol is a selective ____ blocker   alpha-1;   6.1
and non selective ____ blocker.**   beta

**4. List the effects of labetalol on the   6.1
following:**
a. ICP   no change
b. pulse   decrease or no change
c. cardiac output   no change
d. coronary ischemia   no change
e. renal failure   no change

■ Hypotension (Shock)

**5. What is the first sign of hypovolemic   tachycardia   6.2.1
shock?**

**6. Septic shock is most often due to   negative   6.2.1
gram _____ sepsis.**

7. Dopamine is primarily a vaso_____.   constrictor   6.2.2

**8. Characterize the effect of dopamine at   Table 6.1
these doses**
a. 0.5-2.0 mcg/kg/min   dopaminergic
b. 2-10 mcg/kg/min   beta-1
c. > 10 mcg/kg/min   alpha, beta, dopaminergic

9. True or False. Dobutamine   6.2.2
   a. is primarily a vasodilator by beta-1.   true
   b. increases cardiac output by inotropy.   true
   c. may exacerbate myocardial ischemia.   true

10. **Phenylephrine _____ blood pressure**   elevates;   6.2.2
    by _____ SVR, and causes reflex   increasing;
    _____ in parasympathetic tone   increase;
    resulting in _____ pulse.   decreased

11. **For the listed pressors complete the**   6.2.2
    following statements to describe the
    cautions required.
    a. Phenylephrine: avoid in s_____ c_____   spinal cord injury
       i_____
    b. Dopamine: may cause h_____.   hyperglycemia
    c. Dobutamine: may cause dysfunction of   platelets
       p_____.

■ Acid Inhibitors

12. **True or False. Extra CNS risk factor**   6.3.1
    that increase the odds of stress ulcers
    are the following:
    a. burns covering >25% of body surface   true
       area
    b. hypotension   true
    c. renal failure   true
    d. coagulopathies   true

13. **When is the peak time for acid and**   3-5 days after injury 6.3.1
    pepsin production after head injury?

14. **Should prophylactic use of H2 blocker**   no—usually not warranted 6.3.2
    be given when steroids are used?

15. **Gastric pH > 4 may _____ risk of**   increase   6.3.3
    pneumonia from aspiration.

16. **Omeprazole may _____ the**   decrease;   6.3.5
    effectiveness of prednisone and   decrease;
    _____ the clearance of warfarin and   inhibition
    phenytoin due to _____ of hepatic P-
    450 enzymes.

17. **Sucralfate may _____ the incidence of**   lower   6.3.6
    pneumonia and mortality more than
    agents that affect gastric pH.

6

7

Sedatives, Paralytics, Analgesics

■ Sedatives and Paralytics

1. **The Richmond Scale: RASS quantitates** _____ **and** _____ **levels.**   agitation and sedation   7.1.1
   a. Positive numbers for _____   agitation
   b. Negative numbers for _____   sedation

2. **True or False. Indicate whether the following statements are true or false:**   7.1.2, 7.1.3
   a. Methohexital (Brevital) is more potent and shorter acting than thiopental.   true
   b. Remifentanil rapidly crosses BBB.   true
   c. Fentanyl causes dose-dependent respiratory depression.   true
   d. Propofol has better neuroprotection than barbiturates (during aneurysm surgery).   false (barbiturates are better)
   e. Precedex can be used to reduce shivering.   true

3. **True or False. The following sedatives may induce seizure:**   7.1.3
   a. Thiopental   false
   b. Methohexital   true
   c. Fentanyl   false
   d. Propofol   false
   e. Precedex   false

4. **T_____ may cause necrosis when injected intraarterially.**   Thiopental   7.1.3

5. **Complete the following statements about propofol infusion syndrome:**   7.1.3
   a. Characterized by
      i. _____kalemia   hyperkalemia
      ii. _____megaly   hepatomegaly
      iii. m_____ a_____   metabolic acidosis
      iv. r_____   rhabdomyolysis
      v. r_____ f_____   renal failure
      vi. m_____ f_____   myocardial failure
      vii. h_____   hypertriglyceridemia

6. **Complete the following statements about Precedex.**   7.1.3

a. Mechanism of action   alpha-2-adrenoreceptor
                                                       agonist

b. Acts in
    i.   l_____ c_____ and   locus ceruleus
    ii. d_____ r_____ g_____   dorsal root ganglia
c. Has both _____ and _____   sedative and analgesic
    properties.
d. Side effects: h_____, b_____   hypotension, bradycardia

7. **Choose the correct order from long-acting to short-acting for the following neuromuscular agents:**   Table 7.2

a. Pancuronium   Pancuronium: 60 to 180
                                                        minutes
b. Succinylcholine   Vecuronium: 40 to 60
                                                        minutes
c. Rocuronium   Rocuronium: 40 to 60
                                                        minutes (but shorter onset)
d. Vecuronium   Succinylcholine: 20 minutes

■ Paralytics (Neuromuscular Blocking Agents)

8. **S_____ is always required in a conscious patient simultaneously with the use of a paralytic agent and as ventilation is being established.**   Sedation   7.2.1

9. **True or False.**   Table 7.2
a. Pancuronium is long acting.   true
b. Rocuronium is short acting.   true
c. Succinylcholine is a competitive blocker   false (Succinylcholine is
    and is short acting.   noncompetitive blocker and
                                                         is considered the only
                                                         depolarizing ganglionic
                                                         blocker. It has been linked to
                                                         malignant hyperthermia)
d. Sedation is required for conscious   true
    patients.

10. **Which is the only depolarizing ganglionic blocker among the following paralytics:**   a. Succinylcholine   7.2.1
a. Succinylcholine
b. Rapacuronium
c. Mivacuronium
d. Rocuronoium

11. **Complete the following regarding**   7.2.1
    possible side effects of succinylcholine
    a. Increases serum potassium by _____.   0.5 mEq/mL
    b. Causes severe hyperkalemia in patients   neuronal or neuromuscular
       with _____ pathology.   pathology
    c. It is contraindicated in which acute phase   Major burns, multipletrauma
       injuries?
    d. May cause dysrhythmias, especially   sinus bradycardia
       _____ _____.

12. **Which of the following paralytic is**   a. Succinylcholine   7.2.1
    contraindicated in the acute phase of
    injury because of the risk of
    hyperkalemia?
    a. Succinylcholine
    b. Metocurine
    c. Doxacurium
    d. Pancuronium
    e. Vecuronium

13. **Which of these is the shortest acting**   c. Vecuronium   7.2.4
    nondepolarzing blocking agent?
    a. Mivacurium
    b. Rocuronium
    c. Vecuronium
    d. Metocurine
    e. Doxacurium

14. **Which nondepolarzing paralytic does**   a. Vecuronium   7.2.4
    not affect ICP or CPP?
    a. Vecuronium
    b. Pancuronium
    c. Succinylcholine
    d. Rapacuronium
    e. Rocuronium

15. **What is the main difference between**   d. Cistracurium does not   7.2.4
    cistracrium and its isomer atracurium?   release histamine
    a. cost
    b. onset of action
    c. duration
    d. Cistracurium does not release histamine.
    e. none of the above

16. **State if pancuronium increases or**   7.2.4
    decreases the following:
    a. cardiac output   increases
    b. pulse rate   increases
    c. ICP   increases

17. **Complete the following statements about reversal of competitive muscle blockade:**   7.2.5

   a. Reversal is not attempted until patient has at least ____ twitch to _____ stimulus.   1 twitch to train of four

   b. A response of ¼ indicates ____% muscle blockade.   90

   c. What medication is used for reversal?   neostigmine (2.5 mg to 5 mg IV)

   d. What medications can be added to prevent bradycardia?

      i. a_____   atropine (0.5 mg for each mg of neostigmine)

      ii. g_____   glycopyrrolate (0.2 mg for each mg of neostigmine)

■ Analgesics

18. **Metastatic cancer pain can be desensitized by which of these analgesics?**   a, b, c   7.3.3

   a. steroids
   b. aspirin
   c. nonsteroidal anti-inflammatory drugs
   d. acetaminophen

19. **How do NSAIDs work?**   7.3.4

   a. They inhibit _____.   cyclooxygenase
   b. which thereby interferes with the synthesis of p_____   prostaglandins

   c. and t_____.   thromboxanes
   d. This inhibits the function of _____   platelets
   e. and prolongs _____ _____   bleeding time
   f. They may also cause _____.   nephrotoxicity

20. **Complete the following concerning NSAIDS and platelet function:**   7.3.4

   a. The NSAID that results in irreversible binding is _____.   aspirin

   b. Which NSAID results in reversible inhibition of platelet function?   most NSAIDS

   c. The NSAID that does not interfere with platelet function is _____.   Relafen (nabumetone)

21. **List the doses of the following substances:**   Table 7.4

   a. NSAID to use

      i. Naprosyn loading: _____ then _____ every _____ to _____ hours.   500 mg; then 250 mg; 6 to 8

      ii. Motrin no loading: Start dose _____ to _____ mg then _____ times per day.   400 to 800; then 4 times per day

7

b.   Opioid to use (moderate to severe pain)
   i.   Percodan no loading: Start dose   1 to 2 pills;
        _____ to _____ pill(s) every   3 to 4 hours
        _____ to _____ hours.
   ii. Vicodin no loading: Start dose   1 pill;
        _____ pill(s) every _____ hours.   every 6 hours
        Limit to _____ every _____   8 pills every 24 hours
        hours per day.
c.   Opioids use (mild to moderate pain)
   i.   Codeine loading?   no loading;
        Start dose _____ to _____ mg at   30 to 60 mg at 3 hours;
        _____ hours, to _____mg at   60 mg at 3 to 5 hours
        _____ to _____ hours

22.   How much Tylenol is safe?   Table 7.3
   a.   Comes in dosages of _____ or   650 or 1000 mg
        _____ mg.
   b.   Safe up to _____ mg/day   4000 mg/day
   c.   Has a ceiling effect at _____ mg/day 1300 mg/day
   d.   Has hepatic toxicity above   10,000 mg/day
        _____mg/day

23.   A serious side effect of acetaminophen hepatotoxicity   Table 7.3
        is _____.

24.   Complete the following regarding   7.3.4
        ketorolac (Toradol).
   a.   Only _____ NSAID approved for use in parenteral
        pain control in the U.S.
   b.   A_____ effect is more potent than its analgesic;
        ____-_____ effect.   anti-inflammatory
   c.   Half-life is _____ hours   6

25.   True or False. Regarding opioid   7.3.5
        analgesics:
   a.   They have no ceiling effect.   true
   b.   With chronic use, tolerance develops.   true
   c.   Overdose is possible with severe   true
        respiratory depression.
   d.   Treatment of overdose includes   true
        administration of naloxone.
   e.   Flumanezil helps in treatment of   false (Flumanezil is useful on
        overdose.   treatment overdose from
                                                benzodiazepines.)

26.   True or False. Regarding narcotics: 7.3.5
   a.   Some opioids may cause seizures.   true
   b.   Physical and psychological tolerance   true
        develops with chronic use.
   c.   There is a ceiling effect with increasing true
        dosage.
   d.   Overdose can cause respiratory   true
        depression.

27. **Complete the following mnemonic about opioids:**   7.3.5
    a. o_____   overdose is possible
    b. p_____   potential for respiratory
                           depression
    c. i_____   increase dosage = increase
                           effect – no ceiling effect
    d. o_____   small pupils – miosis
    e. i_____   intoxication - treat with
                           Narcan
    f. d_____   develops tolerance with
                           chronic use

28. **To what type of opioid receptor**   μ-opioid receptor   7.3.5
    subtype does tramadol (Ultram) bind?

29. **Ultram acts centrally to inhibit**   7.3.5
    reuptake of
    a. n_____ and   norepinephrine
    b. s_____   serotonin

30. **True or False. OxyContin tablets**   true   Table 7.6
    should never be taken crushed,
    divided or chewed.

31. **What is the intramuscular:per os**   Table 7.7
    (IM:PO) potency ratio for morphine?
    a. single dose   1:6
    b. chronic dosing   1:2 to 3

32. **Indicate the following adjuvant**   7.3.6
    medications' characteristic actions:
    a. Tricyclics   blocks serotonin intake
    b. Tryptophan   precursor of serotonin
    c. Antihistamines   anxiolytic
    d. Phenothiazine   tranquilizing

33. **What craniofacial pain syndromes are**   7.3.6
    responsive to carbamazepine?
    a. t_____ n_____   trigeminal neuralgia
    b. g_____ n_____   glossopharyngeal neuralgia
    c. p_____-_____ n_____   post-herpetic neuralgia

34. **Chronic use of tryptophan may cause**   Vitamin B6 depletion   7.3.6
    _____.

7

8

Endocrinology

■ Corticosteroids

1. **Cortisol is released by the _____ _____ and is stimulated by adrenocorticotrophic hormone (ACTH) from the _____, which in turn is stimulated by corticotropin releasing hormone (CRH) from the _____.**

   adrenal glands; pituitary; hypothalamus

   8.1.1

2. **True or False. The following has to be replaced in adrenal failure:**
   a. Mineralocorticoids — true
   b. Glucocorticoids — true

   8.1.2

3. **True or False. The following has to be replaced in pituitary failure:**
   a. Mineralocorticoids — false
   b. Glucocorticoids — true

   8.1.2

4. **True or False. The following medications have mineralocorticoid potency:**
   a. Cortisone — true
   b. Cortisol — true
   c. Solu-Cortef — true
   d. Prednisone — true
   e. Methylprednisolone — false
   f. Dexamethasone — false

   Table 8.1

5. **Hypothalamic-pituitary-adrenal suppression can occur if a dose**
   a. of 40 mg of prednisone is given for _____ days. — > 7
   b. is given for 7 to 14 days taper over _____. — 1-2 weeks
   c. After a month of steroids, HPA axis may be depressed for as long as _____. — 1 year

   8.1.3

6. **When withdrawal problems develop**   8.1.3
   a. conservative steroid taper includes small decrements equivalent to _____ mg of prednisone   2.5-5
   b. every _____ days.   3-7

7. **List the possible deleterious effects of steroids in alphabetical order.**   8.1.4
   a. a   alkalosis, amenorrhea, avascular necrosis (hip)
   b. b   bone loss
   c. c   cushingnoid features cataracts, compression fractures, chickenpox reactivation
   d. d   diverticular perforation, diabetes
   e. e   epidural lipomatosis
   f. f   fungal infections, fetal adrenal hypoplasia
   g. g   growth suppression in children, GI bleed, glaucoma
   h. h   hypertension, hypokalemia, hyper coagulopathy, hiccups, hirsutism, hyperlipidemia
   i. i   immunosuppression
   j. j
   k. k
   l. l   lipomatosis
   m. m   mental agitation, muscle weakness, myopathy
   n. n   non-ketotic coma, nitrogen metabolism is disturbed
   o. o   obesity
   p. p   progressive multifocal leukoencephalopathy (PML), pseudotumor cerebri, pancreatitis
   q. q
   r. r   reactivation of TB
   s. s   sodium retention, steroid psychosis
   t. t   tissue plasminogen activator inhibition
   u. u
   v. v
   w. w   water retention

8. **What is the best way to test for hypocortisolism?**   8 a.m. cortisol level   8.1.5

8

9. **What are the symptoms of Addisonian crisis?**
(Hint: CLAW)
   a. C_____   Confusion
   b. L_____   Lethargy
   c. A_____   Agitation
   d. W_____   Weakness

8.1.5

10. **What are the signs of Addisonian crisis?**
Start your answers with hypo- or hyper-
   a. blood pressure   hypotension
   b. glucose   hypoglycemia
   c. sodium   hyponatremia
   d. temperature   hyperthermia
   e. potassium   hyperkalemia

8.1.5

■ Hypothyroidism

11. **Levothyroxine is almost pure _____ and contains no T3 because most T3 is produced _____ from T4.**
T4;
peripherally

8.2.3

12. **Signs of myxedema coma include**
   a. h_____   hypotension
   b. h_____   hyponatremia
   c. h_____   hypoglycemia
   d. h_____   hypoventilation
   e. b_____   bradycardia
   f. s_____   seizures

8.2.3

■ Pituitary Embryology and Neuroendocrinology

13. **The posterior pituitary derives from the downward evagination of _____ _____ _____ from the floor of the_____ _____.**
neural crest cells;
third ventricle

8.3.1

14. **The anterior pituitary gland develops from evagination of _____ _____, which is also called _____ _____.**
epithelial ectoderm
Rathke's pouch

8.3.1

15. **The pituitary gland is functionally _____ the blood-brain barrier.**
outside

8.3.1

16. **The pituitary gland releases ____ hormones, _____ from the anterior pituitary and _____ from the posterior pituitary.**
8;
6;
2

8.3.2

17. **Match the hormone and the portion of
    the pituitary where it is produced**
    ① anterior; ② posterior

Fig. 8.1

   a. Thyrotropin releasing hormone   ①
   b. Corticotropin releasing hormone   ①
   c. Oxytocin   ②
   d. Antidiuretic hormone   ②
   e. Somatostatin   ①
   f. Prolactin release inhibitory factor   ①
   g. Gonadotropin releasing hormone   ①

18. **Prolactin is the only pituitary hormone**   inhibitory   8.3.2
    predominantly under _____ control
    from the hypothalamus.

19. **Describe the side effects of ADH.**   8.3.2
   a. _____ the permeability of the distal   increases
      tubules.
   b. _____ reabsorption of water.   increases
   c. _____ circulating blood.   dilutes
   d. Produces _____ urine.   concentrated

20. **What is the most powerful physiologic**   serum osmolality   8.3.2
    stimulus for ADH release?

8

9

Hematology

■ Blood Component Therapy

1. **For an adult, 1 unit of packed red blood cells (PRBCs) should raise the hematocrit by _____%.**   3-4%   9.2.2

2. **Complete the following concerning platelets:**   9.2.3
    a. Normal platelet count is _____ to _____.   150 k-400 k/mm^3
    b. Regarding transfusion of platelets:
        i.   Transfuse if surgery is _____ or   urgent
        ii. patient is on _____ or _____ and can't wait ___ to ___ days.   ASA or Plavix; 5 to 7
        iii. Usual transfusion is _____ of platelets.   an eight pack (=6-10 U)
        iv. One unit raises platelets by _____.   10 k
        v.   Platelet count can be checked in _____ hours.   2
        vi. Retransfusion will be needed in _____ days.   3-5

3. **Complete the following concerning fresh frozen plasma:**   9.2.4
    a. One bag equals _____ cc.   200–250
    b. Risk of acquired immunodeficiency syndrome (AIDS) or hepatitis is the same as _____.   a unit of blood
    c. Use to reverse Coumadin:
        i.   Prothrombin time (PT) greater than _____.   18 seconds
        ii. International normalized ratio (INR) greater than _____.   1.6
        iii. Von Willebrand's disease unresponsive to _____.   DDAVP
        iv. Multiple coagulation dysfunction such as in:
             h_____ _____   hepatic dysfunction;
             v _____ _____ _____   vitamin K deficiency;
             D_____   DIC

4. **True or False. Regarding Prothrombin complex concentrate (PCC):**   9.2.4
    a. Contains clotting factors II, VII, IX, X.   true
    b. Contains protein C & S.   true
    c. Primary indication is to be given for warfarin reversal.   true
    d. Requires higher volume than FFP to work.   false (lower volume)

5. **In regard to the use of anticoagulation in a patient who has**   9.2.5
    a. an unruptured aneurysm < 4 mm, anticoagulation is _____.   ok
    b. a drug eluting cardiac stent – continue _____.   Plavix
    c. At onset of SAH, we would _____ anticoagulation.   reverse
    d. Post-operative craniotomy may start ____ to ____ days after surgery.   3 to 5

6. **Regarding anticoagulation in preparation for surgery. If a patient has:**   9.2.5
    a. a mechanical heart valve
        i.   stop warfarin _____ days before surgery   3
        ii. and begin _____.   Lovenox
    b. chronic atrial fibrillation
        i.   stop warfarin ____ days before surgery.   4 to 5

7. **Complete the following regarding anticoagulation:**   9.2.5
    a. May resume anticoagulation ____ days after craniotomy.   3 to 5
    b. Annual risk of complications while not anticoagulated for a patient with
        i.   mechanical heart valve is ____% per year.   6%
        ii. chronic atrial fibrillation is ____% per year   4-6%

8. **Complete the following regarding neurosurgical procedures:**   9.2.5
    a. PT should be below _____ seconds.   < 13.5
    b. INR should not be above _____.   1.4
    c. For emergencies give _____   2 U FFP
    d. and _____.   vitamin K

9. **Both Plavix and ASA inhibit platelet function for how long?**   permanently   9.2.5

10. **Plavix is more dangerous drug than ASA because it remains**   9.2.5
    a. _____ for up to   active
    b. _____ after the last dose and   several days
    c. can inhibit even those _____ _____ given treatment.   transfused platelets

9

11. Name the commonly used herbal products that may affect platelet aggregation.   9.2.5
- a. g_____   garlic
- b. g_____   ginkgo
- c. g_____   ginseng
- d. f____ _____   fish oil

12. Complete the following concerning warfarin (Coumadin):   9.2.5
- a. Don't start Coumadin until a _____ has been achieved on heparin   therapeutic partial thromboplastin time (PTT)
- b. to reduce the risk of _____ _____.   Coumadin necrosis
- c. For the first 3 days of Coumadin therapy patients are actually _____;   hypercoagulable
- d. therefore patients should be _____ with _____ or _____.   "bridged"; Lovenox or heparin

13. Possible heparin side effects include   9.2.5
- a. t_____   thrombosis
- b. t_____   thrombocytopenia
- c. These side effects are due to
  - i. _____ in heparin induced thrombosis or   consumption
  - ii. _____ formed against heparin platelet.   antibodies

14. Low molecular weight heparins should   9.2.5
- a. have fewer _____ complications.   hemorrhagic
- b. have more predictable _____ levels.   plasma
- c. eliminate the need to _____ biologic activity.   monitor
- d. have a longer _____ life.   half
- e. require _____ doses per day.   fewer
- f. have a lower incidence of _____.   thrombocytopenia
- g. be more effective in _____ prophylaxis than warfarin.   DVT

15. A serious side effect could be spinal _____ _____.   epidural hematoma   9.2.5

16. Regarding dabigatran (Pradaxa).   9.2.5
- a. It is a d_____ t_____ i_____   direct thrombin inhibitor
- b. Can be reversed with _____.   Idarucizumab

17. Regarding fondaparineux (Arixtra)   9.2.5
- a. It _____ factor Xa inhibition   increases
- b. without affecting Factor _____.   Factor IIa (thrombin)
- c. Unlike heparin, it does not cause h____ i____ t_____.   heparin-induced thrombocytopenia

9

18. **Complete the following concerning coagulopathy:**   9.2.5
    a. To reverse Coumadin anticoagulation in a patient who is at the usual therapeutic level, use _____.   2 to 3 units FFP
    b. For severely prolonged coagulation use _____.   6 units FFP
    c. To reverse PT from Coumadin use
       i. _____   vitamin K aqua mephyton
       ii. Administered by what route?   IM
       iii. Administration may be fatal if given _____   IV
       iv. Why?
          h_____   hypotension;
          a_____   anaphylaxis

19. **Matching. Use the numbers of the listed terms to complete the following statements.**   9.2.5
    ① prothrombin complex concentrate;
    ② protamine sulfate; ③ vitamin K;
    ④ AquaMephyton
    a. Coumadin is reversed by
       i. _____ _____ _____   ①
       ii. _____ _____   ③
       iii. _____   ④
    b. Heparin is reversed by _____ _____   ②

20. **Regarding protamine sulfate.**   9.2.5
    a. 1 mg of protamine reverses _____ of heparin.   100 U
    b. ____% of Lovenox can be reversed with 1 mg of protamine for every mg of Lovenox within the last ____ hours.   60%;
8

21. **Significantly elevated pre-op PTT is commonly due to**   9.2.5
    a. f_____ d_____   factor deficiency
    b. l_____ a_____   lupus anticoagulant

22. **Complete the following concerning thromboembolism:**   9.2.5
    a. Risk of embolism from calf-deep-vein thrombosis is ___%   1%
    b. Extends to proximal deep veins in _____%.   30 to 50%
    c. Embolism from thigh veins is _____%.   40 to 50%
    d. Mortality of DVT in legs is _____%.   9 to 50%
    e. DVTs in neurosurgical patients occur in _____%.   19-50%

23. **Conditions that make neurosurgical patients prone to DVTs are**   9.2.5
    a. c_____ _____   concomitant sludging
    b. l___-_____ _____   long-time immobility
    c. o_____ _____/d_____   operating room/dehydration
    d. t_____ _____   thromboplastin release

24. **The best prophylaxis against DVT is**   9.2.5
  a. PCB, which is the abbreviation for _____.   pneumatic compression boots
  b. low _____ _____.   dose heparin (5000 IU subcutaneous every to 8 to 12 hours first postop day)

25. **Matching. One can diagnose DVT with the following tests. Match the finding with its appropriate diagnostic value.** ① gold standard; ② associated with PE and DVT; ③ only 50% accurate; ④ 99% specific   9.2.5
  a. Hot swollen tender calf with positive Homan sign   ③
  b. Contrast venography   ①
  c. Doppler ultrasonography   ④
  d. D-dimer   ②

26. **What is the treatment of DVT?**   9.2.5
  a. b_____   bed rest
  b. e_____ i_____ leg   elevate involved leg
  c. h_____ or L_____   heparin; Lovenox
  d. c_____   Coumadin
  e. Consider G_____ f_____   Greenfield filter
  f. a_____   ambulate
  g. after _____ to _____days   7 to 10
  h. wear _____-_____ _____   anti-embolic stockings
  i. For how long? _____   indefinitely

27. **Regarding pulmonary embolism.**   9.2.5
  a. Generally occurs _____ to ____ ____ following surgery.   10 to 14 days
  b. Common findings include
    i. t_____   tachypnea
    ii. t_____   tachycardia
    iii. f_____   fever
    iv. h_____   hypotension
  c. Classic EKG finding is   S1Q3T3
  d. Test of choice is c_____-e_____ c_____ C_____   contrast-enhanced chest CT

■ Extramedullary Hematopoiesis

28. **Extramedullary hematopoiesis can result in**   9.3.1
  a. abnormal skull x-ray called _____ _____ _____   hair on end
  b. spinal cord compression due to _____ _____ _____   vertebral body thickening

29. **Extramedullary hematopoiesis can be treated with**   9.3.3
  a. r_____ and/or   radiotherapy
  b. s_____   surgery

10

Neurology for Neurosurgeons

■ Dementia

1. What is the definition of dementia?   10.1
a. Loss of i_____ abilities   intellectual
b. severe enough to interfere with _____   social
c. or o_____ functioning.   occupational
d. Cardinal feature is m_____ d_____   memory deficit
e. plus at least one additional i_____.   impairment
f. Affects __ - ___% of persons over 65.   3 to 11%

2. True or False. The following are risk   10.1
factors for dementia:
a. Advanced age   true
b. Family history   true
c. Apolipoprotein E2   false (apolipoprotein E4)

3. True or False. Regarding dementia vs.   10.1
delirium:
a. Patients with dementia are at increased   true
risk of developing delirium.
b. Fifty percent of patients with delirium   true
die within 2 years.
c. Unlike dementia, delirium has acute   true
onset.

■ Headache

4. Regarding unilateral headache. If it   10.2.1
persists
a. for > 1 year an _____ _____ is   MRI scan
recommended
b. because this is _____ for migraine   atypical
c. and may be a hint of an underlying   AVM
_____.

5. **Matching. Match symptoms with category of migraine.**   10.2.2
   Symptoms:
   ① episodic H/A; ② N/V; ③ photophobia;
   ④ aura; ⑤ focal neurologic deficit;
   (a) that resolves within 24 hours;
   (b) slow march-like progression of
   deficit; (c) that resolves within 30 days;
   ⑥ no headache; ⑦ mostly seen in
   children; ⑧ hemiplegia; ⑨ mostly seen
   in adolescents; ⑩ vertigo, ataxia,
   dysarthria, severe HA
   Category of migraine: (a-f) below
   a. Common migraine   ①-②-③
   b. Classic migraine   ①-②-③-④-⑤-⑤a-⑤b
   c. Complicated migraine   ⑤-⑤c-⑥
   d. Migraine equivalent   ②-⑥-⑦
   e. Hemiplegic migraine   ①-⑧
   f. Basilar artery migraine   ⑨-⑩

6. **True or False. Neurological deficits seen in classic migraine typically resolve within**   10.2.2
   a. 1 hour   false
   b. 1 day   true
   c. 1 week   false
   d. 1 month   false
   e. They are permanent false

7. **True or False. Regarding cluster headaches:**   10.2.2
   a. May include partial Horner's syndrome   true
      and autonomic (ptosis, miosis, tearing)
      symptoms, nasal stuffiness.
   b. Are more common in women.   false (5 men to 1 woman)
   c. Occur almost daily.   true
   d. Last 30 to 90 minutes.   true
   e. Continue for 6 to 9 month period.   false (1 to 3 months)

8. **Treatment of acute attacks of cluster headache includes:**   10.2.2
   a. o_____   oxygen 100% by face mask
   b. e_____   ergotamine
   c. s_____   sumatriptan SQ
   d. s_____   steroids

9. **True or false. Basilar artery migraines are essentially restricted to**   10.2.2
   a. geriatric patients   false
   b. postmenopausal women   false
   c. adolescents   true
   d. men   false

10. **True or False. Patients suffering from basilar artery migraine usually have a family history of migraine.**   true (Family history of migraine is present in 86%.)   10.2.2

10

■ Parkinsonism

11. **Matching. Match the symptoms with type of parkinsonism.**
    Symptoms:
    ① gradual onset of bradykinesia;
    ② asymmetric tremor; ③ responds well to levodopa; ④ rapid progression of symptoms; ⑤ equivocal response to levodopa; ⑥ early midline symptoms (i.e., ataxia, gait, balance); ⑦ early dementia; ⑧ orthostatic hypotension; ⑨ extraocular movement abnormalities
    Types of parkinsonism: (a-b) below
    a. Primary idiopathic paralysis agitans (IPA)
    b. Secondary parkinsonism

    ①-②-③
    ④-⑤-⑥-⑦-⑧-⑨

    10.3.2

12. **In parkinsonism, degeneration of substantia nigra cells (pars compacta) results in**

    10.3.2

    a. _____ in D2 dopamine receptors projecting to the globus pallidus interna (GPi)

    decrease

    b. _____ in D1 receptors projecting to the globus pallidus externa (GPe) and subthalamic nucleus (STN)

    increase

13. **The effects noted in question 12 result in increased activity by**

    10.3.2

    a. _____ causing

    GPi

    b. _____ of the thalamus, which then suppresses activity in the

    inhibition

    c. _____ _____ _____.

    supplemental motor cortex

14. **The effects noted in question 13 increase activity by**

    10.3.2

    a. degeneration of pigmented _____ neurons

    dopaminergic

    b. of the pars compacta of the _____.

    substantia nigra

    c. This reduces the levels of _____ in the

    dopamine

    d. neostriatum; that is the:
       i.   c_____

    caudate

       ii. p_____

    putamen

       iii. g_____ p_____

    globus pallidus

    e. This reduces inhibitory D2 receptors to _____.

    GPi

    f. and causes the loss of inhibitory D1 receptors to _____

    GPe

    g. and the s_____ n_____.

    subthalamic nucleus

    h. The net result is an _____ in activity

    increase

    i. of _____.

    GPi

    j. GPi has inhibitory projections to the t_____

    thalamus

    k. Inhibiting the thalamus also suppresses the s_____ m_____ c_____.

    supplemental motor cortex

15. A hallmark of Parkinson's disease   10.3.2
   a. are _____ _____,   Lewy bodies
   b. which are
      i.   e_____ i_____   eosinophilic intraneuronal
      ii. h_____ i_____   hyaline inclusions

16. List secondary parkinsonism examples   10.3.3
   (Hint: p^4 secondary)
   a. p   phenothiazine antiemetics
   b. p   progressive supranuclear
                                             palsy (PSP)
   c. p   poisoning CO, manganese
   d. p   parkinson-dementia complex
                                             of Guam
   e. s   strial nigral degeneration,
                                             Shy-Drager syndrome
   f. e   post-encephaletic
                                             parkinsonism
   g. c   Compazine
   h. o   olivo-ponto-cerebellar
                                             degeneration
   i. n   neoplasms near substantia
                                             nigra
   j. d   dementia pugilistica
   k. a   anti-psychotic drugs
   l. r   Reglan, Reserpine
   m. y   Huntington's Disease (young
                                             people)

17. Multisystem atrophy (i.e., Shy-Drager   10.3.3
   syndrome) is parkinsonism plus
   a. _____ _____ _____   autonomic nervous system
      dysfunction
   b. plus _____ hypotension.   orthostatic
   c. Most don't respond to _____.   drug therapy

18. List the distinguishing features of the   10.3.3
   progressive supranuclear palsy triad
   a. _____ (vertical gaze)   opthalmoplegia
   b. _____ dystonia   axial
   c. _____ palsy   pseudobulbar

19. Characteristics of the early stage of   10.3.3
   progressive supranuclear palsy (PSP)
   include:
   a. Falling due to _____ _____ palsy   downward gaze
      (can't see the floor).
   b. Difficulty eating due to _____ and downward and vertical gaze
      _____ gaze palsy (can't see plate).

20. **Regarding surgical treatment for Parkinson's disease.**   10.3.3
    a. The target site was _____ _____   ventrolateral nucleus
    b. True or False. The surgery worked better for
        i. bradykinesia   false
        ii. tremor   true
    c. True or False. The more disabling symptom is
        i. bradykinesia   true
        ii. tremor   false
    d. The procedure cannot be done bilaterally   speech disturbance
       because of risk of _____ _____.
    e. Current treatment site is the p_____   posteroventral pallidum
       _____.

■ Multiple Sclerosis

21. **Prevalence of multiple sclerosis (MS) per 100,000 is variable.**   10.4.2
    a. Near the equator it is _____ per 100,000.   <1
    b. In Canada and the northern United States it is _____ per 100,000.   30-80

22. **Multiple sclerosis. Study chart**   10.4
    a. M   (de)myelinating
    b. U   urinary symptoms
    c. L   latitudes (northern latitudes affected)
    d. T   time and space dissemination
    e. I   inter-nuclear ophthalmoplegia (INO)
    f. P   paresthesias, peri-ventricular plaques
    g. L   lymphocytes
    h. E   enhancing lesions on MRI
    i. S   scars of the glia
    j. C   cortico spinal tracts involved
    k. L   la belle indifference (euphoria)
    l. E   equator spared
    m. R   remissions
    n. O   optic atrophy
    o. S   sensory loss
    p. I   inflammatory response, IgG elevated
    q. S   shower test (hot causes exacerbation)

23. **The most common category is r_____-r_____.**   relapsing-remitting   10.4.3

10

24. **Name the clinical categories of MS corresponding to their definition.**   Table 10.2
    a. r_____-r_____ (acute episodes with recovery)   relapsing-remitting
    b. s_____-p_____ (gradual deterioration)   secondary-progressive
    c. p_____p_____ (continuous deterioration)   primary-progressive
    d. p_____-r_____ (gradual deterioration with superimposed relapses)   progressive-relapsing
    e. Deficits persist if they remain > _____.   > 6 months   10.4.3

25. **Matching. Match the multiple sclerosis signs and symptoms with anatomic location.**   10.4.4
    Symptoms:
    ① visual acuity; ② diplopia; ③ extremity weakness; ④ quadriplegia; ⑤ spasticity; ⑥ scanning speech; ⑦ loss of proprioception
    Anatomic location: (a-f) below
    a. optic nerve   ①
    b. retro-bulbar region   ①
    c. MLF   ②
    d. pyramidal tract   ③-④-⑤
    e. cerebellum   ⑥
    f. posterior columns   ⑦

26. **Matching. Match anatomic location with multiple sclerosis signs and symptoms.**   10.4.4
    Anatomic location:
    ① optic nerve; ② retro-bulbar region; ③ MLF; ④ pyramidal tract; ⑤ cerebellum; ⑥ posterior columns
    Anatomic location: (a-g) below
    a. visual acuity   ①-②
    b. diplopia   ③
    c. extremity weakness   ④
    d. quadriplegia   ④
    e. spasticity   ④
    f. scanning speech   ⑤
    g. loss of proprioception   ⑥

27. **Provide the frequency of multiple sclerosis signs and symptoms.**   10.4.4
    a. Visual symptoms are among the presenting symptoms of multiple sclerosis in _____%   15%
    b. and occur in multiple sclerosis patients during the course of illness in approximately _____%.   50%
    c. In addition, abdominal cutaneous reflexes are lost in _____%.   70 to 80%

28. **A multiple sclerosis plaque in the medial longitudinal fasciculus (MLF) will cause**   10.4.4
   a. _____ _____, which will result in   internuclear ophthalmoplegia (INO)
   b. _____.   diplopia
   c. This is important because _____ rarely occurs in other diseases.   INO

29. **Indicate the presence or absence of the following reflexes in MS:**   10.4.4
   a. hyperactive muscle stretch reflexes   present
   b. Babinski   present
   c. abdominal cutaneous reflexes   absent

30. **Conditions found in the differential diagnosis of multiple sclerosis include**   10.4.5
   a. _____ _____ _____, generally monophasic and   acute disseminated encephalomyelitis (ADEM)
   b. CNS _____   lymphoma

31. **True or False. In multiple sclerosis the more MRI lesions, the higher the likelihood of a MS diagnosis.**   true (MRI is very specific for MS plaques; specificity is 94%.)   10.4.6

32. **Provide MRI criteria for MS.**   10.4.6
   a. Gadolinium: acute lesions _____   enhance
   b. Size: at least _____ in diameter   3mm
   c. White matter abnormalities: _____%   80%
   d. T2-weighted image: _____ _____   lesions are high signal
   e. Periventricular lesions best seen on ____   proton density
   f. Criterion for dissemination is a _____ _____ _____   new enhancing lesion
   g. or a _____ _____ _____   new T2 WI lesion

33. **True or False. Focal tumefactive demyelination lesions (TDL) can be mistaken for neoplasms because**   10.4.6
   a. they enhance   true
   b. they show perilesional edema   true
   c. they can be solitary   true
   d. they can be in patients known to have MS   true
   e. they can be distinguished from MS   false
   f. a biopsy may be necessary   true
   g. a biopsy results may be confusing   true

34. **Regarding CSF analysis for MS.**   10.4.6
   a. It should include q_____ _____ testing.   qualitative IgG
   b. In 90% of MS patients the CSF _____ is high.   IgG

10

■ Acute Disseminated Encephalomyelitis

35. **True or False. Regarding acute disseminated encephalitis.**   10.5

   a. Associated with recent history of vaccination.   true

   b. May demonstrate oligoclonal bands in CSF.   true

   c. Is generally monophasic.   true

   d. Has good response to high dose IV corticosteroids.   true

■ Motor Neuron Diseases

36. **Complete the following regarding amyotrophic lateral sclerosis:**   10.6.2

   a. aka m_____ n_____ disease   motor neuron

   b. aka L_____ G_____ disease   Lou Gehrig

   c. a mixed _____ and _____   upper and lower

   d. m_____ n_____ disease   motor neuron

   e. degeneration of a_____ h_____ cells and   anterior horn

   f. c_____ t_____ in the cervical spine and medulla   corticospinal tracts

37. **True or False. Regarding clinical characteristics of ALS.**   10.6.2

   a. There is no cognitive, sensory, or autonomic dysfunction.   true

   b. Spares voluntary eye muscles and urinary sphincter.   true

   c. Presents initially with weakness and atrophy of hands, spasticity and hyperreflexia.   true

38. **The common condition that must be distinguished from ALS is _____ _____.**   cervical myelopathy   10.6.2

39. **R_____ inhibits presynaptic release of g_____, and increases tracheostomy-free survival at _____ and _____ months.**   Riluzole; glutamate; 9 and 12 months   10.6.2

10

■ Guillain-Barré Syndrome

40. Regarding Guillain-Barré Syndrome (GBS).   10.7.1

  a. Involves a____ onset of peripheral neuropathy with — acute

  b. p_____ muscle weakness with a_____. — progressive; arreflexia

  c. Reaches maximum over ____ days to __ weeks. — 3 days to 3 weeks

  d. Little or no _____ involvement. — sensory (but paresthesias are not uncommon)

41. What is albuminocytologic dissociation? — Elevated CSF protein without pleocytosis   10.7.1

42. What infectious organism is commonly involved? — Campylobacter jejuni   10.7.1

43. Features casting doubt on the diagnosis   10.7.1

  a. asymmetry of _____ — weakness

  b. dysfunction of _____ — bladder

  c. more than 50 _____ in CSF — monocytes

  d. any _____ in CSF — PMNs

  e. sharp _____ level — sensory

44. Complete the following about Miller-Fisher variant of GBS: 10.7.3

  a. Describe the triad

    i. a_____ — ataxia

    ii. a_____ — arreflexia

    iii. o_____ — ophthalmoplegia

    iv. Serum biomarker: anti-_____ antibodies — anti-GQ1b

45. Complete the following about CIDP: 10.7.4

  a. Stands for c_____ i_____ d_____ p_____. — chronic immune demyelinating polyradiculoneuropathy

  b. Symptoms must be present for more than _____ _____. — 2 months

  c. Cranial nerves are usually _____. — spared

  d. Balance difficulties are _____. — common

  e. Electrodiagnostic and nerve biopsy findings are indicative of d_____. — demyelination

  f. CSF findings are similar to _____. — GBS

  g. Most respond to _____ and _____. — prednisone and plasmapharesis

10

■ Myelitis

46. **True or False. Regarding Acute Transverse Myelitis**   10.8.3

a. The most common sensory level in acute transverse myelitis is thoracic. — true (68% thoracic sensory level in ATM)

b. ATM progresses rapidly. — true (66% reach maximal deficit by 24 hours)

c. CSF can be normal in the acute phase. — true (38%, remainder can have elevated protein or pleocytosis or both)

d. An emergency MRI is the first test of choice — true (if not available a myelogram with CT to follow)

47. **True or False. Regarding treatment of ATM.**   10.8.5

a. No treatment has been studied in a randomized controlled trial. — true

b. High dose IV methylprednisolone for 3-5 days can be administered. — true

c. Plasma exchange can be given for those who do not respond to steroids. — true

48. **True or False. Regarding prognosis of ATM.**   10.8.6

a. There is 15% mortality. — true

b. 62% of survivors are ambulatory. — true

c. Recovery occurs between 1 month to 2 years — false (1 to 3 months)

d. No improvement occurs after 3 months. — true

■ Neurosarcoidosis

49. **Regarding sarcoidosis. Complete the following:**   10.9.1

a. The most common manifestation is _____ _____. — diabetes insipidus

b. Treat with _____. — corticosteroids

50. **CNS sarcoidosis involves the l_____.** — leptomeninges   10.9.1

a. M_____-e_____ may occur as well as — meningo-encephalitis

b. b_____ m_____ — basal meningitis

c. T_____ ventricle and h_____ may also be involved. — Third; hypothalamus

51. Complete the following statements about neurosarcoidosis
10.9.2, 10.9.4

a. Microscopically we see features of n_____ g_____.   non-caseating granulomas

b. Clinical findings include
i. c_____ n_____ p_____   cranial nerve palsies
ii. p_____ n_____   peripheral neuropathy
iii. m_____   myopathy
iv. h_____   hydrocephalus
c. Diabetes insipidus from involvement of the _____.   hypothalamus

52. Regarding laboratory findings in neurosarcoidosis.
10.9.5

a. Serum test that is positive in 83% of cases is _____   ACE
b. CSF test that is helpful is _____.   ACE
c. How frequently is it positive?   55%
d. CSF suggests _____.   meningitis
e. ACE stands for _____ _____ _____.   angiotensin converting enzyme

53. List the test performed with the results in sarcoidosis.
10.9.6

a. Chest X-ray
i. H_____ a_____   hilar adenopathy
ii. M_____ l_____ n_____   mediastinal lymph nodes
b. MRI
i. Enhancement of l_____   leptomeninges
ii. Enhancement of o_____ n_____   optic nerve
iii. Best seen on _____ sequence   FLAIR
c. Gallium scan (nuclear medicine). Useful in neurosurgery for:
i. s_____   sarcoidosis
ii. c_____ v_____ o_____   chronic vertebral osteomyelitis

10

11

Neurovascular Disorders and Neurotoxicology

■ Posterior Reversible Encephalopathy Syndrome (PRES)

1. PRES:

a. PRES stands for _____ _____ _____ _____.
   posterior reversible encephalopathy syndrome
   11.1.1

b. Characterized by v_____ b_____ e_____ on CT or MRI with some predominance in _____ and _____ regions.
   vasogenic brain edema; parietal; occipital

c. Associated conditions include h_____, e_____, s_____, a_____ d_____, and t_____.
   hypertension, eclampsia, sepsis, autoimmune disease, transplantation
   11.1.2

d. Treatment involves control of _____ _____ and of underlying cause.
   blood pressure
   11.1.3

■ Vasculitis and Vasculopathy

2. Giant cell arteritis:
11.3.2

a. Also known as _____ _____.
   temporal arteritis

b. Involves branches of the _____ _____ artery.
   external carotid

c. Seen almost exclusively in _____ older than _____, with a female:male ratio of _____.
   caucasians; 50; 2:1

d. The most common presenting symptom is _____.
   headache

e. Most serious consequence is _____, which occurs in _____% and is not _____.
   blindness; 7%; reversible

f. The warning symptom that precedes permanent visual loss is _____ _____, which occurs in _____%.
   amaurosis fugax; 44%

g. Giant cell arteritis is associated with _____ _____ _____, which is _____ times as likely in this disease.
   thoracic aortic aneurysms; 17 times

h. ESR > _____ mm/hr is suspicious.
   40

i. ESR > _____ mm/hr is highly   80
    suggestive.
j. ESR may be normal in _____% with   22.5%
    giant cell arteritis.
k. Diagnosed via _____ _____   temporal artery
    biopsy.
l. Optimal length of STA biopsy is   4-6 cm
    _____ cm.
m. Spare _____ and _____ branch   main trunk; parietal
    of STA during biopsy.
n. Manage with _____ for _____   steroids; 6-24 months
    months.

3. Behcet's syndrome consists of the   11.3.6
    following:
    (Hint: Behcet's)
a. B_____   Behcet
b. e_____   eye lesions
c. h_____   headache
d. c_____, c_____   cerebellar signs, CSF
                                               pleocytosis
e. e_____   erosions of mouth and
                                               genitals
f. t_____, t_____   thrombophlebitis, thrombosis
                                               of dural sinuses
g. s_____, s_____   skin lesions, seizures

4. Fibromuscular dysplasia: 11.3.9
a. The most common vessel involved is the   renal, 85%
    r_____ artery, _____%.
b. The second most common vessel   carotid
    involved is the c_____ artery.
c. The incidence of aneurysms with FMD is   20-50%
    _____%.
d. Presenting symptoms include:
    i.   H_____ in _____%   headache; 78%
    ii.   u_____   unilaterally
    iii. can be mistaken for t_____   typical migraine
          m_____.
    iv.   S_____ in _____%   syncope; 31%
    v.   due to involvement of the   carotid sinus
          c_____ s_____.
    vi.   T_____ changes in _____%   T-wave; 33%
    vii. due to involvement of the   coronary arteries
          c_____ a_____.
    viii. H_____ syndrome in   Horner's;
          _____%.   8%
    ix.   T_____ or i_____ in up to   TIA; infarction;
          _____%.   50%
e. Gold standard for diagnosis is _____   DSA;
    where the most common finding is   "string of pearls"
    "_____" appearance.
f. The recommended treatment is   aspirin
    _____.

11

5.   CADASIL: 11.3.6
   a.   CADASIL stands for _____   Cerebral autosomal dominant
        _____ _____ _____ with   arteriopathy with subcortical
        _____ _____ and _____.   infarcts and
                                                 leukoencephalopathy
   b.   _____ _____ inheritance   Autosomal dominant;
        pattern mapped to chromosome   19
        _____.
   c.   MRI findings similar to multiple   hypertension
        subcortical infarcts from hypertension,
        except there is no evidence of
        _____.

■ Neurotoxicology

6.   Ethanol toxicity: 11.4.1
   a.   The primary effect of ethanol on the CNS   neuronal excitability, impulse
        is depression of n_____   conduction, neurotransmitter
        e_____, i_____ c_____,   release
        and n_____ r_____.
   b.   Mellanby effect: the severity of   rising
        intoxication is greater when blood
        alcohol level is _____.
   c.   Blood alcohol level of 25 mg/dL causes   mild intoxication
        _____ _____.
   d.   Blood alcohol level of 100 mg/dL causes   cerebellar dysfunction
        _____ _____.
   e.   Blood alcohol level of 500 mg/dL causes   respiratory depression
        _____ _____.
   f.   Legal intoxication in most jurisdictions is   100 mg/dL
        a blood alcohol level of _____.
   g.   As alcohol levels fall, _____ may   hyperactivity;
        occur as a compensation for the   CNS depressant
        _____ effects of chronic alcohol
        use.
   h.   Mainstay of treatment for alcohol   Benzodiazepines
        withdrawal syndrome are _____.
   i.   They reduce a_____ h_____   autonomic hyperactivity;
        and may prevent s_____ and or   seizures;
        _____ _____.   delirium tremens
   j.   For alcohol withdrawal also use   Thiamine;
        _____ for _____ days and   3 days;
        _____ for seizures.   Dilantin
   k.   Delirium tremens occurs within   4 days
        _____ days of alcohol withdrawal.
   l.   Symptoms include a_____,   agitation, confusion,
        c_____, and a_____   autonomic instability
        i_____.
   m.   Mortality is _____% if untreated.   5-10%
   n.   Treatment includes _____.   benzodiazepines
   o.   Classic triad of Wernicke's   encephalopathy,
        encephalopathy is e_____,   ophthalmoplegia, ataxia
        o_____, and a_____.

11

p. Due to _____ deficiency.   thiamine
q. Eye signs occur in _____%.   96%
r. Gait disturbance occurs in _____.   87%
s. Memory disturbance is called _____   Korsakoff's;
    syndrome and occurs in _____%.   80%
t. Atrophy of the _____ _____   mammillary bodies
    may be seen on MRI.
u. It is a medical emergency and should be   thiamine, 100 mg;
    treated with _____, _____ mg   5 days
    daily for _____ days.
v. Thiamine administration improves   eye signs;
    _____ _____ but not   Korsakoff's
    _____ syndrome.

7. **Opioid toxicity:**   11.4.2
a. Opioids include h_____ and   heroin;
    _____ drugs.   prescription
b. Produce _____ pupils.   small
c. Reversal of toxicity is achieved with   Naloxone
    _____.

8. **Cocaine:**   11.4.3
a. Prevents reuptake of the   norepinephrine
    neurotransmitter _____.
b. Produces _____ pupils.   large
c. Can be associated with _____.   stroke

9. **Amphetamines:**   11.4.4
a. Toxicity is similar to _____.   cocaine
b. Their use can result in stroke due to   vasculitis
    _____.

10. **Carbon monoxide poisoning:**   11.4.5
a. The largest source of death from   carbon monoxide
    poisoning in the U.S. is from _____
    _____.
b. It poisons by binding to _____,   hemoglobin;
    thereby displacing _____.   oxygen
c. "_____" color of blood occurs in   Cherry-red;
    _____%.   6%
d. In severe cases, CT scan may show   low attenuation;
    l_____ a_____ in the   globus pallidus
    g_____ p_____.
e. _____% die.   40%
f. _____% have persistent sequelae.   10-30%
g. _____% make full recovery.   30-40%

11

12

Plain Radiology and Contrast Agents

■ C-Spine X-rays

1. **A lateral C-spine x-ray has four contour lines:**   12.1.1
   a. along anterior surface of vertebral bodies: a_____ m_____ l___   anterior marginal line
   b. along the back surface of the vertebral bodies: p_____ m_____ l___   posterior marginal line
   c. along the posterior margin of the spinal canal: s_____ l_____ l___   spino-laminar line
   d. along the posterior margin of the spinous process: p_____ s_____ l___   posterior spinous line

2. **Complete the following about spine films:**   12.1.4
   a. Cervical spine normal canal diameter is _____ mm.   17 +/- 5mm
   b. Stenosis is present when the anteroposterior diameter is less than _____ mm.   12 mm

3. **Complete the following about normal prevertebral soft tissue:**   12.1.4
   a. anterior C1 _____mm   10
   b. anterior C2,3,4 _____mm   7
   c. anterior C5-C6 _____mm   22

4. **Interspinous distances:**   12.1.4
   a. Are abnormal if it is _____ times the adjacent level on AP film.   1.5
   b. True or false. If present they represent:
      i. fracture   true
      ii. dislocation   true
      iii. ligament disruption   true
   c. This is called _____ on lateral x-ray.   fanning

5. **C1 has how many ossification centers?** 3   12.1.5

6. **C2 has how many ossification centers?** 4   12.1.5

■ Lumbosacral (LS) Spine X-rays

7. Complete the following regarding lumbosacral spine films.   12.2

a. The disc space with the greatest height is   L4-5
at _____.

b. AP view. Look for "owl eyes."
   i.   These correspond to the _____.   pedicles
   ii. Can be eroded in _____ disease.   metastatic

c. Oblique views. Look for the neck of the scotty dog.
   i.   It corresponds to the _____.   pars interarticularis
   ii. Discontinuity occurs in a _____.   fracture

■ Skull X-rays

8. Matching. Match the following skull film findings with their characteristics: 12.3.1
① enlarged sella; ② J-shaped sella; ③ symmetrical ballooning; ④ erosion of posterior clinoids

a. craniopharyngioma   ④
b. pituitary adenoma   ①
c. optic glioma   ②
d. empty sella   ③

9. True or False. On a skull x-ray, erosion of the posterior clinoids would most often be seen in the setting of   12.3.1

a. craniopharyngioma   true
b. empty sella syndrome   false
c. pituitary adenoma   false
d. Hurler syndrome   false
e. optic glioma   false

10. True or False. The most common congenital anomaly of the craniocervical junction is: 12.3.1

a. Chiari malformation   false
b. basilar impression   true
c. os odontoideum   false
d. incomplete arch C1   false
e. C1-C2 subluxation   false

11. What are the types of basilar invagination?   12.3.2

a. Type I: _____   BI without Chiari malformation

b. Type II:_____   BI with Chiari malformation

12. Regarding basilar invagination: 12.3.2

a. In Type I ____% can be reduced with traction.   85%

b. In Type II, f_____ m_____ d_____ is appropriate.   foramen magnum decompression

12

13. **True or False. In the evaluation of basilar invagination, in the normal patient, no part of the odontoid should be above the McRae line.**

true

12.3.2

14. **True or False. A line used in the evaluation of the craniocervical junction is**

12.3.2

a. McRae line   true
b. Chamberlain line   true
c. Wackenheim line   true
d. Maginot line   false
e. Fischgold line   true

15. **True or False. Basilar invagination is seen in**

12.3.2

a. hypoparathyroidism   false
b. Paget's disease   true
c. osteogenesis imperfecta   true
d. osteomalacia   true
e. hyperparathyroidism   true

■ Contrast Agents in Neuroradiology

16. **Characteristics of iodinated contrast agents**

12.4.1

a. may delay excretion of _____,   metformin
b. which is an _____ _____ agent   oral hypoglycemic
c. used in _____ _____ _____   diabetes type 2
d. and can be associated with l_____   lactic acidosis
   a_____
e. and r_____ f_____.   renal failure
f. It should be held for _____ hours before   48
   and after administration of contrast
   agent.

17. **The primary approved agent for intrathecal use is _____, trade name _____.**

iohexol;
Omnipaque

12.4.1

18. **Use Omnipaque cautiously in patients who have**

12.4.1

a. s_____ h_____   seizure history
b. c_____-v_____ d_____   cardio-vascular disease
c. c_____ a_____   chronic alcoholism
d. m_____ s_____   multiple sclerosis
e. and stop _____ medications at least   neuroleptic;
   _____ hours before procedure.   48

12

19. **Complete the following regarding iodinated contrast allergy prep:**   12.4.1
   a. Prednisone
      i.   Pretest timing in hours   20 to 24 hours, 8 to 12 hours, 2 hours
      ii. Dose in mg   50
      iii. Route   PO
   b. Benadryl
      i.   Pretest timing in hours   1
      ii. Dose in mg   50
      iii. Route   IM
   c. Cimetidine
      i.   Pretest timing in hours   1
      ii. Dose in mg   300
      iii. Route   PO or IV

20. **_____ may increase the risk of contrast media reactions**   Beta blockers   12.4.2
   a. and may mask manifestations of a_____ reaction.   anaphylactoid

21. **Describe some idiosyncratic reactions to contrast media.**   12.4.2
   a. Anaphylactoid reaction
      i.   h_____   hypertension
      ii. t_____   tachycardia
   b. Vasovagal reaction
      i.   h_____   hypotension
      ii. b_____   bradycardia
   c. Facial or laryngeal angioedema
      i.   Treat with _____.   epinephrine (0.3 – 0.5 mL of 1:1000 SQ)
      ii. If respiratory distress, i_____.   intubate

■ Radiation Safety for Neurosurgeons

22. **Characterize radiation safety.**   12.5.2
   a. Rem is the absorbed dose in rads multiplied by _____.   Q
   b. Q "is the quality factor": the Q of x-ray is _____.   1
   c. 1 rem causes _____ cases of cancer in every 1 million people.   300   12.5.3
   d. Spine x-rays with obliques is _____ rem.   5
   e. Cerebral angiogram is _____rem.   10 to 20
   f. Cerebral embolization is _____ rem.   34

23. **Complete the following regarding occupational radiation exposure:**   12.5.4
   a. It is advised to keep below _____ rem per year,   2
   b. averaged over a _____ year period.   5

12

24. Provide the precautions advised.   12.5.4

a. Increase the _____ from the radiation   distance
    source.

b. Exposure is proportional to the _____   inverse square
    of the distance.

c. Stay at least _____ feet, preferably   6;
    _____ feet away.   10

d. Double the distance and get _____ of   1/4
    the radiation.

e. What is better: lead "doors" or lead   doors
    aprons?

13

Imaging and Angiography

■ CAT Scan (AKA CT Scan)

1. For measurement on a CT scan

13.1.1

a. Give Hounsfield units for
   i. air — 1000
   ii. water — 0
   iii. bone — +1000
   iv. blood clot — 75-80
   v. calcium — 100-300
   vi. disc material — 55-70
   vii. thecal sac — 20-30

b. Effect of anemia on an acute subdural hematoma (SDH) in a patient with less than 23% HCT will look _____. — isodense

2. Indications for Non-contrast vs. IV contrast enhanced CT scan (CECT):

13.1.2

a. Noncontrast:
   i. Excels in demonstrating a_____ b_____, f_____, f_____ b_____, p_____ and h_____ — acute blood, fractures, foreign bodies, pneumocephalus and hydrocephalus
   ii. Weak in demonstrating a____ s____ and has poor signal quality in the p____ f____. — acute stroke; posterior fossa

b. CECT: Excels in demonstrating n____ and v_____ m_____ — neoplasms and vascular malformations

3. Abnormalities that can be demonstrated by CT perfusion (CTP):

13.1.4

a. f____ s____ s_____ — flow significant stenosis
   i. decreased C__ & C__ — decreased CBV & CBF
   ii. increased M__ and T___ — increased MTT (mean transit time) and TTP (time to peak)

b. s___: after A__ c_____, — steal: after ACZ (acetazolamide) challenge
   i. decreased C__ & C__ — decreased CBV & CBF
   ii. increased c_____ c_____ t____ & M__ — increased corresponding contralateral territory and MTT

■ Magnetic Resonance Imaging (MRI)

4. **Matching. Match the best completion for each of the following:**
① short TE, short TR; ② short TE, long TR; ③ long TE, short TR; ④ long TE, long TR

a. T1-weighted MRI has _____, _____   ①
b. T2-weighted image has _____, _____   ④

13.2.1

5. **Complete the following about magnetic resonance imaging (MRI):**

a. List the four materials that appear white on T1-weighted imaging (T1WI) MRI.   fat, melanin, and subacute blood (3-14 days), Onyx
b. What color is pathology on T1WI?   low signal on T1 (dark)
c. What color is pathology on T2WI?   high signal on T2 (white)

13.2.2

6. **Matching. Match the phrases with the appropriate signal.**
① high signal (bright); ② low signal (dark); ③ intermediate signal

a. Fat on T1 is _____   ①
b. Fat on T2 is _____   ②
c. 7- to 14-day-old blood on T2-weighted MRI is _____   ①
d. 7- to 14-day-old blood on T1-weighted MRI is _____   ①
On T1 both fat and 7-to14-day-old blood are high signal (white). On T2 fat drops out (i.e., is dark); blood remains white.

13.2.2, 13.2.3

7. **Complete the following about MRI:**
a. The best sequence for CVA is _____, which stands for _____-_____ _____ _____.   FLAIR; fluid-attenuated inversion recovery
b. Cerebrospinal fluid (CSF) is _____.   black
c. Most lesions appear _____ in this sequence.   bright
d. Most lesions are more _____.   conspicuous

13.2.5

8. **The best MRI sequence for**
a. acute SAH is _____.   FLAIR   13.2.5
b. old blood is _____ _____.   gradient echo   13.2.7

9. **Gradient echo:**
a. aka _____ _____   T2 star   13.2.7
b. aka _____   grass
c. CSF and flowing blood appear _____.   white
d. In cervical spine produces a _____ effect.   myelographic
e. Improves delineation of _____ _____.   bone spurs
f. Also shows small old _____.   hemorrhage
g. It is the most sensitive MRI sequence for i_____ b_____.   intraparenchymal blood

13

10. **Complete the following about MRI:**   13.2.8
   a. An MRI sequence that summates T1 and   STIR
      T2 signals and causes fat to be
      suppressed is called the _____
      sequence.
   b. STIR stands for _____ _____   short tau inversion recovery
      _____ _____.   (summates T1 and T2
                                                 images)
   c. Use it to see tissues that _____ in   enhance
      areas of fat.

11. **Name two contraindications to MRI.**   13.2.9
   a. Patients who contain _____ or   ferro metals or cobalt (i.e.,
      _____   cardiac pacemaker,
                                                 implanted neurostimulators,
                                                 cochlear implants,
                                                 ferromagnetic aneurysm
                                                 clips, foreign bodies with a
                                                 large component of iron or
                                                 cobalt, metallic fragments in
                                                 the eye, placement of stent,
                                                 coil, or filter within past 6
                                                 weeks)
   b. A relative contraindication to MRI is   claustrophobia
      _____

12. **Complete the following regarding**   13.2.9
    programmable valves and MRI:
   a. Can such patients have MRI studies?   yes
   b. You may need to check the _____   pressure setting
      _____ after the MRI.

13. **Hemorrhage on MRI. Related to time.**   13.2.10
    T1.
    Hint: George Washington Bridge
   a. acute g_____   gray
   b. subacute w_____   white
   c. chronic b_____   black

14. **Hemorrhage on MRI. Related to time.**   13.2.10
    T2.
    Hint: layers of Oreo cookie
   a. acute b_____   black
   b. subacute w_____   white
   c. chronic b_____   black

15. **Hemorrhage on MRI. Related to time.**   13.2.10
    Hint: i - baby, i - di, bi - di, ba - by, da - da
   a. hyper-acute
      i.   T1: i_____   isodense
      ii. T2: b_____   bright
   b. acute
      i.   T1: i_____   isodense
      ii. T2: d_____   dark
   c. subacute early
      i.   T1: b_____   bright
      ii. T2: d_____   dark

13

d. subacute late
  i.   T1: b_____   bright
  ii. T2: b_____   bright
e. chronic
  i.   T1: d_____   dark
  ii. T2: d_____   dark

16. **Age of hemorrhage**   13.2.10
  a. hyper acute: <24 hours
  b. acute: 1 to 3 days
  c. subacute early: 3 to 7 days
  d. subacute late: 7 to 14 days
  e. chronic: >14 days

17. **If MRI contrast is given to patients**   nephrogenic systemic fibrosis   13.2.11
    with severe renal failure, a rare
    condition called n_____ s_____
    f_____ may occur.

18. **Complete the following regarding**   13.2.13
    diffusion weighted images (DWI):
  a. Its primary use is to detect
    i.   _____   ischemia
    ii. and a_____ MS p_____.   active; plaques
  b. It first generates on _____ map.   ADC
  c. On DWI, freely diffusible water is
     _____.   dark
  d. Restricted diffusion is _____.   bright
  e. Which is abnormal?   restricted diffusion

19. **Characterize DWI.**   13.2.13
  a. Restricted perfusion usually indicates   cell death
     _____ _____.
  b. DWI abnormally will be present for   1 month
     _____.
  c. DWI abnormalities can light up within   minutes
     _____ of ischemia.

20. **The most sensitive study for ischemia**   PWI (Perfusion Weighted   13.2.13
    of the brain is the _____.   Imaging)

21. **DWI and PWI mismatch identifies**   13.2.13
    penumbra.
    Hint: DWI death PWI penumbra
  a. Which modality shows irreversible cell   DWI
     injury (death)?
  b. Which modality shows reversible cell   PWI
     injury (penumbra)?

22. **The important peaks in MRS are:**   13.2.14
    Hint: li-la-Na-crea-chol
  a. li_____   lipid
  b. la_____   lactate
  c. N a_____   N acetyl aspartate
  d. crea_____   creatine
  e. chol_____   choline

13

23. **The significance of important peaks in MRS are**   13.2.14
    a. hypoxia   lactate
    b. a couplet peak   lactate
    c. nerve and axons   NAA
    d. a reference for choline   creatinine
    e. membrane synthesis   choline
    f. increased in tumor   choline
    g. increased in developing brain   choline
    h. reduced in CVA   choline

24. **The test that may help distinguish hemangiopericytoma**   13.2.14
    a. from meningioma is the _____;   MRS
    b. specifically the presence of a large   inositol
       _____ peak.

25. **The test that may help a surgeon avoid critical white matter**   13.2.15
    a. tracts during brain surgery is _____,   DTI
    b. which stands for d_____ t_____   diffusor tensor imaging
       i_____.

■ Myelography

26. **True or False. The risk of postlumbar puncture headache is higher with**   13.4
    a. water-soluble contrast.   false
    b. non-water-soluble contrast.   true

27. **Matching. Match each of the following two statements with answers ①, ②, ③, or ④.**   13.4
    ① 10%; ② 35%; ③ 65%; ④ 90%
    a. In lumbar disc disease, what percentage   ②
       of free fragments move inferiorly?
    b. In lumbar disc disease, what percentage   ③
       of free fragments move superiorly?

■ Radionuclide Scanning

28. **Applications for bone scans include:**   13.5.1
    a. i_____   infection
    b. t_____   tumor
    c. d_____ involving a_____ b_____   diseases involving abnormal
       m_____   bone metabolism
    d. c_____   craniosynostosis
    e. s_____ or s_____ f_____   spine or skull fractures
    f. "l_____ b_____ p_____"   "low back problems"

29. **Applications for Gallium scan are**   13.5.2
    a. s_____   sarcoidosis
    b. c_____ v_____ o_____   chronic vertebral
                                       osteomyelitis

13

14

Electrodiagnostics

■ Electroencephalogram (EEG)

1. True or False. Periodic epileptiform discharges (PLEDs) may be produced by

14.1.1

a. herpes simplex encephalitis — true
b. brain abscess — true
c. embolic infarct — true
d. brain tumor — true
e. any acute focal cerebral insult — true

2. Matching. Match the following EEG patterns and their probable diagnostic pathology:

14.1.1

① Creutzfeldt-Jakob disease; ② hepatic encephalopathy, post anoxia and hyponatremia; ③ SSPE-subacute sclerosing panencephalitis

a. triphasic waves — ②
b. body jerks plus high-voltage periodicity with 4-15 second separation; no change with pain — ③
c. myoclonic jerks, bilateral sharp waves 1.5-2/sec, react to painful stimulation — ①

3. What is the frequency of the following EEG rhythms?

Table 14.1

a. Delta — 0-3 Hz
b. Theta — 4-7 Hz
c. Alpha — 8-13 Hz
d. Beta — >13 Hz

■ Evoked Potentials

4. Complete the following statements about evoked potentials:

14.2.3

a. Evoked potentials offer limited usefulness in avoiding _____ intraoperative injury because they are _____. — acute; delayed

b. Criteria for significance:
i. Increased latency of ____%. 10%
ii. Decreased amplitude of ____%. 50%

5. **Intraoperative SSEP may localize the primary sensory cortex by _____ potential across the central sulcus.** phase reversal 14.2.3

6. **When testing brainstem auditory evoked responses (BAER):** Table 14.5
a. Prolongation in peak I-III suggests lesion between p____ and i_____ c_____. pons and inferior colliculus
b. Prolongation in peak III-V suggests lesion between l____ p____ and m_____. lower pons and midbrain

7. **Evoked potentials during spine surgery:** 14.2.3
a. May remain unchanged by injury to the _____ cord anterior
b. but are sensitive to injury to the _____ columns of the _____ cord. posterior, dorsal

8. **True or false. Regarding transcranial (i.e., motor evoked) potentials:** 14.2.3
a. Too painful to do on the awake patient. true
b. Feedback is prompt, almost immediate. true
c. Can't record continuously because of muscle contractions. true
d. Useful for cervical spine surgery. true
e. Useful for thoracic spine surgery. true
f. Useful for lumbar spine surgery. false
g. Have more special anesthetic requirements. true

9. **Provide the SSEP deterioration plan.** 14.2.4
a. R_____ remove hardware
b. R_____ reposition patient
c. R_____ release retraction
d. S_____ sixty Hz
e. S_____ steroids
f. S_____ stop surgery
g. T_____ temperature
h. A_____ anemia
i. H_____ hypotension
j. E_____ electrode contact

■ NCS/EMG

14

10. **Name the parts of the EMG examination.** 14.3.2
a. I_____ a_____ insertional activity
b. S_____ a_____ spontaneous activity
c. V_____ a_____ volitional activity

11. **How long following denervation of muscle after nerve injury do you want to see fibrillation potentials on electromyography (EMG)?**   14.3.2
    a. The earliest is _____, but   10 days
    b. reliably not until _____.   3 to 4 weeks
    c. Therefore, don't order EMG until at least   4 weeks
       _____weeks after the injury.

12. **SNAP:**   14.3.2
    a. aka_____ _____ action potential.   sensory nerve
    b. Ganglion lies within the _____ _____.   neural foramen
    c. Herniated disc is preganglion; therefore,   not affected
       SNAP is _____ _____.

13. **F wave:**   14.3.2
    a. May be_____ in multilevel   prolonged
       radiculopathy.
    b. Most helpful in evaluating _____ root   proximal
       slowing.

14. **H reflex:**   14.3.2
    a. Is practical only regarding the _____   S1
       root.
    b. Has similar information to the ____   Ankle jerk
       _____.

15. **True or False. Regarding EMG:**   14.3.2
    a. Is low yield for radiculopathy.   true
    b. Best reserved for patients with weakness.   true
    c. Pain without weakness, EMG has low   true
       yield.

16. **True or False. Radiculopathy EMG is:**   14.3.2
    a. Reliable if negative   false – EMG is not sensitive
                                                     for radiculopathy
    b. Reliable if positive   true – when positive very
                                                     specific.

17. **The earliest possible finding in EMG for radiculopathy is _____ _____**   reduced recruitment (2-3 days)   14.3.2

18. **Findings with healing radiculopathy:**   14.3.2
    a. _____ potentials return first.   Motor
    b. If lost, _____ return last or may not   Sensory
       return.

14

15

Primary Intracranial Anomalies

■ Arachnoid Cysts, Intracranial

1. Characterize intracranial arachnoid cysts. · 15.1.1
a. Origin: c_____ · congenital
b. Arise from splitting of a_____ m_____. · arachnoid membrane
c. Contain fluid identical to _____. · CSF
d. Incidence per 1000 autopsies: · 5
e. More common in male or female? · male
f. Most are a_____. · asymptomatic
g. If symptomatic, typical symptoms are:
   i. i_____ h_____ · intracranial hypertension
   ii. s_____ · seizures

2. True or False. Acute deterioration in patients with known arachnoid cysts usually signifies · 15.1.4
a. rapid increase in cyst size. · false
b. postictal state. · false
c. rupture into subdural space. · false
d. rupture of bridging veins and cyst bleed. · true

3. Complete the following about arachnoid cysts:
a. The location of the only extradural type of arachnoid cyst is in the _____ cyst. · intrasellar · 15.1.3
b. A retrocerebellar arachoid cyst might mimic a _____-_____ syndrome. · Dandy-Walker
c. The most common location for an arachnoid cyst is the _____ _____. · Sylvian fissure · Table 15.1
d. The next most common location is the _____ _____. · cerebellopontine angle
e. They are associated with ventriculomegaly in _____%. · 64% · 15.1.5
f. The best treatment is probably c_____ s_____. · cyst shunting · 15.1.6

15

■ Craniofacial Development

4. Complete the following about craniofacial development: 15.2.1

a. The anterior fontanelle closes by age _____.   2.5 years

b. Head size is 90% of adult size at age _____.   1 year

c. The head stops enlarging by age _____.   7 years
d. The skull is _____ at birth.   unilaminar
e. Diploe appears by the _____ year and   4th
f. Reaches a maximum at age _____.   35
g. Diploic veins form at age _____.   35
h. Air cells in the mastoid occur in _____ year.   6th

5. True or False. Craniosynostosis   15.2.2
a. has been proven to occur after shunting.   false
b. of one suture does not cause increased ICP.   false (11% have high ICP)

6. Complete the following about craniofacial development: 15.2.2
a. The most common craniosynostosis is _____.   sagittal

b. The male to female ratio is _____.   80:20
c. The resulting skull shape is _____.   dolichocephalic/ scaphocephalic/boat shape

d. Surgery should be done within the age range of _____.   3 to 6 months
e. The strip craniectomy should be _____ cm wide.   3 cm

7. Complete the following regarding coronal synostosis   15.2.2
a. Incidence of patients with craniosynostosis who have coronal synostosis is _____%.   18%

b. In which is it more common, males or females?   females

8. Complete the following regarding coronal suture synostosis (CSS):   15.2.2
a. Plus syndactyly is called _____ syndrome.   Apert's syndrome
b. Unilateral CSS is called _____.   plagiocephaly
c. CSS plus hypoplasia of the face is called _____ disease.   Crouzon's disease
d. Plagiocephaly
   i.   Forehead on affected side is _____ or _____.   flattened; concave
   ii. Supraorbital ridge has a _____ margin.   higher

9. Regarding harlequin eye sign   15.2.2

15

a. Occurs in u_____ c_____ suture   unilateral coronal
    closure
b. seen on _____ _____ _____.   anteroposterior skull X-ray
c. The abnormal bony structure is the   supraorbital margin
    _____ _____,
d. which is _____ than the normal side.   higher

10. **Complete the following about**   15.2.2
    craniofacial development:
    a. What suture is closed to produce   metopic
        trigonocehaly?
    b. It is usually associated with an   19 p
        abnormality of the _____
        chromosome.

11. **Characterize lambdoid synostosis.**   15.2.2
    a. Male to female ratio is _____.   4:1
    b. Side involved most frequently is _____. right side
    c. The frequency of involvement is   70%
        _____% right.
    d. Does it have a ridge or an indentation to indentation (Not a ridge like
        palpation?   the sagittal or coronal
                                                  synostosis)

12. **Considering lambdoid synostosis:**   15.2.2
    a. Differentiate from positional flattening top of the head
        by looking at the ears from the
        _____.
    b. In lambdoid synostosis you will see the   lags behind
        ipsilateral ear _____ _____.
    c. In positional flattening you will see the pushed forward (If flat side of
        ipsilateral ear is _____ _____.   occipital bone is same side as
                                                  the posteriorly positioned ear
                                                  it is a case of lamboid
                                                  synostosis; if not it is a case of
                                                  positional flattening)

13. **Answer the following concerning**   15.2.2
    lambdoid synostosis treatment:
    a. True or False. All require surgery.   False (15% won't respond to
                                                  repositioning.)
    b. True or False. Surgery is indicated early False (one can observe for 3
        (i.e., 3 to 6 months).   to 6 months for
                                                  improvement)
    c. Ideal age for surgery is _____ to _____ 6 to 18
        months.
    d. Early surgery is indicated for s_____ severe disfigurement and
        d_____ and e_____ i_____   elevated intracranial pressure
        p_____.

14. **Complete the following about**   15.2.3
    encephalocele:
    a. Incidence of basal form of encephalocele 1.5%
        is _____%.
    b. May exit the skull via a defect in

15

i.   c_____ p_____   cribriform plate
ii. f_____ c_____   foramen cecum
iii. s_____ o_____ f_____   superior orbital fissure

■ Dandy Walker Malformation

15. **To differentiate DWM from   15.3.2
retrocerebellar arachnoid cyst observe
for**
  a. v_____ a_____   vermian agenesis
  b. cyst opens into f_____ v_____   fourth ventricle
  c. enlarged p_____ f_____   posterior fossa
  d. elevation of the t_____ h_____ torcular herophili

16. **What is Dandy-Walker pathogenesis?**   15.3.3
  a. D   dilation of 4th ventricle
  b. A   agenesis of vermis
  c. N(m)   membrane of 4th ventricle
  d. D   dysembryo genesis
  e. Y   hydrocephalus

17. **Complete the following regarding
Dandy-Walker malformation (DWM):**
  a. It is caused by a _____ of the f_____   atresia of the foramina;   15.3.5
     of M_____ and L_____.   Magendie and Luschka (old
                                            theory)
  b. Results in   15.3.3
     i.   agenesis of _____   vermis
     ii. large _____ _____ _____ which   posterior fossa cyst
          communicates with the
     iii. _____ _____, which becomes   fourth ventricle;
          _____.   enlarged

18. **What is Dandy-Walker pathogenesis?**
  a. Hydrocephalus is present in _____%   70 to 90%   15.3.3
  b. and _____% of hydrocephalus patients   2 to 4%
     have DWS.
  c. A common associated abnormality is   15.3.5
     i.   a_____ of the c_____ c_____   agenesis of the corpus
                                            callosum
     ii. in _____ %.   17%
  d. and c_____ a_____.   cardiac abnormalities
  e. If treatment is necessary, you must shunt   cyst   15.3.6
     the ventricle, the cyst, or both?
  f. If aqueductal stenosis you should shunt   ventricle
     _____ also.
  g. But shunting the lateral ventricle alone
     i.   is _____   contraindicated
     ii. because it might cause _____   upward herniation
          _____.
  h. To avoid _____ herniation,   upward
  i. you must not shunt the _____ alone.   ventricle

19. **What is the prognosis of DWM?**   15.3.7

a. Seizures occur in _____%.   15%
b. Mortality occurs in _____ to _____%   12 to 50%
c. Normal IQ is _____%.   50%

■ Aqueductal Stenosis

20. **True or False. Aqueductal stenosis is**   False (Adults can present with   15.4.1
    seen only in children.   symptoms as well.)

21. **What are the causes of aqueductal**   15.4.2
    stenosis?
   a. A   astrocytoma of brain stem
   b. Q   quadrigeminal plate mass
   c. E(i)   inflammation infection
   d. C   congenital atresia
   e. T   tumor
   f. A   arachnoid cyst
   g. L   lipoma

22. **Complete the following concerning**   15.4.3
    aqueductal stenosis:
   a. It is associated with congenital   70%   15.4.4
      hydrocephalus in _____%.
   b. MRI may show absence of
      i.   n_____ f_____ v_____ in the   normal flow void
      ii. a_____ of S_____   aqueduct of Sylvius
   c. MRI with contrast should be used to rule   tumor
      out _____.
   d. Follow-up should be for at least _____.   2 years
   e. In order to rule out _____.   tumor

23. **True or False. A patient with**   15.4.4
    aqueductal stenosis of adulthood may
    have the following symptoms:
   a. Headache   true
   b. Visual disturbances   true
   c. Decline of mental function   true
   d. Gait disturbance   true
   e. Papilledema (sign)   true
   f. Ataxia   true
   g. Urinary incontinence   true

24. **What are the treatment options for**   15.4.4
    aqueductal stenosis?
   a. Ventriculoperitoneal _____ _____   CSF shunting
   b. T_____ _____ _____ _____   Torkildsen shunt in adults
   c. ETV = _____ _____ _____   endoscopic third
                                                     ventriculostomy

---

■ Agenesis of the Corpus Callosum

15

25. **Agenesis of the corpus callosum forms**   2 weeks;   15.5.1
    at age _____ after conception and   rostrum to splenium
    forms from _____ to _____.

26. **Complete the following concerning the bundles of Probst:**   15.5.3
   a. They are aborted beginnings of the   corpus callosum
       _____ _____
   b. bulging into the _____ _____.   lateral ventricles

27. **Complete the following regarding agenesis of the corpus callosum:**   15.5.4
   a. Does it always have clinical significance?   No, it may be an incidental finding
   b. Underlying cause may be an abnormality   chromosome
       of a _____.

■ Absence of the Septum Pellucidum

28. **One possible cause of absence of septum pellucidum is**   15.6
   a. s_____-o_____ d_____   septo-optic dysplasia
   b. aka _____ _____,   de Morsier syndrome
   c. which produces h_____ of o_____   hypoplasia of optic nerve
       n_____
   d. and o_____ c_____ as well as   optic chiasm
   e. p_____ i_____.   pituitary infundibulum

■ Intracranial Lipomas

29. **Intracranial lipomas**   15.7.2
   a. are usually found in the _____   midsagittal plane
       _____
   b. especially in the _____ _____.   corpus callosum
   c. They are frequently associated with   agenesis
       _____
   d. of the _____ _____.   corpus callosum
   e. They may less frequently involve the
       i.   t_____ c_____   tuber cinereum
       ii. and the _____ _____.   quadrigeminal plate

30. **True or False. Characteristics of intracranial lipomas include**   15.7.3
   a. association with _____ abnormalities   congenital
   b. on CT they have a _____ density.   low
   c. Differential diagnosis is
       i.   d_____ c_____   dermoid cyst
       ii. t_____   teratoma
       iii. g_____   germinoma
   d. On MRI they have a _____ intensity on   high
       T1.
   e. On MRI they have a _____ intensity on   low
       T2.

15

31. **Intracranial lipomas may present clinically with**   15.7.4
    a. s_____   seizures
    b. h_____ d_____   hypothalamic dysfunction
    c. h_____   hydrocephalus
    d. m_____ r_____   mental retardation

■ Hypothalamic Hamartomas

32. **Hypothalamic hamartomas**   15.8.1
    a. are frequent or rare?   rare
    b. are neoplastic or nonneoplastic?   nonneoplastic
    c. consist of a mass of _____ _____   neuronal tissues
    d. that arises from the
        i.   in_____ h_____ or   inferior hypothalamus
        ii. t_____ c_____   tuber cinereum

33. **Hypothalamic hamartomas clinically**   15.8.2
    a. may present with a special type of   gelastic; laughing
        seizure called _____, which means
        _____ seizure.
    b. may also have _____ attacks.   rage
    c. may also present with p_____   precocious puberty
        p_____
    d. due to release of g_____ r_____   gonadotropin releasing
        h_____   hormone
    e. formed within the _____ cells.   hamartoma

15

16

Primary Spinal Anomalies

■ Spinal Dysraphism (Spina Bifida)

1. Study sheet. Spinal bifida occulta 16.2.2

a.	B	bifida
b.	I	incidental
c.	F	foot deformity
d.	I	innocuous
e.	D	diastematomyelia
f.	A	atrophy of leg
g.	O	occurs in 20 to 30%
h.	C	cutaneous stigmata
i.	C	clinical importance nil
j.	U	urinary incontinence
k.	L	lipoma leg weakness
l.	T	tethered cord
m.	A	absent spinous process

2. Complete the following regarding myelomeningocele (MM): 16.2.3

a. The anterior neuropore closes at gestational age day _____.   25

b. The posterior neuropore closes at gestational age day _____.   28

3. Complete the following regarding myelomeningocele (MM): 16.2.3

a. Incidence if no previous child has MM equals ____% or _____ per 1000.   0.2% or 2%

b. One previous MM child: _____% or _____ per 1000.   2%, 20

c. Two previous MM children: _____% or _____ per 1000.   6%, 60

d. Associated hydrocephalus: incidence of _____%.   80%

e. Associated Chiari II occurs in _____ children with MM.   most

4. **Answer the following about myelomeningocele:**   16.2.3
    a. What is the incidence of meningocele or myelomeningocele?   1 to 2/1000 live births (0.2%)
    b. Does the risk increase in families with one affected child?   Yes (The risk does increases to 2 to 3% in families with one previous myelomeningocele child.)
    c. Does the risk increase in families with two affected children?   Yes (It further increases to 6 to 8% in families with two previous affected children.)

5. **True or False. All children born with myelomeningocele have an associated Chiari II malformation.**   false (Not all, but most, have Chiari II.)   16.2.3

6. **True or False. Closure of myelomeningocele may result in the need for CSF shunting.**   true   16.2.3

7. **Meningomyelocele patients develop allergy to _____.**   latex   16.2.3

8. **True or False or Uncertain. Intrauterine closure of mm defect reduces**   16.2.3
    a. Chiari II defect   true
    b. hydrocephalus   uncertain
    c. neurological dysfunction   false

9. **Complete the following concerning myelomeningocele:**   16.2.3
    a. If ruptured, start _____ (n_____ and g_____).   antibiotics (nafcillin and gentamicin)
    b. Perform surgery within _____ to _____ hours.   24 to 36 hours
    c. Better functional outcome occurs if children have spontaneous _____ of _____ _____.   movement of lower extremities
    d. Do multiple anomalies occur in myelomeningocele?   Yes (average 2 to 2.5 additional anomalies in myelomeningocele)

10. **Complete the following about myelomeningocele and early closure:**   16.2.3
    a. True or False. Results in improvement of neurological functions.   false
    b. True or False. Results in lower infection rate.   true
    c. Myelomeningocele should be closed within 12, 24, or 36 hours?   24 hours

16

11. **Considering late problems in myelomeningocele repair. Possible late problems include:**   16.2.3
    a. brain: hydrocephalus – malfunctioning shunt
    b. cervicomedullary junction: Chiari II compressing medulla
    c. cord: Syrinx
    d. cauda: tethered cord

12. **Characterize myelomeningocele outcome without treatment and with treatment.**   16.2.3
    a. Survive infancy without treatment ___ - ___%; with treatment ____%.   15 to 30%; 85%
    b. Normal IQ without treatment _____%; with treatment _____%   70%; 80%
    c. Ambulatory without treatment ____%; with treatment ____ - ____%   50%; 40 to 85%
    d. Continence without treatment _____; with treatment ____ - ____%.   rare; 3 to 10%

13. **For each of the following, what are the facts to know concerning lipomeningocele?**   16.2.4
    a. age for surgery   2 months is appropriate
    b. band   thick fibrovascular band
    c. conus   is split
    d. dura   is dehiscent
    e. epidural fat versus _____   lipoma (is distinct from epidural fat)
    f. placode   attached to neural placode
    g. neuro exam   is normal in 50%
    h. sensory loss   most common neurological abnormality
    i. stigmata   cutaneous
    j. urologic exam   should be done pre-op

14. **True or False. Lipomyelomeningocele is associated with tethered cord.**   true   16.2.4

15. **Study Chart. Lipomeningocele:**   16.2.4
    a. Steps in surgical management (Courtesy of Dr. David Frim):
       1. Untether the cord using Xomed CUSA and recording from anal sphincter
       2. Free up sides from attachment to dura.
       3. Reduce the bulk of fat using CUSA in the midline.
       4. Tie dura open to sides.
       5. Place bovine pericardial graft as dural substitute.

16. **True or False. The most common location of a dermal sinus tract is the:**   16.2.5
   a. occipital region   false
   b. cervical region   false
   c. thoracic region   false
   d. lumbosacral region   true

17. **What is the most likely cause of dermal sinus?**   16.2.5
   a. Failure of the _____ ectoderm   cutaneous
   b. to_____   separate
   c. from the _____-ectoderm   neuro
   d. at the time of _____   closure
   e. of the _____ _____.   neural groove

18. **Dermal sinus facts to know include:**   16.2.5
   a. Most commonly located in the _____ area.   lumbosacral
   b. Results from _____ of _____ of _____ _____   failure of separation of cuteanous ectoderm
   c. from _____ _____.   neural ectoderm
   d. Appears as a _____: dimple
      i.   Hair?   With or without
      ii. Midline?   Close to midline
      iii. Skin stigmata?   yes
   e. First manifestation is _____.   bladder dysfunction
   f. Tract always courses _____ from lumbosacral area.   cephalad

19. **True or False. An epidermoid cyst contains hair follicles and sweat glands.**   false   16.2.5

20. **What is the major difference between epidermoid cyst and dermoid cyst?**   16.2.5
   a. Epidermoid cyst is
      i. lined with s_____ s_____ e_____   stratified squamous epithelium
      ii. and contains only _____   keratin
   b. Dermoid cyst is
      i.   lined with _____   dermis
      ii. and contains _____ _____ such as   skin appendages
      iii. hair follicles?   yes
      iv. sebaceous glands?   yes

21. **True or False. A dermal sinus tract is a potential pathway for intradural infection such as meningitis or abscess.**   true   16.2.5

22. **Radiologic evaluation of dermal sinus.**   16.2.5
   a. If seen at births do _____.   ultrasound
   b. If first seen later do _____.   MRI

16

23. **Given the above, indicate whether the dermal sinus tract should be excised at the given locations.**   16.2.5
    a. lumbar   yes
    b. sacral   yes
    c. coccygeal   no

24. **Complete the following concerning the cranial dermal sinus:**   16.2.5
    a. The track extends _____   caudally
    b. If the dermal sinus tract enters the skull   caudal
       it does so _____ to the torcula.

■ Klippel-Feil Syndrome

25. **True or False. Klippel-Feil syndrome results from failure of**   16.3.1
    a. primary neurulation   false
    b. secondary neurulation   false
    c. dysjunction   false
    d. segmentation   true

26. **Klippel-Feil syndrome**   16.3.1
    a. Results from failure of _____ of   segmentation of cervical
       _____ _____ at gestational age of   somites
    b. ___ to ___ weeks.   3 to 8 weeks
    c. Clinical triad   16.3.2
       i.   Hairline is _____.   low
       ii. Neck is _____.   short
       iii. Motion is _____.   limited
    d. Limitation of range of motion of the neck   3
       occurs only if more than _____
       segments are fused.
    e. True or false. Other congenital   true
       abnormalities may also be present.
    f. True or false. Klippel-Feil causes   false
       symptoms related to fused vertebrae.

27. **True or False. Anomalies seen associated with Klippel-Feil include**   16.3.2
    a. Sprengel deformity   true
    b. webbing of the neck   true
    c. basilar impression   true
    d. unilateral absence of the kidney   true

28. **Possible systemic congenital abnormalities include**   16.3.2
    a. g_____   genitourinary – absence of
                                             one kidney
    b. c_____   cardiopulmonary

16

■ Tethered Cord Syndrome

29. **List the six presenting signs and symptoms of tethered cord syndrome.**
    a. c_____
    b. s_____
    c. b_____
    d. s_____
    e. g_____
    f. p_____

    cutaneous (54%)
    scoliosis (29%)
    bladder (40%)
    sensations (70%)
    gait (93%)
    pain (37%)

    Table 16.2

30. **True or False. Regarding tethered cord syndrome.**
    a. Progressive scoliosis is not seen in conjunction with tethered cord syndrome.

    false

    b. Early untethering may result in improvement in scoliosis.

    true

    16.4.4

31. **True or False. The following is associated with adult tethered cord syndrome:**
    a. Foot deformities
    b. Pain
    c. Leg weakness
    d. Urological symptoms

    false
    true
    true
    true

    16.4.5

32. **True or False. Urological symptoms are not common in the adult tethered cord syndrome.**

    false

    16.4.5

33. **True or False. A tethered conus lies distal to L2 on radiographic evaluation.**

    true

    16.4.5

34. **Complete the following concerning tethered cord syndrome:**
    a. Name two criteria.
       i. Conus below level _____
       ii. Thick filum greater than _____
    b. A preop test that is strongly recommended is a _____.

    L2
    2mm diameter
    cystometrogram

    16.4.5

    16.4.6

35. **Indicate the characteristics used to identify the filum.**
    a. The vessel on the surface is _____.
    b. The color of the filum is _____ _____ than nerve roots

    squiggly
    more white

    16.4.6

36. **Complete the following outcome from tethered cord:**
    a. In meningomyelocele it is usually _____ to permanently _____.
    b. Repeated untethering is advised till patient stops _____.

    impossible; untether

    growing

    16.4.6

16

37. **Symptoms of untethering are especially likely during the a_____ g_____ s_____.**

    adolescent growth spurt   16.4.6

38. **Surgical release in an adult is**
    16.4.6
 a. good for _____ _____ and   pain relief
 b. poor for return of _____ _____.   bladder function

■ Split Cord Malformation

39. **True or False. Diastematomyelia is associated with nonrigid bony septum that separates two durally unsheathed hemicords.**

    false (septum is rigid)   16.5.2

40. **Complete the following concerning diastematomyelia:**
    16.5.2
 a. Cutaneous stigmata are h_____ tuft or hypertrichosis.   hair
 b. True or false. There are foot abnormalities,   true
 c. specifically n_____ h_____-a_____ f_____.   neurogenic high-arched foot

16

17

Primary Craniospinal Anomalies

■ Chiari Malformations

1. Compare Chiari types I and II.   Table 17.1
a. medulla-caudal dislocation   Chiari I, no;
                                              Chiari II, yes
b. into cervical canal   Chiari I, tonsils;
                                              Chiari II, vermis, medulla,
                                              fourth ventricle
c. myelomeningocele   Chiari I, no;
                                              Chiari II, yes
d. hydrocephalus   Chiari I, no;
                                              Chiari II, yes
e. medullary kink   Chiari I, no;
                                              Chiari II, 55%
f. cervical nerves   Chiari I, normal;
                                              Chiari II, upward
g. age at presentation   Chiari I, adult;
                                              Chiari II, infant
h. symptoms   Chiari I, neck pain;
                                              Chiari II, hydrocephalus,
                                              respiratory distress

2. Complete the following about Chiari   17.1.2
   malformation:
a. Chiari I has how many abnormalities?   1—with many names
b. List four names this abnormality has
    been called.
    i.   t_____ h_____   tonsillar herniation
    ii. c_____ d_____ of c_____   caudal displacement of
                                              cerebellum
    iii. p_____ e_____ of t_____   peglike elongation of tonsil
    iv. c_____ e_____   cerebellar ectopia

3. Chiari I   17.1.2
a. has how many deformities?   1
b. is known by the following names
    i.   e_____   ectopia
    ii. e_____   elongation
    iii. d_____   displacement
    iv. h_____   herniation

17

c. symptoms
    i.   o_____ h_____   occipital headaches
    ii. c_____ p_____   cervical pain

4. **What is the particular eye sign**   Downbeat nystagmus is   17.1.2
   associated with Chiari I?   considered a characteristic of
                                              this condition in 47%, but it
                                              can also occur in Chiari II.

5. **What percentage of Chiari I patients**   20 to 30% of Chiari I patients   17.1.2
   have hydrosyringomyelia?   have a syrinx.

6. **Characterize the location of tonsils**   Table 17.4
   and Chiari I.
   a. Normal range related to foramen
      magnum
      i.   high   8 mm above
      ii. low   5 mm below
      iii. mean   1 mm above
   b. Chiari I range is
      i.   high   3 mm below
      ii. low   29 mm below
      iii. mean   13 mm below
   c. Symptoms can occur with tonsils at   2
      _____ mm below.
   d. Usual level considered cutoff for   5
      diagnosis is _____ mm below.

7. **Possible better correlation with**   17.1.2
   symptoms of tonsillar herniation is the
   degree of brain stem compression
   a. at the _____ _____   foramen magnum
   b. as seen on the _____   axial
   c. T_____ W1 MRI.   2
   d. The best results from surgery occur if 2
      treated within _____ years of onset
      of symptoms.

8. **Complete the following concerning**   17.1.2
   Chiari I:
   a. The most common postop complication   respiratory depression in 15%
      is _____ _____ in _____ %.
   b. Occurs within how many days of   5
      surgery?
   c. Occurs mostly at what time of day?   night
   d. Death can occur from s_____   sleep apnea
      a_____.
   e. Other risks of surgery include
      i.   c_____ f_____ l_____   cerebrospinal fluid leak
      ii. injury to p_____ i_____   posterior inferior cerebellar
           c_____ a_____   artery (PICA)
      iii. h_____ of c_____ h_____   herniation of cerebellar
                                              hemispheres

17

9. **Complete the following concerning Chiari I:**   17.1.2
   a. Operative results
      i.   Main benefit may be to a_____   arrest progression
           p_____.
      ii. Best results in patients with   cerebellar
           _____ syndrome
      iii. which consists of
           t_____ a_____   truncal ataxia
           l_____ a_____   limb ataxia
           n_____   nystagmus
           d_____   dysarthria
   b. Which responds better: pain or   pain
      weakness?

10. **Factors that correlate with a worse outcome are**   17.1.2
    a. a_____   atrophy
    b. s_____   scoliosis
    c. symptoms that are lasting more than   2 years
       _____ _____

11. **Which Chiari malformation is associated with myelomeningocele?**   Chiari II   17.1.3

12. **Study Chart. Chiari II anatomical abnormalities: A to Z.**   17.1.3

    *a*tlas assimilation
    *b*eaking of tectum, *b*ony abnormalities
    *c*erebellar folia poorly myelinated, *c*ervical medullary junction compression, *c*raniolacunia, *c*orpus callosum agenesis
    *d*egenerated lower CN nuclei
    *e*nlarged massa intermedia
    *f*alx hypoplasia, *f*ourth ventricle trapped, *f*usion of cervical vertebrae
    *g*yri miniaturized
    *h*ydrocephalus, *h*eterotopia, *h*ydromyelia
    *K*lippel-Feil deformity
    *l*ow attachment of tentorium
    *m*assa intermedia enlarged
    *m*edulla oblongata "z" bend
    *m*icrogyria
    *n*uclei of lower CN degenerated
    *p*latybasia, *p*eg of cerebellar tonsils
    *s*eptum pellucidum absent, *s*yringomyelia
    *t*ectum beaking, *t*entorium low attachment
    Z-shaped bend of medulla

17

13. **Finding on presentation of Chiari II.**   17.1.3
Hint: n^2 chiari two

a. n_____   nystagmus—down beat
b. n_____ _____   nasal regurgitation
c. c_____   cyanosis
d. h_____   hoarseness
e. i_____ _____ _____   impaired ventilatory drive
f. a_____ _____, _____   apneic spells, aspiration
g. r_____, _____ _____   regurgitation, respiratory
                                        arrest
h. i_____ _____   inspiratory stridor
i. t_____ _____ _____   tenth nerve (vagus) vocal
    _____ _____   cord paralysis
j. w_____ _____   weak arm—weak cry
k. o_____   opisthotonus

14. **Complete the following regarding**   17.1.3
Chiari II.

a. The most common cause of mortality is   respiratory arrest
    _____ _____.

b. The mortality at 6 years follow-up is   40%
    _____%.

c. Range of mortality
    i.   Infants in poor condition (i.e.,   71%
         cardiopulmonary arrest, vocal cord
         paralysis, and/or arm weakness
         mortality) is _____%.

d. If there is gradual onset of symptoms,   23%
    mortality is _____%.

e. The worst prognostic factor for response   bilateral vocal cord paralysis
    to surgery is b_____ v_____
    c_____ p_____.

■ Neural Tube Defects

15. **With neural tube defects there are**   17.2.1
classification systems. Give examples
of

a. neurulation defects
    i.   a_____   anencephaly
    ii. m_____   myelomeningocele
b. postneurulation defects
    i.   m_____   microcephaly
    ii. h_____   hydranencephaly
    iii. h_____   holoprosencephaly
    iv. l_____   lissencephaly
    v.   s_____   schizencephaly
c. spinal defects
    i.   d_____   diastematomyelia
    ii. s_____   syringomyelia

16. **Complete the following about neural tube defects:**   17.2.1
   a. Failure to fuse the anterior neuropore results in _____.   anencephaly
   b. Failure to fuse the posterior neuropore results in _____.   myelomeningocele
   c. The definition of microcephaly is head circumference _____ _____ _____ below the mean.   2 standard deviations
   d. In hydranencephaly the cortex is replaced by _____.   CSF
   e. Failure to cleave can result in _____.   holoprosencephaly

17. **Complete the following about neural tube defects:**   17.2.1
   a. Give examples of neurulation defects.
       i.   a_____   anencephaly
       ii. c_____   craniorachischisis
       iii. m_____   myelomeningocele
   b. These defects are due to _____ of the neural tube.   nonclosure

18. **Complete the following about neural tube defects:**   17.2.1
   a. Name five postneurulation defects.
       i.   h_____   hydranencephaly
       ii. l_____   lissencephaly (most severe)
       iii. h_____   holoprosencephaly
       iv. a_____ of _____ _____   agenesis of corpus callosum
       v.   d_____   diastematomyelia
   b. Which is the most severe?   lissencephaly

19. **Complete the following regarding lissencephaly:**   17.2.1
   a. It is an example of an abnormality of neuronal _____.   migration
   b. It results in an abnormality of the _____ _____   cortical convolutions
   c. called _____   agyria

20. **Name the key features of schizencephaly.**   17.2.1
   a. _____ which communicates with _____   cleft; ventricle
   b. lined with _____ _____   gray matter
   c. Two types are
       i.   o_____ l_____   open lipped
       ii. c_____ l_____   close lipped

21. **Complete the following about neural tube defects:**   17.2.1
   a. In schizencephaly, the cleft wall is lined with cortical _____ _____.   gray matter
   b. In porencephaly, the cystic lesion is lined with _____ or _____ tissue.   connective or glial

22. Hydranencephaly   17.2.2
   a. is a _____ defect.   post-neurulation
   b. Cranium is filled with _____.   CSF
   c. Is there a small or large head?   large (macrocrania)
   d. Most common etiology is _____   bilateral ICA infarcts

      _____ _____.

   e. Angiography
      i.   of anterior circulation shows   no flow

          _____ _____.

      ii. of posterior circulation shows   normal flow

          _____ _____.

23. Complete the following about neural   17.2.2
   tube defects:
   a. What are the three types of
      holoprosencephaly? Please list in order
      of decreasing severity.
      i.   a_____   alobar (single ventricle, most
                                               severe)
      ii. s_____   semilobar
      iii. l_____   lobar (least severe)
   b. They occur because of
      i.   failure to _____   cleave
      ii. of the _____ _____.   telencephalic vesicle

24. List the risk factors for neural tube   17.2.3
   defects.
   a. B_____ i_____   B12 insufficiency
   b. c_____   cocaine—maternal use
   c. D_____   Depakene—use during
                                               pregnancy
   d. f_____ a_____ i_____   folic acid insufficiency
   e. f_____   fever in first trimester
   f. h_____ e_____   heat exposure—maternal hot
                                               tub, sauna
   g. o_____   obesity before and during
                                               pregnancy
   h. v_____ a_____   valproic acid use during
                                               pregnancy
   i. v_____   vitamins—prenatal lack of
                                               folic acid and B12

25. What are the tests for prenatal   17.2.4
   detection of neural tube defects?
   a. Serum _____ _____.   alfa fetoprotein (If high at 15
                                               to 20 weeks be suspicious for
                                               neural tube defects.)
   b. U_____,   ultrasonography
   c. which can detect what % of spina bifida 90%
      cases?
   d. a_____   amniocentesis

26. **Regarding prenatal detection of neural tube defects.**   17.2.4

   a. Test mother's serum for _____   alpha fetoprotein
      _____,

   b. which has a sensitivity rate for spina   91%; 100%
      bifida _____% and for anencephaly
      _____%.

   c. Closed spinal dysraphism _____   may be missed
      _____ _____.

   d. An overestimate of gestational age will   normal
      make us think that a high alpha
      fetoprotein level is _____.

   e. Real-time imaging through _____.   ultrasonography

   f. Identifies _____% of s _____   90% of spinal bifida
      b_____.

   g. Obtaining fluid from the womb is called   amniocentesis
      _____.

   h. It carries a risk of fetal loss of   6%
      _____%.

■ Neurenteric Cysts

27. **Complete the following about neurenteric cysts:**   17.3.1

   a. A neurenteric cyst is a central nervous   endothelium
      system (CNS) cyst lined with _____

   b. resembling the _____ or _____   gastrointestinal or respiratory
      tract.

   c. Regions affected are usually the   cervical or thoracic
      _____ or _____ areas.

   d. Histologically, cyst lined with   cuboidal-columnar   17.3.2
      c_____-c_____ e_____   epithelium

   e. with m_____-s_____ g_____   mucin-secreting goblet cells
      c_____.

18

Coma

■ General Information

1. **Write out the Glascow Coma Scale (GCS) and indicate the score assigned to each point on the scale.**
   a. Eyes
      i. e___   4 spontaneous
      ii. y___   3 to speech
      iii. e___   2 to pain
      iv. s___   1 nil
   b. Verbal
      i. v___   5 oriented
      ii. o___   4 confused
      iii. i___   3 inappropriate
      iv. c___   2 incoherent
      v. e___   1 nil
   c. Motor
      i. m___   6 obeys
      ii. o___   5 localizes
      iii. v___   4 withdrawal
      iv. i___   3 decorticate
      v. n___   2 decerebrate
      vi. g___   1 nil

   18.1

2. **True or False. A patient with a GCS score E2 V1 M2 (GCS 5) is in a coma.**

   false (Whereas 90% of patients with GCS < 8 are in a coma, coma is defined as the inability to obey commands, speak or open the eyes even to pain.)

   18.1

3. **Define coma.**

   A GCS less than 8 is a generally accepted operational definition of coma.

   18.1

4. **List the three locations of brain lesions that produce coma.**
   a. u_____ p____ and m_____   upper pons and midbrain
   b. d_____   diencephalic
   c. b_____ c_____ h_____   bilateral cerebral hemisphere

   18.1

■ Posturing

5. Disinhibition by removal of the corticospinal pathways above the midbrain typically results in _____ (f_____) posturing.

decorticate (flexion)   18.2.2

6. Disinhibition by removal of the vestibulospinal tract and pontine reticular formation by removing inhibition of medullary reticular formation typically results in _____ (e_____) posturing.

decerebrate (extension)   18.2.3

7. Complete the following about coma in general:
   a. In a decorticate posturing
      i. the upper extremities are in _____.
      ii. the lower extremities are in _____.

18.2.3

flexion
extension

   b. In decerebrate posturing
      i. the upper extremities are in _____.
      ii. the lower extremities are in _____.

extension
extension

■ Etiologies of Coma

8. A patient is brought to the ER in a coma after being found down. Pupils are equal and reactive. Painful stimulus elicits no movement. No signs of trauma are evident. Studies show Na 130, K 4.9. C 1-100, HCO$_3$ 2-15, BUN 30, Cr 1.2, Glu 440. The likely cause of coma is _____ _____.

diabetic ketoacidosis   18.3.1

9. Indicate the effect of midline shift on level of consciousness.
   a. 0 to 3 mm:
   b. 3 to 4 mm:
   c. 6 to 8.5 mm:
   d. 8 to 13 mm:

Table 18.3

alert
drowsy
stuporous
comatose

10. The three categories of disorders in the different diagnosis of pseudocoma are:
   a. l_____-i_____ s_____ and v_____ p_____ i_____

18.3.3

locked-in syndrome; ventral pontine infract

   b. p_____ d_____, c_____, and c_____ r_____

psychiatric disorders, catatonia; conversion reaction

   c. n_____ w_____ and m_____ g_____, G_____-B_____ s_____

neuromuscular weakness; myasthenia gravis; Guillain-Barré syndrome

18

18

11. **A patient presents with coma. Your first move is to assess and secure the _____.**   airway   18.3.4

12. **Complete the following about approach to the comatose patient:**   18.3.4
    a. What percentage of patients with Wernicke's encephalopathy present with coma?   3%
    b. You would initially treat those patients with _____.   thiamine

13. **Matching. Match the respiratory pattern with the location of the lesion.** ① medullary; ② pontine; ③ bilateral cerebral hemisphere; ④ high medulla or lower pons   18.3.4
    a. Cheyne-Stokes   ③
    b. hyperventilation   ②
    c. cluster breathing   ④
    d. apneustic   ②
    e. ataxic   ①

14. **What is the significance of equal, reactive pupils in a comatose patient?**   Indicates toxic metabolic cause.   18.3.4

15. **What is the most useful sign in distinguishing metabolic from structural coma?**   the light reflex   18.3.4

16. **The only metabolic causes of fixed/dilated pupils are**   18.3.4
    a. a_____ e_____   anoxic encephalopathy
    b. g_____ t_____   glutethimide toxicity
    c. a_____ u_____   anticholinergic use (i.e., atropine)
    d. b_____ t_____ p_____   botulin toxin poisoning

17. **In a third nerve palsy**   18.3.4
    a. the pupil is _____   dilated
    b. and the eye looks _____ and _____.   down and out

18. **True or False. The following ocular finding can be seen in comatose patients with pontine lesions:**   18.3.4
    a. pinpoint pupils   true
    b. periodic alternating gaze   false (usually indicates bilateral cerebral dysfunction)
    c. ocular bobbing   true
    d. bilateral conjugate deviation to cold caloric   false

18

19. In frontal lobe lesions patient looks   18.3.4
   a. _____ the side of the destructive   toward;
      lesions that is _____from the   away
      hemiparesis.
   b. _____ from the side of the irritative   away;
      lesions (seizures) that is _____ the   toward
      jerking side.

**20. In a pontine lesion the eyes deviate   hemiparetic   18.3.4
   towards the _____ side.**

**21. Name three causes of bilateral   18.3.4
   downward gaze deviation.**
   a. t_____ l_____   thalamic lesion
   b. m_____ p_____ l_____   midbrain pretectal lesion
   c. b_____   barbiturates

**22. Complete the following concerning   18.3.4
   internuclear opthalmoplegia:**
   a. Is due to a lesion in the _____ _____   medial longitudinal fasciculus
      _____.
   b. Fibers are interrupted that go to the   contralateral 3rd nerve
      _____ _____ _____.   nucleus
   c. Results in
      i.   loss of _____   adduction
      ii. of the _____ eye   ipsilateral
      iii. on _____ _____ _____   spontaneous eye movement
      iv. or in response to _____ _____.   reflex movement (doll's,
                                                  calorics)
      v.   and convergence is ____ _____.   not impaired

**23. Complete the following regarding   18.3.4
   oculo-vestibular reflex:**
   a. A comatose patient with an intact   tonic; towards
      brainstem will have _____ conjugate eye
      deviation _____ the side of the cold
      stimulus,
   b. which may be delayed up to _____   1
      minute.
   c. Will there be nystagmus?   No

**24. In a normal ciliospinal reflex, the pupil   dilates   18.3.4
   _____ to noxious cutaneous
   stimulus.**

**25. True or False. The ciliospinal reflex is   18.3.4
   indicative of**
   a. parasympathetic pathways   false
   b. spinothalamic pathways   false
   c. integrity of the periaqueductal gray   false
   d. sympathetic pathway   true

■ Herniation Syndromes

26. **True or False. Subfalcine herniation is of concern because:**   18.4.2
   a. Anterior cerebral artery territory infarcts may occur.   true
   b. Transtentorial herniation may occur.   true
   c. There is no obvious concern.   false

27. **True or False. Decreased consciousness occurs early in uncal herniation.**   false (It occurs late in uncal and early in central herniation.)   18.4.2

28. **True or False. Uncal herniation rarely gives rise to decorticate posturing.**   true   18.4.2

29. **Upwards cerebellar herniation**   18.4.3
   a. can occlude the _____,   SCA
   b. resulting in _____ infarction   cerebellar

30. **Tonsillar herniation**   18.4.3
   a. can compress the _____,   medulla
   b. resulting in _____.   respiratory arrest

31. **Central herniation**   18.4.4
   a. can occlude the _____,   PCA
   b. resulting in _____.   cortical blindness
   c. It can shear the basilar artery _____ and cause D _____ hemorrhages.   perforators; Duret

32. **True or False. This stage of central herniation is reversible.**   18.4.4
   a. medullary stage   false
   b. diencephalic stage   true
   c. lower pons   false
   d. upper pons   false

33. **List the distinguishing features of pupils and respiratory rate in the following injuries.**   18.4.4
   a. Injury at the diencephalon:
      i. Pupils _____ to _____   react to light
      ii. Respiratory pattern is _____.   Cheyne-Stokes
   b. Injury at the midbrain:
      i. Pupils are in _____.   midposition
      ii. Respiratory pattern is _____.   hyperventilation
   c. Injury at the pons:
      i. Pupils_____.   pin-point
      ii. Respiratory pattern is_____.   apneustic
   d. Injury at the medulla oblongata:
      i. Pupils are _____.   dilated, fixed
      ii. Respiratory pattern is _____.   ataxic

34. **True or False. Internuclear ophthalmoplegia is prominent at the "lower pons" stage of central herniation.**   false (at the upper pons stage)   18.4.4

35.	**Why does injury to the pons result in pinpoint pupils?**	Sympathetics are lost.	18.4.4

| 36. | **Why does injury of midbrain herniation result in moderately dilated, fixed pupils?** | Sympathetics and parasympathetics are lost. | 18.4.4 |

18

37. **What percentage of patients with central herniation symptoms had:**   18.4.4
   a. good outcome?   9%
   b. functional outcome?   18%
   c. died?   60%

38. **True or False. Regarding uncal herniation:**   18.4.4
   a. The earliest consistent sign is
      i.   impaired consciousness   false
      ii. unilateral dilated pupil true

39. **What shape is the suprasellar cistern?**   pentagonal   18.4.4

40. **During uncal herniation, Kernohan's phenomenon occurs**   18.4.4
   a. when the _____ cerebral peduncle   contralateral
   b. is compressed against the _____   tentorial edge

      _____,
   c. causing _____ hemiplegia.   ipsilateral
   d. Kernohan's phenomenon is designated   false
      as a _____ localizing sign

■ Hypoxic Coma

41. **Regarding the most vulnerable cells in anoxic encephalopathy.**   18.5
   a. Cortex
      i.   _____ cortical layer   3rd
      ii. _____ horn   Ammon's
   b. Basal ganglia
      i.   g_____ p_____   globus pallidus
      ii. c_____   caudate
      iii. p_____   putamen
   c. Cerebellum
      i.   P_____ cells   Purkinje
      ii. d_____ nucleus   dentate
      iii. i_____ o_____   inferior olive
   d. What tissue is more sensitive to anoxia,   gray (has greater O_2
      gray or white matter?   requirement)
   e. Are steroids useful after cardiac arrest?   no

19

Brain Death and Organ Donation

■ Brain Death in Adults

1. **True or False. According to the Uniform Determination of Death Act of 1980, an individual is dead if they have sustained**

   19.1

   a. irreversible cessation of circulatory and respiratory functions.

   true

   b. irreversible cessation of all functions of the entire brain, including brain stem.

   true

■ Brain Death Criteria

2. **The basic requirements and clinical findings that may be used in determining brain death include:**

   Table 19.1

   a. Core temperature _____.   > 36 C (96.8F)

   b. Systolic blood pressure _____.   > 100 mmHg

   c. Blood alcohol level _____.   < 0.08 %

   d. Absence of b_____ r_____.   brainstem reflexes

   e. No response to d____ c____ p_____.   deep central pain

   f. Failed a_____ c_____.   apnea challenge

3. **When testing oculovestibular reflex you should**

   19.2.3

   a. instill ___ - ___ mL of ice water into one ear   60-100

   b. with HOB at ____,   30 degrees

   c. wait ___ minute for response and   1

   d. > ___ minutes before testing the opposite side.   5

4. **The apnea test:**

   19.2.3

   a. Assesses f_____ of m_____   function of medulla

   b. to be valid test for brain death, the $PaCO_2$ must reach _____ without any respirations.   > 60 mmHg

   c. This usually takes ____ minutes.   6

5. **True or False. The apnea test should be aborted if:**   19.2.3

a. the patient has chest or abdominal movement.   true

b. SBP < 90 mmHg   true

c. SaO_2 drops < 80% for > 30 seconds.   true

6. **True decerebrate or decorticate posturing or seizures are _____ with the diagnosis of brain death.**   incompatible   19.2.3

7. **Spinal cord mediated reflex movements are _____ with the diagnosis of brain death.**   compatible   19.2.3

8. **Name five complicating conditions that must not be present to declare an adult brain dead.**   19.2.3

a. h_____   hypothermia: core temperature < 32.2 (90F)

b. i_____   intoxication (i.e. paralytics, barbiturates, benzodiazepines)

c. p_____   post-resuscitation (i.e., could be in shock, or atropine may have been used in resuscitation, causing fixed dilated pupils)

d. p_____   pentobarbital (> 10 ug/mL)

e. s_____   shock (SBP < 90 mmHg)

9. **Cerebral angiography is compatible with brain death when there is _____ of intracranial flow at the level of the c_____ b _____ or the c_____ of W_____.**   absence; carotid bifurcation; circle of Willis   19.2.5

10. **True or False. Regarding the use of EEG as an ancillary confirmatory test.**   19.2.5

a. It is able to detect brainstem activity.   false

b. It does not exclude the possibility of reversible coma.   true

c. It requires electro-cerebral silence.   true (no electrical activity > 2mcV)

11. **When performing a cerebral radionuclide angiogram for brain death confirmation, the finding of no uptake in brain parenchyma is also called h____ s_____ p_____.**   hollow skull phenomenon   19.2.5

19

■ Brain Death in Children

19

12. **Current guidelines for diagnosis of brain death in children are not supported for infants ____ week gestational age due to insufficient data.**

< 37

19.3.1

13. **Recommended observation periods to declare brain death in children:**
    a. Term newborn – 30 days of age   24 hours
    b. Infants and children   12 hours

19.3.2

■ Organ and Tissue Donation

14. **Brain death can result in the following physiologic aberration:**
    a. h_____   hypotension
    b. h_____   hypothermia
    c. d_____ i_____   diabetes insipidus

19.4.3

15. **True or False. Candidates for organ donation by cardiac death:**
    a. Are ventilator dependent.   true
    b. Their family has decided to withdraw support. true
    c. Further treatment would improve outcome.   false (it would be futile)

19.4.5

20

Bacterial Infections of the Parenchyma and Meninges and Complex Infections

■ Meningitis

1. True or false. Regarding meningitis.

a. Community acquired meningitis is typically more fulminant than meningitis following a neurosurgical procedure or trauma.

true

20.1.1

b. Focal neurological signs are common in acute meningitis

false

2. What syndrome describes large petechial hemorrhages in the skin and mucous membranes, fever, septic shock, adrenal failure, and DIC in children with disseminated meningococcal infection?

Waterhouse-Friderichsen syndrome

20.1.1

3. Regarding treatment of meningitis.

a. What is empiric antibiotic coverage for post-neurosurgical procedure meningitis?

Vancomycin (MRSA coverage), 15mg/kg q 8 – 12 hrs to achieve a trough level of 15 – 20 mg/dl + cefepime 2gm IV q 8 hrs

20.1.2

b. If the patient has a severe PCN allergy, what antibiotics can be used instead?

Aztreonam 2gm IV q 6 – 8 hrs or Ciprofloxacin 400 mg IV q 8 hrs

c. What are the three phases of antifungal treatment for cryptococcal meningitis?

Induction therapy: liposomal amphotericin B 3-4 mg/kg IV daily + flucytosine 25 mg/kg PO QID for at least two weeks followed by
Consolidation therapy: fluconazole 400mg PO daily for at least 8 weeks followed by
Chronic maintenance therapy: fluconazole 200mg PO daily

20

4. **What are the most common causal organisms in post-neurosurgical procedure meningitis?**   20.1.2
   a. C_____-n_____ S_____   Coagulase-negative staphylococci
   b. S_____ a_____   S. aureus
   c. E_____   Enterobacteriaceae
   d. P_____ sp.   Pseudomonas sp.
   e. P_____   Pneumococci (usually with basilar skull fractures and otorhinologic surgery)

5. **In immunocompromised patients, what additional organisms must be considered in the differential diagnosis?**   20.1.2
   a. C_____ n_____   Cryptococcus meningitis
   b. M_____ t_____   Mycobacterium tuberculosis
   c. H_____ a_____ m_____   HIV aseptic meningitis
   d. L_____ m_____   Listeria Monocytogenes

6. **True or false. Regarding post-traumatic meningitis.**   20.1.3
   a. Most cases will have a basal skull fracture.   true
   b. Most patients have obvious CSF rhinorrhea.   true
   c. Most infections are from organisms indigenous to the nasal cavity.   true
   d. Surgical treatment is preferred to conservative management.   false
   e. Ciprofloxacin or Imipenem is the treatment for gram-negative organisms.   true
   f. Penicillin is the treatment of choice for gram-positive organisms.   false
   g. Antibiotics should be continued for 1 week after CSF is sterilized.   true

7. **Patients with recurrent meningitis must be evaluated for the presence of the following etiologies of an abnormal communication between the environment and the intraspinal/intracranial compartment.**   20.1.4
   a. d_____ s_____   dermal sinus
   b. C__ f_____   CSF fistula
   c. n_____ c___   neuroenteric cyst

8. **Differential diagnosis for chronic meningitis:**   20.1.5
   a. t_____   tuberculosis
   b. f_____ i_____   fungal infections
   c. n_____   neurocysticercosis
   d. s_____   sarcoidosis
   e. m_____ c_____   meningeal carcionmatosis

9. **List the favored antibiotic for each of**   20.1.6
    the following organisms:
    a. S. pneumonia   PCN G
    b. N. meningitidis   PCN G
    c. H. influenza   ampicillin (beta lactamase
                                           neg) or ceftriaxone (beta
                                           lactamase pos)
    d. Group B Strep   ampicillin
    e. L. monocytogenes   ampicillin ± IV gentamicin
    f. S. auerus   oxacillin (MSSA) or
                                           vancomycin ± rifampin
                                           (MRSA)
    g. aerobic gram negative bacilli   ceftriaxone
    h. P. aeruginosa   ceftazidime or cefepime
    i. Candida spp.   Liposomal amphotericin B +
                                           flucytosine

20

■ Cerebral Abscess

10. **True or false. Regarding brain**   20.2.1
    abscesses.
    a. Are most commonly polymicrobial.   true
    b. Staphylococcus is the most common false
        organism isolated.
    c. CRP is typically normal.   false
    d. Symptoms are similar of other mass true
        lesions by progress rapidly.

11. **The incidence of brain abscesses is** higher   20.2.2
    _____ in developing countries.

12. **What are the risk factors for a brain**   20.2.3
    abscess?
    a. p_____ a_____   pulmonary abnormalities
    b. c_____ c_____ h_____   congenital cyanotic heart
        d_____   disease
    c. b_____ e_____   bacterial endocarditis
    d. p_____ h_____ t_____   penetrating head trauma
    e. c_____ s_____   chronic sinusitis
    f. o_____ m_____   otitis media
    g. i_____ h____   immunocompromised host

13. **Complete the following about sources**   20.2.4
    of brain abscesses:
    a. For what percentage of cerebral   25% of cases
        abscesses is no source found?
    b. Where is the most common origin for chest
        hematogenous spread?
    c. Ethmoidal and frontal sinusitis leads to frontal lobe
        an abscess in which lobe?
    d. Why are infants less likely to develop a Lack of aerated sinuses and
        brain abscess following purulent   air cells.
        sinusitis?
    e. After penetrating trauma, open surgical remove foreign matter and
        debridement is required to _____.   devitalized tissue

20

14. **Complete the following about causative pathogens of brain abscesses:**   20.2.5

   a. What percentage of cerebral abscesses fail to grow an organism on culture?   25%

   b. The most common organism is _____.   Streptococcus

   c. The most common orgamisms in frontal-ethmoid sinusitis are _____ _____ and _____ _____.   Streptococcus milleri and Streptococcus anginosus

   d. The most common organism in traumatic causes is _____ _____.   Streptococcus auerus

   e. The most common organisms in transplant patients are _____ _____.   fungal infections

   f. The most common organisms following neurosurgical procedures are _____ _____ and _____ _____.   Staphylococcus epidermidis and Staphylococcus aureus

   g. The most common type of organism in infants is _____ _____.   gram negative

   h. The most common organism from a dental source is _____.   actinomyces

   i. The most common organisms in AIDS patients are _____ _____.   toxoplasmosis nocardia

15. **The symptoms of a brain abscess in adults are largely the result of?**   Edema surrounding the lesion causing increased ICP (headache, nausea/vomiting, lethargy) and a rapid progression of symptoms   20.2.6

16. **Describe the four stages of a cerebral abscess.**   20.2.7

   a. Stages
      i. stage 1 e_____ c_____   early cerebritis
      ii. stage 2 l_____ c_____   late cerebritis
      iii. stage 3 e_____ c_____   early capsule
      iv. stage 4 l_____ c_____   late capsule
   b. Number of days
      i. stage 1   1 to 3
      ii. stage 2   4 to 9
      iii. stage 3   10 to 13
      iv. stage 4   > 14
   c. Histologic characteristics
      i. stage 1   inflammation
      ii. stage 2   developing necrotic center
      iii. stage 3   neovascularity, reticular network
      iv. stage 4   gliosis around collagen capsule
   d. Resistance to needle aspiration
      i. stage 1   intermediate resistance
      ii. stage 2   no resistance
      iii. stage 3   no resistance
      iv. stage 4   firm resistance

17. **Indicate the value of the following diagnostic tests in the work up for a brain abscess?**   20.2.8

  a. blood work   WBC may be normal or mildly elevated; blood cultures should be obtained but are often negative; ESR may be normal or elevated; CRP is typically elevated

  b. lumbar puncture (LP)   very dubious and not routinely done – may cause herniation

  c. computed tomography (CT)   excellent (sensitivity ≈ 100%)

  d. MRI   good for staging cerebral abscesses

  e. MRS   presence of amino acids and either acetate or lactate are diagnostic for abscess

  f. leukocyte scan   excellent although infrequently used

  g. effect of steroids   tests become less positive - may mislead

18. **How long should antibiotics be used for treating brain abscesses?**   Often IV x 6-8 wks followed by oral x 4-8 wks, although duration should be guided by clinical and radiographic response (note: CT improvement may lag behind clinical improvement (neovascularity remains) so it is okay to d/c antibiotics even if the CT abnormalities persist.   20.2.9

19. **Medical therapy alone is more successful for the treatment of abscesses if:**   20.2.9

  a. it is in the _____ stage.   cerebritis stage (before complete encapsulation)

  b. the abscess is less than ___ cm in diameter.   3

  c. symptom duration is less than ___ wks.   2

20. **What antibiotics are used in AIDS patients with Toxoplasma gondii?**   Sulfadiazine + pyrimethamine + leucovorin   20.2.9

21. **General management of brain abscesses includes:**   20.2.9

  a. b_____ c_____   blood cultures
  b. e_____ a_____   empiric antibiotics
  c. a_____   anticonvulsants (optional)
  d. s_____   steroids (controversial)

22. **The surgical mainstay of treatment for a brain abscess is _____ _____.**   needle aspiration   20.2.9

23. **Complete the following regarding outcomes for patients with brain abscesses?**   20.2.10
    a. mortality (in the CT era)   0 – 10%
    b. neurologic disability   45%
    c. late focal or generalized seizures   27%
    d. hemiparesis   29%
    e. mortality for transplant patients with fungal abscesses?   approaches 100%

20

■ Subdural Empyema

24. **Why is a subdural empyema (SDE) typically more emergent than a brain abscess?**   No anatomic barrier to spread of a SDE, no surrounding tissue reaction to contain the infection, and poor antibiotic penetration into the space   20.3.1

25. **Where are SDE typically located?**   70-80% over the convexity, 10-20% are parafalcine   20.3.2

26. **List the most common etiologies of SDE:**   20.3.3
    a. p_____ s_____ (especially f_____)   paranasal sinusitis (esp. frontal)
    b. o_____ (usually c_____ o_____ m_____)   otitis (usually chronic otitis media)
    c. p____ s_____ (neuro or ENT)   post surgical
    d. t_____   trauma

27. **Causative organisms in SDE:**   20.3.4
    a. Associated with sinusitis? a_____ and a_____ s____   aerobic and anaerobic strep
    b. Following trauma or procedures? s____ and g___-n____   staph and gram-negatives
    c. Sterile cultures are more common following _____.   previous antibiotic exposure

28. **Neurological findings in SDE include:**   20.3.5
    a. f_____   fever
    b. h_____   headache
    c. m_____   meningismus
    d. h_____   hemiparesis
    e. a_____ m_____ s_____   altered mental status
    f. s_____   seizures (usually occur late)
    g. s_____ t_____   sinus tenderness
    h. n_____/v_____   nausea/vomiting
    i. h_____ h_____   homonymous hemianopsia

29. True or False. Evaluating SDE with a LP is potentially hazardous and rarely positive.

true

20.3.6

30. True or False. Burr holes are more effective for SDEs early in the course when the pus tends to be more fluid and fewer loculations have developed.

true

20.3.7

31. Fatal cases of SDE have been associated with v_____ i_____ of the b_____.

venous infarction of the brain

20.3.8

■ Neurologic Involvement in HIV/AIDS

32. **Regarding patients with AIDS.**

20.4.1

  a. What percentage will present initially with a neurological complaint?

33%

  b. How many patients that die with AIDS have a normal brain at autopsy?

5%

33. **The most common conditions producing focal CNS lesions in AIDS are:**

20.4.1

  a. t_____

toxoplasmosis

  b. p_____ C__ l_____

primary CNS lymphoma

  c. p_____ m_____ l_____

progressive multifocal leukoencephalopathy (PML)

  d. c_____

cryptococcus

  e. t_____

tuberculoma (TB)

34. **Infection with HIV itself can have direct neurological involvement such as:**

20.4.1

  a. A____ e_____

AIDS encephalopathy (most common)

  b. A____ d_____

AIDS dementia

  c. a_____ m_____

aseptic meningitis

  d. c_____ n_____

cranial neuropathies (e.g. Bell's palsy)

  e. A____-r_____ m_____

AIDS-related myelopathy

  f. p_____ n_____

peripheral neuropathy

35. **Complete the following about CNS diseases in AIDS:**

20.4.1

  a. Does CNS toxoplasmosis occur early or late in the course of HIV infection?

late (typically CD4 counts < 200 cells/mm3)

  b. What causes PML?

JC virus

  c. What virus is associated with primary CNS lymphoma (PCNSL)?

EBV

  d. How quickly can AIDS patients develop neurosyphilis?

as little as 4 months following infection

36. **Complete the following chart by**   20.4.2
   listing the CT and MRI findings in each
   of the following:
a. Toxo
   i.   number   > 5 lesions
   ii. enhance   ring
   iii. location   basal ganglia and grey-white
                                  junction
   iv. mass effect   mild-moderate
   v.   miscellaneous   surrounded by edema
b. PCNSL
   i.   number   < 5 lesions
   ii. enhance   homogenous
   iii. location   subependymal
   iv. mass effect   mild
   v.   miscellaneous   may cross corpus callosum
c. PML
   i.   number   may be multiple
   ii. enhance   none
   iii. location   white-matter
   iv. mass effect   none-minimal
   v.   miscellaneous   high signal on T2WI, low
                                  signal on T1W1

37. **Complete the following about the**   20.4.3
   management of AIDS-related
   intracerebral lesions:
a. Treatment for toxoplasmosis
   i.   p_____   pyrimethamine
   ii. s_____   sulfadiazine
   iii. l_____   leucovorin
b. How promptly should we see   2 to 3 weeks
   improvement clinically and
   radiologically?
c. If successful, how long should   Patients need lifetime meds
   toxoplasmosis be treated?
d. biopsy should be considered if there is   3 weeks
   no response in _____ _____.
e. True or false. Toxo cannot be
   radiologically distinguished from
   i.   PCNSL.   true
   ii. PML.   usually
f. For diagnosis, check:
   i.   for toxo   serum toxo titers
   ii. for lymphoma   OP of LP and cytology; PCR
                                  amplification of EBV DNA

38. Considerations for performing a biopsy of a brain lesion in an HIV+ patient?

20.4.3

a. If toxo titers are _____.   negative

b. If no response to toxo meds in _____.   3 weeks

c. True or false. Biopsy is equally valuable in lesions that enhance or don't enhance.   false (more valuable in enhancing lesions to differentiate toxo from lymphoma)

d. Technique for biopsy: stereotactic

e. What two areas should be sampled?   enhancing rim and center

f. Positive biopsy can be expected in _____%   96

39. Indicate the survival times for AIDS patients with the following conditions:

20.4.4

a. CNS toxo _____   15 months

b. PML _____   15 months

c. lymphoma _____   3 months (1 month w/o treatment)

d. lymphoma in nonimmunosuppressed patients _____   13.5 months

■ Lyme Disease – Neurologic Manifestations

40. Lyme disease is caused by _____ and transmitted by the _____ tick.   Borrelia spirochetes; Ixodes   20.5.1

41. Regarding clinical findings of Lyme disease.   20.5.2

a. classic rash e_____ c_____ m_____   erythema chronicum migrans ("bulls-eye" rash)

b. clinical triad of neurological manifestations

   i. c_____ n_____   cranial neuritis (bilateral "Bell's palsy")

   ii. m_____   meningitis

   iii. r_____   radiculopathy

c. neurological findings frequently m_____   migrate

d. cardiac c_____ d_____ and m_____   conduction defects; myopericarditis

e. in the late stage: a_____ and c____ n_____ s_____   arthritis; chronic neurological syndromes

42. True or false. Regarding diagnosis of Lyme disease.   20.5.3

a. No test is indicative of active infection.   true

b. Antibodies can be seen on serology immediately after initial infection.   false (typically requires 2-3 weeks for antibodies to be detected in untreated patients)

c. CSF studies may be compatible with aspectic meningitis or MS.   true (oligoclonal bands may be seen)

20

■ Nocardia Brain Abscess

43. **Complete the following regarding Nocardia:**   20.6.1
   a. It arises from the _____.   soil
   b. It is a _____.   bacteria (not a fungus)
   c. Seen in patients with c_____ d_____ i___.   chronic debilitating illness

44. **Nocardia is typically diagnosed with a b____ b_____.**   brain biopsy   20.6.2

45. **The treatment regimen for Nocardia is:**   20.6.3
   a. T___-S___   TMP-SMX
   b. i_____   imipenem
   c. Duration?   > one year or life-long

21

Skull, Spine, and Post-Surgical Infections

■ Shunt Infection

1. **Regarding shunt infection.**   21.1.1
   a. Acceptable infection rate?   < 5 – 7%
   b. Risk of early infection after surgery?   7%
   c. ___% of Staph infections occur within 2   70% (> 50% within the first
      mos.   two weeks)
   d. Most common source is _____   patients' skin
      _____.

2. **Mortality ranges from __ to __% for**   10 to 15%   21.1.2
   children after a shunt infection.

3. **Risk factors for shunt infection:**   21.1.3
   a. y_____ a___ of p_____   young age of patient
   b. l_____ of p_____   length of procedure
   c. o____ n_____ t____ d_____   open neural tube defect

4. **Causal pathogens of shunt infections:**   21.1.4
   a. Early infection
      i. S____ e_____ (most common)   Staph. epidermidis
      ii. S. a_____   Staph. aureus
      iii. g___-n_____ b_____   gram-negative bacilli
      iv. in neonates: E____ c___ and S_____   E. coli and Strep. hemoliticus
          h_____
   b. Late infection (> 6 months after
      procedure)
      i. risk?   2.7 – 31% (typically 6%)
      ii. most common organism?   Staph. epidermidis
   c. Fungal infections
      i. most common: C_____ spp.   Candida

5. **What are the common characteristics**   21.1.5
   of shunt nephritis?
   a. v_____v_____ shunt   ventriculovascular
   b. c_____ l___ l_____ infection   chronic low level
   c. i_____ c_____ deposition in   immune complex; glomeruli
      g_____
   d. p_____ and h_____   proteinuria; hematuria

21

6. **Gram negative bacillus (GNB) shunt infection compared with gram positive bacillus (GPB):**   21.1.5
   a. morbidity — higher in GNB
   b. Following a shunt tap
      i. Gram stains — more than 90%+ Gram stain (in contrast to only 50% in GPB)
      ii. protein — higher in GNB
      iii. glucose — lower in GNB
      iv. neutrophils — higher in GNB

7. **True or False. Regarding treatment of shunt infections.**   21.1.5
   a. Remove shunt. — true
   b. Treatment with antibiotics without shunt removal is only recommended when patients are terminally ill, is a poor anesthetic risk, or has ventricles that may be difficult to catheterize. — true
   c. Place EVD. — true
   d. Intraventricular injection of preservative-free antibiotics in addition to IV therapy is never indicated. — false
   e. Antibiotics should be continued 7 days after sterilization of the CSF. — false (10-14 days)
   f. Patients with peritonitis and a VP shunt will often have ascending infection into the CNS. — false
   g. VP shunts must be immediately removed following peritonitis. — false

■ External Ventricular Drain (EVD)-Related Infection

8. **The diagnosis of an EVD-related infection is suggested by:**   21.2.1
   a. h_____ — hypoglycorrhea (CSF glucose/blood glucose < 0.2)
   b. r_____ c____ i_____ — rising cell index
   c. C__ p_____ > ____ — CSF pleocytosis > 1000
   d. in the presence of p_____ C___ c_____ — positive CSF cultures

9. **What is the formula for cell index?**   21.2.2

   $$\text{Cell index} = \frac{CSF_{leukocytes}/CSF_{erythrocytes}}{Blood_{leukocytes}/Blood_{erythrocytes}}$$

10. **Contamination in the context of EVD-infection is**   21.2.2
    a. P_____ CSF c_____ and/or g____ s_____. — positive CSF culture and/or gram stain
    b. No attributable s_____ or s_____. — No attributable symptoms or signs

11. Risk factors for EVD infections: 21.2.3
  a. d_____ of EVD   duration
  b. s___ l_____   site leakage
  c. b_____ in CSF (IVH and SAH)   blood
  d. i_____ and f_____   irrigation and flushing

12. The usual organisms that cause EVD-   21.2.4
   related infections are
  a. s_____ f_____   skin flora (coagulase-negative
                                                staph, P. acnes)
  b. present in the h_____ e_____   healthcare environment
  c. May form a b_____ that increases   biofilm
      antimicrobial resistance.

13. Management of an EVD infection: 21.2.7
  a. empiric antibiotics:
      i.   v_____ +   vancomycin
      ii.   c_____ or c_____   ceftazidime or cefepime
  b. r_____ catheter   remove (if it is safe to do so)
  c. add i_____ a_____   intrathecal antibiotics
  d. by clamping _____ for _____ minutes   EVD; 15 – 60 min
  e. wait at least _____ days after CSF   7 – 10 days
      sterilizes to implant new shunt

14. Prevention of EVD infections.   21.2.7
  a. tunneling _____ away from the burr hole > 5 cm
  b. a_____ c_____ c_____   antibiotic coated catheters
                                                (rifamipin+ minocycline)
  c. do NOT
      i.   e_____ the catheter at day 5   exchange
      ii.   give p_____ a_____ p_____   prolonged antibiotic
                                                prophylaxis

■ Wound Infections

15. Laminectomy superficial wound   21.3.1
   infection management:
   Hint: bcdefgh
  a. b_____   bacitracin (half-strength)
                                                followed by normal saline
  b. c_____   culture
  c. d_____ w_____   debride wound
  d. e_____ use v_____ + c_____   empirically; vancomycin +
                                                cefepime
  e. f_____   fill with iodoform ¼ inch
  f. g_____   gradually trim 0.5-1 inch of
                                                packing with each dressing
                                                change
  g. h_____   change q8 hrs for hospitalized
                                                patients, BID for patients at
                                                home

16. **Regarding post-operative discitis.**   21.3.1
a. _____ _____ is the most   Staph aureus
    common pathogen.
b. ___% present by 3 weeks post-op   80%
c. ____ _____ at the site of the operation is   back pain
    the most common symptom.
d. Management includes:
    i.   a_____ + m_____ r_____   analgesics + muscle relaxants
    ii. a_____   antibiotics
    iii. a_____ r_____   activity restriction
    iv. c_____ if radiographs are   culture
         suspicious

21

■ Osteomyelitis of the Skull

17. **Complete the following concerning**
Pott's puffy tumor:
a. Treatment   21.4.4
    i.   f_____ r_____   flap removal
    ii. d_____   debridement
    iii. antibiotics for _____ weeks. ___ for   6 to 12; IV
         first week
    iv. wait approx. ____ months for   6
         cranioplasty
b. Most common organism is _____   Staphlococcus aureus   21.4.2
    _____.

■ Spine Infections

18. **What are the main categories of spine**   21.5
infections?
a. v_____ o_____   vertebral osteomyelitis
b. d_____   discitis
c. s____ e_____ a_____   spinal epidural abscess
d. s____ s_____ e_____   spinal subdural empyema
e. m_____   meningitis
f. s_____ c_____ a_____   spinal cord abscess

19. **Describe a spinal epidural abscess.**   21.5.1
a. Most common site for spinal epidural   thoracic level; 50%
    abscess is the _____ _____ at ____%
b. The next most common is _____ at   lumbar;
    _____%, followed by _____ at _____%   35%; cervical; 15%
c. Symptoms include:
    i.   s____ t_____   spine tenderness
    ii. f_____   fever
    iii. b____ p____   back pain
d. Co-morbid conditions
    i.   d____ m_____   diabetes mellitus
    ii. I_ d____ a_____   IV drug abuse
    iii. a_____   alcoholism
    iv. c___ r____ f_____   chronic renal failure
    v.   i_____ c_____   immune compromised

e.   ____ _____ is the most common organism cultured.

Staph. aureus

f.   ____ is the imaging study of choice.

MRI

g.   Treatment consists of _____ _____ + _____

surgical evacuation + antibiotics

20.   **Describe the pathophysiology of spinal cord dysfunction.**   21.5.1
a.   Compression by
   i.   m_____ of a_____

mass of abscess

   ii.   b____ by c_____ of o_____ v_____ b____

bone by collapse of osteomyelitic vertebral body

b.   Infarction by v_____ t_____

venous thrombophlebitis

c.   Direct spread to the cord can cause m_____.

myelitis

21.   **Complete the following regarding causes of spinal epidural abscess:**   21.5.1
a.   Hematogenous – most commonly from
   i.   f_____

furuncle

   ii.   IV d_____ a____

IV drug abuse

b.   d____ e_____

direct extension (e.g. psoas abscess)

c.   Spinal procedures
   i.   d_____

discectomy (incidence of SEA is 0.67%)

   ii.   n_____

needles (catheters)

22.   **Cultures from spinal epidural abscess patients can be expected to show the following:**   21.5.1
a.   Staphlococcus aureus: ___%

50 – most common organism

b.   no growth: ___ to ___%

30 to 50%

c.   Streptococcus (frequency)

second most common organism

d.   TB associated with ___ disease: ___%

Pott's disease; 25%

e.   multiple organisms: ___%

10%

23.   **Complete the following regarding spinal epidural abscess (SEA):**   21.5.1
a.   If during a spinal tap you encounter pus, what should you do?

Stop advancing the needle and culture the pus.

b.   Empiric antibiotics for SEA
   i.   c_____

ceftriaxone or cefepime (if pseudomonas is a concern)

   ii.   v_____

vancomycin (until MRSA can be ruled out)

   iii.   m_____

metronidazole

   iv.   ±r_____

rifampin PO

c.   The length of time IV antibiotics should be administered for SEA is ____.

min. 6 weeks with immobilization

d.   Mortality is ____%

4 to 31%

e.   Recovery of severe neurologic deficit is _____ ____.

very rare

f.   An exception to this rule is ____ - __% improve neurologically.

Pott's disease – 50% improve neurologically

21

21

24. Complete the following regarding vertebral osteomyelitis: 21.5.2

  a. Risk factors
     i.   d_____   drug abuse
     ii. d_____   diabetes mellitus
     iii. h_____   hemodialysis
     iv. a_____   advanced age
  b. What condition in renal patients can mimic infection on MRI?   destructive spondyloarthropathy
  c. Sources of infection are never found in _____%.   37% (consider urinary tract infection (UTI; most common source), respiratory tract, teeth)
  d. Neurologic deficits occur in _____ to _____% of Pott's disease patients   10 to 47%
  e. How long does it take for plain x-rays to demonstrate changes?   2 to 8 weeks
  f. Best imaging test?   MRI with and without contrast

25. True or False. Regarding the treatment of vertebral osteomyelitis.   21.5.2

  a. Instrumented fusion is contraindicated.   false
  b. It is permitted even in pyogenic infections.   true
  c. 90% of cases can be successfully managed nonoperatively.   true
  d. TLSO brace has no role in nonoperative management.   false

26. One differentiates spinal destruction from   21.5.3

  a. infection: i_____ the d_____   involves the disc
  b. metastases: m_____ the d_____   miss the disc and involve the vertebral body

27. What is the MRI triad of infection in discitis?   21.5.3

  a. a_____ p_____ p_____   annulus posterior portion
  b. b_____ m_____   bone marrow
  c. d_____ s_____   disc space

28. What is the CT triad of infection in discitis?   21.5.3

  a. e_____ p_____ f_____   end plate fragmentation
  b. p_____ s_____   paravertebral swelling
  c. p_____ a_____   paravertebral abscess

29. Complete the following regarding discitis: 21.5.3

  a. Cultures are positive
     i. from the disc space in _____%.   60%
     ii. from the blood in _____%.   50%
  b. The usual pathogen is _____.   Staphlococcus aureus
  c. Special staining is required to detect _____, and should be done in ___ cases.   TB; all

30. **Complete the following about discitis:**

a. In children, discitis manifests itself by the child's refusal to _____ or _____ or ____.   walk or stand or sit   21.5.3

b. Postop discitis is suggested when the   21.3.1

    i. ESR is raised to _____ and does not come down.   20 mm/hr

    ii. CRP is above __ mg/L at ____wks post-op.   10; 2

c. Interval between surgery and radiological changes in discitis:

    i. plain x-rays: _____ weeks   12 (1 to 8 months range)

    ii. polytomography: ___ weeks   3 to 8 weeks

31. **Regarding the treatment of discitis.**   21.5.3

a. a_____   antibiotics

b. i_____   immobilization

c. Approaches for surgery (only needed in 25% of cases)

    i. a_____ in the cervical or thoracic regions   anterior

    ii. p_____ l_____ in lumbar region   posterior laminectomy

32. **Complete the following concerning psoas abscess:**   21.5.4

a. Psoas extends from ___ to ___.   T12 VB to L5 VB

b. Psoas is the primary hip _____   flexor

c. innervated by _____.   L2-4

d. Pain on hip _____.   flexion

e. CT shows _____ of psoas shadow   enlargement

f. inside the ____ wing.   iliac

21

22

Other Nonbacterial Infections

■ Viral Encephalitis

1. Complete the following regarding herpes simplex:

22.1.1

a. HSE stands for _____ _____ _____.
herpes simplex encephalitis

b. b. It has a predilection for the t_____, o_____ l_____ and l_____ s_____.
temporal, orbitofrontal lobes and limbic system

c. Definitive diagnosis requires b_____ b_____ and v_____ i_____.
brain biopsy and virus isolation

d. Treat promptly with _____.
Acyclovir

2. HSE has the following characteristics:

22.1.1

a. CSF: _____-_____
leukocytosis-monocytes

b. EEG: p_____ l_____ e_____ discharges on electroencephalography.
periodic lateralizing epileptiform

c. CT: e_____ in t_____ l_____
edema in temporal lobes

d. Hemorrhage on _____ means _____ _____.
CT; poorer prognosis

e. MRI shows t_____ s_____.
transsylvian sign

f. Significance: If bilateral it is highly suggestive of _____.
HSE

3. Transsylvian sign

22.1.1

a. indicates temporal lobe e_____
edema

b. that extends across the s_____ f_____.
Sylvian fissure

4. General treatment for intracranial pressure (ICP) elevation involves the following:

22.1.1

a. e_____ h_____ of b_____
elevate head of bed

b. m_____
mannitol

c. h_____
hyperventilate

5. **Complete the following concerning acyclovir treatment:**   22.1.1
    a. The dose is _____   30 mg/kg/day (is divided every 8 hours)
    b. for a duration of _____ days.   14 to 21
    c. If you identify HSE before GCS drops, you can l_____ m_____.   limit mortality

6. **Which inclusion body identifies VZV on brain biopsy?**   Cowdry type A   22.1.2
    a. VZV stands for v_____ z_____ v_____   varicella zoster virus

■ Creutzfeldt-Jakob Disease

7. **Complete the following about Creutzfeldt-Jakob disease:**   22.2.1
    a. CJD stands for _____ _____ _____.   Creutzfeldt-Jakob disease
    b. The prognosis is _____ _____.   invariably fatal
    c. The EEG shows _____.   characteristic bilateral sharp waves 0.5 to 2.0 per second
    d. Prion stands for _____ _____ _____.   proteinaceous infectious particles
    e. Classic histologic triad   22.2.8
        i.   n_____ l_____   neuronal loss
        ii. a_____ p_____   astrocytic proliferation
        iii. s_____ s_____   status spongiosus
    f. Diagnostic triad   22.2.10
        i.   d_____   dementia
        ii. E_____   EEG
        iii. m_____   myoclonus

8. **Detection of protein _____ in the CSF has _____% sensitivity and specificity for CJD among patients with dementia.**   14-3-3; 96%   22.2.10

9. **What is the biopsy procedure in suspected CJD?**   22.2.10
    a. Use a _____ cranial saw.   manual
    b. to avoid _____ of the infection.   aerosolization
    c. Avoid cutting the _____ with the saw.   dura
    d. Clearly _____ containers.   label
    e. Fix in _____% phenolized formalin.   15%

22

■ Parasitic Infections of the CNS

10. Regarding cysticercosis.   22.3.2
   a. Caused by which organism?   Taenia solium
   b. At which life cycle stage?   larval stage
   c. The life cycle stages (4) include the
      following:
      i.   e_____   embryo
      ii. a_____   adult
      iii. e_____   eggs
      iv. l_____   larva
   d. The current best test is _____-   enzyme-linked
      _____ _____ _____.   immunoelectrotransfer blot

**11. Complete the following statements
     about parasitic infections of the CNS:**
   a. Cysticercosis is caused by   22.3.2
      i.   the p_____ t_____   pork tapeworm
      ii. T_____ s_____   Taenia solium
   b. Echinococcus is caused by   22.3.3
      i.   the d_____ t_____   dog tapeworm
      ii. E_____ g_____   Echinococcus granulosa
   c. What is hydatid sand?   germinating parasitic
                                            scoleces
   d. Caution is advised during removal not to   rupture the Echinococcus cyst
      _____.   and contaminate adjacent
                                            tissues

12. Describe the life cycle of cysticercosis.   22.3.2
   a. Pig contains _____ _____ in its   encysted embryo
      flesh.
   b. Humans eat undercooked _____ with   pork; embryo
      _____ in it.
   c. Embryo matures to an _____.   adult
   d. The _____ produces eggs.   adult
   e. Eggs are released in the _____ of the   feces
      human.
   f. The same or a different human _____   ingests the eggs (from
      the _____.   contaminated fingers,
                                            vegetables, or water)
   g. Eggs in this host release _____   larvae
   h. which burrow through the _____   small bowel wall to
      _____ _____ to _____.   circulation
   i. Larva lands and develops a _____   cyst wall
      _____
   j. and becomes an _____ _____   encysted embryo
   k. in _____ months.   4

13. Answer the following concerning   22.3.2
    neurocysticercosis
   a. What is the permanent host for the adult   human
      tapeworm?
   b. What is the intermediate host?   human or animal (pig)

22

14. **Answer the following concerning neurocysticercosis**

    a. What is the significance of CT scan with   22.3.2

       i. low-density cysts with eccentric punctate high-density spots in an enhancing ring?   living cysticerci

       ii. above plus edema?   dying cysticerci

       iii. intraparenchymal punctate calcifications?   dead parasites

    b. What may soft tissue x-rays show?   calcifications in thigh or shoulder

    c. What might MRI show?   intraventricular or cisternal cysts

15. **Complete the following regarding CT in cysticercosis:**

    a. Ring-enhancing cysts suggest _____ _____.   living cysticerci   22.3.2

    b. Intraparenchymal punctate calcifications suggest _____ _____.   dead parasites

    c. Ring-enhancing cyst with edema suggests

       i. r_____ d_____ or d_____ p_____ with   recently dead or dying parasite

       ii. i_____ r_____   inflammatory reaction

■ Fungal Infections of the CNS

16. **What organism can cause a cerebral abscess in an organ transplant patient?**   Aspergillus fumigatus   22.4.1

17. **Name the most common fungal infection of the CNS diagnosed in the living patient.**   cryptococcosis   22.4.2

    a. Lumbar puncture usually shows _____ opening pressure in _____% of patients.   elevated, 75%

    b. Serum cryptococcal antigen is _____ with CNS involvement.   elevated

■ Amoebic Infections of the CNS

18. **Describe amoebic infections of the CNS.**   22.5.1

    a. The only amoeba known to cause infection is _____ _____.   Naegleria fowleri

    b. Infection occurs 5 days after exposure in warm _____.   freshwater

    c. The amoeba gains entry to the CNS via o_____ m_____.   olfactory mucosa

    d. 95% fatal within _____   1 week

    e. due to _____.   ↑ICP

    f. Treat with _____ _____.   amphotericin B

22

23

Cerebrospinal Fluid

■ General Information

1. The volume (mL) of cerebrospinal fluid (CSF) in   Table 23.1
   a. a newborn is _____.   5
   b. an adult is _____.   150

2. What is the intracranial:spinal ratio of distribution of CSF in adults?   50:50   Table 23.1

■ Production

3. What percentage of CSF is produced in the lateral ventricles?   80%   23.2.1

4. Where is CSF produced other than in the choroid plexus?   23.2.1
   a. i_____ s_____   interstitial space
   b. e_____ l_____ of the v_____   ependymal lining of the ventricles
   c. d_____ of n_____ r_____ s_____ in s_____   dura of nerve root sleeves in spine

5. The amount of CSF volume produced per day for   23.2.2
   a. adults is _____.   450 to 750 mL/d
   b. newborns is _____.   25 mL/d

6. What is the rate of CSF formation mL/min in adults?   0.3 to 0.5   23.2.2

7. What is the CSF pressure in a patient in lateral decubitus position in the following age groups?   Table 23.1
   a. newborn   9 to 12 cm H_2O
   b. 1 to 10 years old   < 15
   c. young adult   < 18 to 20
   d. adult   < 18 (7 to 15)

8. Complete the following concerning CSF: 23.2.2
   a. What is the rate of CSF production?   0.3 to 0.5 mL/min
   b. That equals how many mL per day?   450 to 750

c.   Normal CSF has
   i.   _____ lymphocytes   0 to 5
   ii. _____ polymorphonuclear   0
        leucocytes (PMN)
   iii. _____ red blood cells (RBCs)   0
d.   White blood cells (WBCs) above   5 to 10
     _____ is suspicious.
e.   WBCs above _____ is definitely   10 WBCs per cubic mm
     abnormal.
f.   Subtract _____ WBC for every   1; 700
     _____ RBCs.
g.   Subtract _____ mg protein for every   1; 1000
     _____ RBCs.

9. **Does intracranial pressure (ICP) have**   no (The rate of formation is   23.2.2
    any effect on CSF formation?   *independent* of CSF pressure
                                                        except if the ICP is so high
                                                        that it causes *reduction* in
                                                        cerebral blood flow [CBF].)

■ Absorption

10. **Complete the following concerning**   23.3
     CSF:
a.   True or False. CSF absorption is a   true
     pressure-dependent phenomenon.
b.   Where does it take place?
   i.   a_____ v_____   arachnoid villi → dural venous
                                                        sinuses
   ii. c_____ p_____   choroid plexus
   iii. l_____   lymphatics

■ CSF Constituents

11. **True or False. The composition of CSF**   false (It differs slightly.)   23.4.1
     is exactly the same in the ventricles as
     in the lumbar subarachnoid space.

12. **True or False. The following are**   23.4.1
     normally found in CSF:
a.   lymphocytes   true
b.   mononuclear cells   true
c.   polymorphonuclear leucocytes   false
d.   RBCs   false

13. **True or False. CSF osmolarity and**   23.4.2
     plasma osmolarity are equal, with a
     ratio 1:1. What is the other
     constituent that is also equal among
     the following?
a.   Na   true
b.   K+   false
c.   Cl−   false
d.   IgG   false

23

14. **True or False. CSF proteins**   23.4.4
   a. are equal in adults and children.   false (30 mg/dL in adults and
                                              20 mg/dL in children)
   b. in prematures are ~60 mg/dL.   false (in prematures 150
                                              mg/dL)
   c. in newborn are ~40 mg/dL.   false (about 80 mg/dL in
                                              newborn)
   d. normally rise ~1 mg/dL/yr of age in   true
       adults.

15. **How do you differentiate true**   Table 23.4
   leukocytosis from normal white blood
   cell count included in the traumatic
   tap?
   a. ratio of _____ to _____   RBC to WBC
   b. normal is _____   700:1
   c. or subtract 1 WBC for every _____ 700 RBCs
       _____

16. **What conditions would affect the**   Table 23.4
   WBC:RBC ratio of 1:700?
   a. a_____   anemia
   b. p_____ l_____   peripheral leukocytosis

17. **How would you estimate the correct**   Table 23.4
   protein in the CSF of a traumatic tap?
   a. Subtract _____ mg of protein   1
   b. for every _____ RBCs/mm3.   1000

18. **Answer the following about**   Table 23.4
   subarachnoid hemorrhage:
   a. How long does it take for RBC to   2 weeks
       disappear?
   b. How long does it take for xanthochromia many weeks
       to disappear?

■ Cranial CSF Fistula

19. **Rosenmüller's fossa is located just**   inferior to the cavernous   23.5.2
   _____ to the _____ _____.   sinus (Rosenmüller's fossa is
                                              located just inferior to the
                                              cavernous sinus exposed by
                                              drilling the anterior clinoid in
                                              a paraclinoid aneurysm.
                                              Upper lateral pharyngeal
                                              recess. Limited above by the
                                              sphenoid and occipital bone
                                              communicates with the nasal
                                              cavities.)

20. **True or False. The following are**   23.5.3
   characteristics of traumatic CSF fistula:
   a. They occur in 2 to 3% of all patients with true
       head injury.
   b. 60% are noted within days of trauma. true
   c. 95% occur within 3 months of trauma. true

d. < 5% of cases of CSF rhinorrhea stop within 1 week.

false (70% of cases stop within 1 week.)

e. Adult:child ratio is 1:10.

false (adult:child ratio is 10:1)

f. Occurrence is common before age 2 years.

false (occurrence uncommon prior to 2 years of age)

g. Anosmia is common.

true (78% have anosmia.)

h. Most CSF otorrhea ceases in 5 to 10 days.

true

21. Complete the following concerning posttraumatic CSF fistula:

23.5.3

a. Rhinorrhea stops within _____ week in _____%.

1; 70%

b. Otorrhea stops within _____ to _____ days in _____ to _____%. .

5 to10; 80 to 85%

22. True or False. Regarding CSF fistulas.

23.5.3

a. Anosmia is common in traumatic leaks.

true (78% in traumatic leaks)

b. Anosmia is common in spontaneous leaks.

false (rare inspontaneous leaks; approximately 5%)

23. Study Chart.

23.5.3

a. Regarding spontaneous CSF fistula: (Hint: spontaneous fistula h)

*s*ense of smell preserved
*p*neumocephalus is not common
*o*titis media
*n*eck stiffness
*t*umor-pituitary-meningioma
*a*llergic rhinitis
*m*eningitis
*e*mpty sella syndrome
*o*titis media may result in CSF leak
*u*ndeveloped floor of anterior fossa
*s*ense of smell preserved cribriform plate
agenesis sinusitis (paranasal sinusitis)
*f*oot plate of stapes is dehiscent—CSF into eustachian tube facial canal fistula into middle ear insidious,
*I*CP is high
intermittent *s*erous effusion
*t*ranssphenoidal surgery consequence
*u*nable to hear due to Mundini dysplasia
*l*abyrinthine anomalies
*a*denoma of pituitary
*h*ydrocephalus

23

■ Meningitis in CSF Fistula

24. The infection rate for   23.7
   a. penetrating injuries and CSF fistulas is   50%
      _____%.
   b. penetrating injuries without fistula is   4.6%
      _____%.

25. **Complete the following concerning**   23.7
   meningitis in CSF fistula:
   a. Posttraumatic CSF leak has an incidence   5 to 10%
      of meningitis of _____ to _____%.
   b. Does CSF leakage after surgery have a   higher
      higher or lower incidence of meningitis?
   c. If the leakage site is not identified before   30% (recurrent leak postop)
      surgery, failure to close CSF leaks is
      _____%.
   d. The most common pathogen is   Pneumococcus; 83%
      _____ and its percentage is
      _____%.

■ Evaluation of the Patient with CSF Fistula

26. **What are the characteristics of the**   23.8.1
   fluid suggesting the presence of
   rhinorrhea or otorrhea resulting from
   a CSF fistula?
   a. CSF fluid is _____.   as clear as water (unless
      infected or blood present).
   b. True or False. Fluid causes excoriation.   false (Fluid doesn't cause
      excoriation of the nose.)
   c. Fluid tastes _____.   salty (in rhinorrhea).
   d. Glucose is greater than _____ mg %.   normal CSF glucose > 30 mg
      %.
   e. It contains a special chemical called β_2-transferrin (present in CSF)
      _____.
   f. The special sign when it drops on a sheet   ring sign (An old but
      is called a _____.   unreliable sign. Described as
      a ring of blood surrounded by
      a larger concentric ring of
      clear fluid [suggests the
      presence of CSF] seen when
      blood-tinged fluid allowed to
      drip onto linen [sheet or
      pillowcase].)

27. **Name five characteristics of fluid that**   23.8.1
   suggest the presence of CSF fistula.
   Hint: bcsfg
   a. B_____ β_2-transferrin
   b. c_____   clear
   c. s_____   salty taste
   d. f_____   fluid does not excoriated
   e. g_____   glucose

23

■ Treatment for CSF Fistula

28. **True or False. The procedure of choice**   23.9.2
   to localize the site of CSF fistula is
   a. magnetic resonance imaging   false
   b. iohexol cisternography   true
   c. computed tomography with intravenous   false
       contrast
   d. plain x-ray   false

■ Intracranial Hypotension (Spontaneous)

29. **Spontaneous intracranial hypotension**   23.10.1
   is characterized by
   a. o_____ h_____   orthostatic headache
   b. l_____ c_____ p_____   low CSF pressure
   c. d_____ p_____ e_____   diffuse pachymeningial
                                          enhancement

30. **Characteristics on imaging that**   23.10.1
   suggest intracranial hypotension
   (Hint: SEEPS)
   a. S_____ b_____   sagging brain
   b. E_____   enhancement
                                          (pachymeningeal)
   c. E_____ v_____   engorged veins
   d. P_____ h_____   pituitary hyperemia
   e. S_____ f_____   subdural fluid

31. **True or False. Epidural blood patch**   true   23.10.1
   provides relief for the majority of
   patients.

32. **Conservative management for**   23.10.1
   intracranial hypotension includes
   a. b_____ r_____   bed rest
   b. h_____   hydration
   c. a_____   analgesics
   d. c_____   caffeine
   e. a_____ b_____   abdominal binder

23

24

Hydrocephalus – General Aspects

■ Etiologies of Hydrocephalus

1. Complete the following statements about hydrocephalus: 24.3.1
a. Incidence of congenital hydrocephalus is _____%.   0.2%
b. Due to either _____ CSF resorption or   subnormal
c. CSF _____.   overproduction

2. True or False. Indicate if the following are considered "true" hydrocephalus: 24.3.1
a. hydrocephalus ex vacuo   false
b. obstructive hydrocephalus   true
c. communicating hydrocephalus   true

3. Regarding the characteristics of the etiology of hydrocephalus.   24.3.2
a. True or False. There is excess production of CSF.   true
b. True or False. There is impaired absorption of CSF.   true
c. True or False. It is congenital without myelomeningocele.   true
d. Congenital with myelomeningocele usually occurs with_____.   Chiari II
e. Chiari I, if a cause, has _____ _____ _____ _____.   fourth ventricle outlet obstruction
f. Aqueductal stenosis presents symptoms in _____.   infancy
g. Secondary aqueductal stenosis is due to _____ _____, _____, or _____.   intrauterine infection, hemorrhage, or tumor
h. Atresia of foramina of Luschka and Magendie is called _____-_____ _____.   Dandy-Walker syndrome

4. **Complete the following concerning etiologies of hydrocephalus:**   24.3.2
   a. _____% of post-op pediatric post-fossa tumor patients develop hydrocephalus and need a shunt.   20%
   b. This may be delayed for up to _____.   1 year
   c. Dandy-Walker malformation occurs in what percentage of patients with hydrocephalus?   2.4%

■ Signs and Symptoms of HCP

5. **List the signs and symptoms of active hydrocephalus in older children/adults with rigid cranial vault.**   24.4.1
   a. h_____   headache
   b. n_____   nausea
   c. v_____   vomiting
   d. changes in g_____ and b_____ c_____   gait; bladder control
   e. p_____   papilledema
   f. u_____ g_____ p_____   upward gaze palsy

6. **List signs and symptoms of hydrocephalus in young children.**   24.4.2
   (Hint: hydrocephalusss)
   a. h_____   hydrocephalus
   b. y_____   young (children)
   c. d_____   diplopia (on lateral gaze; abducens palsy)
   d. r_____   respiratory pattern (irregular)
   e. o_____   outward protrusion of fontanelle
   f. c_____   cracked pot sound of Macewen
   g. e_____   enlargement of cranium
   h. p_____   poor head control, Parinaud syndrome
   i. h_____   hyperactive reflexes
   j. a_____   apneic spells, abducens nerve palsy
   k. l_____   large head
   l. u_____   upward gaze palsy
   m. s_____   scalp veins prominent
   n. s_____   setting sun sign
   o. s_____   splaying of cranial sutures (seen on plain skull x-rays)

7. **Occipital frontal circumference (OFC) in the normal child should equal the distance from crown to _____.**   rump   24.4.2

24

8. **For the indicated ages give the expected normal head circumference pattern.**
   (Hint: At 33 weeks the circumference is 33 cm. In a child younger than 33 weeks the head circumference is greater in cm than the age of the child in weeks old. After 33 weeks head circumference growth slows so that at 40 weeks of age the head circumference is 36 cm.)

Fig. 24.1

   a. Premature (ages in weeks)
      i.   28   29 cm
      ii.   29   30 cm
      iii. 30   31 cm
      iv.   31   31.5 cm
      v.   32   32 cm
      vi.   33   33 cm
      vii. 34   33.5 cm
      viii. 35   34 cm
      ix.   36   34.5 cm
      x.   37   35 cm
      xi.   38   35 cm
      xii. 39   35.5 cm
      xiii. 40   36 cm
   b. Full term (ages in months)
      (Hint: Note the pattern; with each month head circumference increases by 1 cm.)
      i.   1   40 cm
      ii.   2   42 cm
      iii. 3   43 cm
      iv.   4   44 cm
      v.   5   45 cm
      vi.   6   46 cm
   c. What is the upper limit of head circumference for a baby?
      i.   28 weeks gestational age   29 cm
      ii.   33 weeks gestational age   33 cm
      iii. 2 months old   42 cm
      iv.   3 months old   43 cm
      v.   4 months old   44 cm
      vi.   6 months old   46 cm

9. **Blindness in hydrocephalus may be due to:**
   (Hint: pop)

24.4.3

   a. p_____   papilledema (chronic—optic atrophy—damage to optic disc)

   b. o_____ c_____ c_____   optic chiasm compression (due to dilation of third ventricle)

   c. p_____ c_____ a_____   posterior cerebral artery
      o_____   occlusion (compressed at tentorial edge due to downward herniation)

10. **Types of blindness from hydrocephalus are _____ _____ and _____ _____.**   pregeniculate blindness and postgeniculate blindness   24.4.3
   a. Characteristics for pre_____   pregeniculate blindness
     b_____
      i. o_____ n_____ a_____ s_____ —   optic nerve atrophy—severe
      ii. p_____ r_____ —p_____   pupillary reflexes—poor
      iii. due to p_____, h_____, a_____   pressure, hypotension, anemia
   b. Characteristics for post_____   postgeniculate blindness
     b_____
      i. o_____ n_____ a_____ m_____ —   optic nerve atrophy—minimal
      ii. p_____ r_____ —n_____   pupillary reflexes—normal
      iii. due to _____ or _____   hypoxia or trauma (macular sparing in PCA occlusion, no macular sparing in trauma to occiput)

11. **Cortical blindness may be associated with**   24.4.3
   a. Anton's syndrome = d_____ of v_____ d_____   denial of visual deficit
   b. Ridoch's phenomenon = a_____ of m_____ o_____, but n___ a_____ of s_____ o_____   appreciation of moving objects, but no appreciation of stationary objects

24

■ CT/MRI Criteria for Hydrocephalus

12. **Hydrocephalus-radiologic criteria:**   24.5.2
   a. Temporal horns' width is >_____mm.   2 mm
   b. Frontal horns ballooning look like M_____ M_____.   Mickey Mouse
   c. Transependymal _____   edema
   d. Ratio of frontal horns to internal diameter of brain.   50%
   e. Anteroposterior (AP) view shows _____.   disproportion of ventricle size and cortical sulci
   f. Third ventricle on AP view shows _____ _____.   bowing laterally
   g. Evans ratio > _____.   0.3
   h. Corpus callosum is _____   thin/atrophic
   i. and shows _____and _____ _____.   stretching and upward bowing

■ Chronic HCP

13. **Characteristics of chronic HCP:**   24.7
   a. Inner table shows _____ _____.   beaten copper cranium
   b. Sella shows _____.   erosion
   c. Corpus callosum shows _____.   atrophy

■ External Hydrocephalus (AKA Benign External Hydrocephalus)

14. Complete the following about external hydrocephalus: 24.8.1
  a. Malignant or benign?   benign
  b. Enlarged s_____ spaces over the   subarachnoid
  c. f_____ poles in the   frontal
  d. f____ year of life.   first
  e. Resolves by age _____.   2 years of age

15. External hydrocephalus may be   cortical vein sign   24.8.1
  distinguished from subdural hematoma by the presence of c_____ v_____ s_____.

16. The cortical vein sign shows _____   veins; inner table   24.8.1
  extending from the brain to the i____ t_____ of the skull on CT or MRI.

■ X-linked Hydrocephalus

17. X-linked hydrocephalus
  a. is a type of h_____ that is   hydrocephalus; inherited   24.9.1
     _____.
  b. occurs in _____% of patients with   2%
     hydrocephalus.
  c. Gene is located on _____.   Xq28
  d. It causes abnormality in m_____   membrane receptor and   24.9.2
     r_____ and L_____.   L1CAM
  e. produces classical syndromes   24.9.3
     (Hint: crash)
     i.   c_____ c_____ h_____   corpus callosum hypoplasia
     ii. r_____   retardation
     iii. a_____ t_____   adducted thumbs
     iv. s_____ p_____   spastic paralysis
     v.   h_____   hydrocephalus

18. Complete the following regarding radiographic finding of L1 syndrome:
  a. Large   24.9.3
     i.   p_____ h_____   posterior horn
     ii. m_____ i_____   massa intermedia
     iii. q_____ p_____   quadrigeminal plate
  b. Small (hypoplastic)
     i.   c_____ c_____   corpus callosum
     ii. c_____ v_____   cerebellar vermis
  c. Rippled
     i.   v_____ w_____   ventricular wall
  d. Which feature is pathognomonic?
     i.   r_____ v_____ w_____   rippled ventricular wall
  e. Available treatment for retardation?   none

■ "Arrested Hydrocephalus"

19.	**True or False. With regard to "arrested hydrocephalus":**	24.10.1
a.	It is interchangeable with the term "uncompensated hydrocephalus."	false
b.	Arrested hydrocephalus satisfies the following criteria in the absence of a cerebrospinal fluid (CSF) shunt:	
	i. ventriculomegaly nonprogressive	true
	ii. normal head growth curve	true
	iii. continued psychomotor development	true
20.	**True or False. When deemed "arrested," no further follow-up is needed.**	false (deterioration can still occur) · 24.10.2
21.	**True or False. Shunt dependency is likely in hydrocephalus due to**	24.10.2
a.	aqueductal stenosis	true
b.	spina bifida	true
c.	communicating hydrocephalus (i.e., secondary to arachnoidal adhesions	false (shunt independence more likely to occur)
22.	**True or False. With respect to a disconnected or nonfunctioning shunt:**	24.10.3
a.	A disconnected shunt may continue to function by CSF flow through a subcutaneous fibrous tract.	true
b.	If in doubt, better to watch, not shunt.	false
c.	Patients with a nonfunctioning shunt should not be followed with serial CT scans but possibly with serial neuropsychological evaluations.	false

24

■ Entrapped Fourth Ventricle

23.	**Complete the following about entrapped fourth ventricle.**	
a.	Usually seen with c_____ s_____ of the l_____ v_____.	chronic shunting of the lateral ventricles · 24.11.1
b.	Possibly due to a_____.	adhesions
c.	Occurs in ___ to ___% of patients with shunts.	2 to 3%
d.	True or False. May be treated with a separate VP shunt or by linking into an existing shunt.	true · 24.11.3

■ Normal Pressure Hydrocephalus (NPH)

24. **What are the symptoms of normal pressure hydrocephalus?**   24.12.1
(Hint: dig)
  a. d_____   dementia (wacky)
  b. i_____   incontinence of urine (wet)
  c. g_____   gait disturbances (wobbly)

25. **What is the etiology?**   24.12.1
(Hint: mistapa)
  a. m_____   meningitis
  b. i_____   idiopathic
  c. s_____   subarachnoid hemorrhage
  d. t_____   trauma
  e. a_____   aqueductal stenosis
  f. p_____   posterior fossa surgery
  g. A_____   Alzheimer's disease

26. **In clinical triad, which symptom precedes the others?**   gait disturbance   24.12.3

27. **Note the clinical features of NPH as expected (+) or not expected (−).**   Table 24.3
  a. wide-based gait   +
  b. shuffling steps   +
  c. unsteadiness on turning   +
  d. difficult initiating steps   +
  e. feel glued to the floor   +
  f. ataxia of limbs   −
  g. slowness of thought   +
  h. unwitting urinary incontinence −
  i. papilledema   −
  j. seizure   −
  k. headaches   −

28. **What is the upper limit opening pressure suggested for the definition of NPH?**   24 cm H_2O 24.12.5

29. **What is the tap test?**   LP with removal of CSF and assessment of response.   24.12.5
  a. How much CSF is withdrawn?   40 to 50 mL of CSF

30. **What is the procedure of choice for treatment of NPH?**   VP shunt   24.12.8
  a. Complication rates may be as high as _____%.   35%
  b. Complications include:
    i. s_____ h_____ or h_____   subdural hematoma or hygroma
    ii. s_____ i_____   shunt infection
    iii. i_____ h_____   intracerebral hemorrhage
    iv. s_____   seizures

31. **In NPH what is the sequence in which symptoms are likely to improve with shunting?**
    24.12.9
    Hint: igd
    a. i_____   incontinence
    b. g_____   gait
    c. d_____   dementia

■ Hydrocephalus and Pregnancy

32. **Patients with shunt for hydrocephalus should, prior to conception,**
    24.13.1
    a. have up-to-date _____ or _____.   CT or MRI
    b. have assessment of any m_____.   medications
    c. If prospective mother's hydrocephalus is   2 to 3%
       accompanied by a neural tube defect
       (NTD), her child could be born with an
       NTD incidence of _____ to
       _____%.
    d. have genetic c_____.   counseling
    e. start taking v_____.   vitamins
    f. avoid excessive h_____.   heat

33. **If shunt malfunctions during pregnancy, shunt revision is performed**
    24.13.3
    a. in the first two trimesters using a   revised VP shunt
       _____
    b. in the third trimester using a _____-   ventriculo-atrial or ventriculo-
       _____ or a _____-_____   pleural
       shunt.

34. **During labor and delivery**
    24.13.4
    a. use p_____ a_____.   prophylactic antibiotics
    b. If patient is asymptomatic, _____   vaginal
       delivery is performed.
    c. If patient is symptomatic, deliver via   cesarean
       _____.
    d. In light of increased cranial pressure   epidurals
       avoid _____.

24

25

Treatment of Hydrocephalus

■ Medical Treatment of Hydrocephalus

1. **Answer the following about the treatment of hydrocephalus:**
   a. True or False. Hydrocephalus is a medically treated condition.

   false (mainly to be treated surgically)   25.1

   b. Diuretic therapy can include a_____ and f_____.

   acetazolamide and furosemide   25.1.1

   c. Be sure to watch for the complication of _____ _____.

   electrolyte imbalances

   d. Role of spinal taps in hydrocephalus is to t_____.

   temporize (Hydrocephalus after intraventricular hemorrhage may be only transient, and serial taps [ventricular or lumbar] may temporize until resorption resumes, but lumbar taps can be performed only for communicating hydrocephalus.)   25.2

   e. Critical protein level of CSF is _____.

   100 mg/dL (If reabsorption does not resume when protein content of CSF is <100 mg/dL, then it is unlikely that spontaneous resorption will occur and a shunt will usually be necessary.)

■ Spinal Taps

2. **Complete the following concerning spinal taps and hydrocephalus:**   25.2
   a. Protein above _____ CSF will not be absorbed.

   100 mg/dL

   b. Protein below _____ CSF may be absorbed.

   100 mg/dL

■ Endoscopic Third Ventriculostomy

3. **Complete the following concerning surgery and hydrocephalus:**

a. Third ventriculostomy when looking into ventricle   25.4.3

   i. Where is thalamostriate vein?   lateral wall

   ii. Where is septal vein?   medial wall

   iii. Where is choroid plexus?   enters foramen of Monro

b. Where is puncture of third ventricle to occur?   anterior to mammillary bodies

c. Into the _____   interpeduncular cistern

d. Watch out for _____.   basilar artery

e. Success rate is _____% for a_____ s_____,   approximately 56% for aqueductal stenosis   25.4.5

f. but only 20% for p_____ p_____.   preexisting pathology

■ Shunts

4. **Concerning shunts and hydrocephalus, what type of shunts do you know?**   25.5.1

   (Hint: palmt)

a. v_____p_____   ventriculoperitoneal

b. v_____-a_____   ventriculo-atrial

c. l_____   lumboperitoneal

d. m_____ s_____   miscellaneous shunts– ventriculopleural

e. T_____ s_____   Torkildsen shunt (ventricle–cisterna magna)

5. **What is shunt usage priority?**   25.5.1

a. most often used: _____ _____   ventriculoperitoneal shunt

b. abdominal abnormality: _____ _____   ventriculoatrial shunt; Surgery; peritonitis; morbid obesity

c. pseudotumor cerebri: _____ _____   lumboperitoneal shunt–small ventricles

d. alternative: _____ _____   miscellaneous shunts

e. acquired obstructive hydrocephalus: _____ _____   Torkildsen shunt

25

6. **Which are the miscellaneous shunts?**   25.5.1
   Hint: gupc
   a. g_____   ventricle to gall bladder shunt
   b. u_____   ventricle to ureter or bladder
                               shunt
   c. p_____   ventriculopleural shunt
   d. c_____   cyst shunt (arachnoid cyst or
                               subdural Hygroma cavity to
                               peritoneum)

7. **Name six possible shunt**   25.5.2
   complications.
   Hint: odesma
   a. o_____   obstruction
   b. d_____   disconnection of shunt parts
   c. e_____   erosion through skin
   d. s_____   seizures–5.5% first year, 1.1%
                               after 3 years
   e. m_____   metastases of tumor cells
   f. a_____   allergy to silicone

8. **What are ventriculoperitoneal shunt**   25.5.2
   complications?
   Hint: h^2alo^3mvps
   a. h_____   hernia–inguinal 17%
   b. h_____   hydrocele
   c. a_____   CSF ascites
   d. l_____   lengthen catheter with
                               growth (preventable)
   e. o_____   obstruction by omentum or
                               debris, peritoneal cyst
                               (infection or talc from
                               surgical gloves), severe
                               peritoneal adhesions,
                               malposition of catheter tip,
                               collapsed ventricular wall,
                               choroid
   f. o_____   obstruction or strangulation
                               of intestine
   g. o_____   overshunting
   h. m_____   migration of tip to: scrotum
                               perforation of stomach,
                               bladder, diaphragm
   i. v_____   volvulus
   j. p_____   peritonitis
   k. s_____   subdural hematoma

25

9. **What are ventriculoatrial shunt complications?**   25.5.2
   (Hint: liverssh)
   a. l_____   lengthening in children
   b. i_____   infection
   c. v_____   vascular perforation
                                           thrombophlebitis pulmonary
                                           microemboli
   d. e_____   shunt embolus
   e. r_____   retrograde blood flow
   f. s_____   superior vena cava
                                           obstruction
   g. s_____   subdural hematoma
   h. h_____   hypertension (pulmonary)

10. **What are lumboperitoneal shunt complications?**   25.5.2
    (Hint: Carols)
    a. C_____   Chiari I malformation (70%
                                           made worse)
    b. a_____   arachnoiditis and adhesions
    c. r_____   radiculopathy (from tube
                                           hard to control)
    d. o_____   overshunting (sixth and
                                           seventh cranial nerve
                                           dysfunction)
    e. l_____   leakage of CSF
    f. s_____   scoliosis due to laminectomy
                                           (14% in children)

25

■ Shunt Problems

11. **What are the two most common shunt problems?**   25.6.1
    a. u_____   undershunting
    b. i_____   infection

12. **True or False.**   25.6.3
    a. Radiographic shunt evaluation involves   true ("shunt series")
        plain x-rays.
    b. "Shunt series" is used to rule out   true
        disconnection or migration of tip.
    c. "Shunt-o-gram" is used if shunt function   true
        cannot be reliably ascertained by other
        imaging.

13. **When do you tap the shunt?**   25.6.3
    a. To study CSF for
        i.   i_____   infection
        ii. c_____   cytology
        iii. b_____   blood
    b. To assess function:
        i.   measure p_____   pressure
        ii. instill c_____   contrast
        iii. inject m_____   medication

14. **When tapping a shunt, what is normal CSF pressure measured from the ventricle?**

less than 15 cm of CSF in relaxed recumbent position

Table 25.2

15. **What are acute symptoms of under-shunting?**
(Hint: salvadibh)

a.	s_____	seizures
b.	a_____	ataxia
c.	l_____	lethargy
d.	v_____	vomiting
e.	a_____	apnea
f.	d_____	diplopia
g.	i_____	irritability
h.	b_____	bradycardia
i.	h_____	headache

25.6.3

16. **What are signs of acute increase in intracranial pressure?**
(Hint: p^4b^2)

a.	p_____	Parinaud's syndrome
b.	p_____	palsy of abducens
c.	p_____	papilledema
d.	p_____	prominent scalp veins
e.	b_____	blindness or field cut
f.	b_____	bulging fontanelle

25.6.3

17. **What are complications of overshunting?**
(Hint: s^4i)

a.	s_____	slit ventricles 12%
b.	s_____	subdural hematoma/hygroma
c.	s_____	sylvian aqueduct occlusion
d.	s_____	skull changes—craniosynostosis or microcephaly
e.	i_____	intracranial hypotension

25.6.6

18. **Regarding intracranial hypotension.**
   a. When patient is erect, column of CSF produces a s_____ e_____.

   siphon effect

   b. Diagnose by documenting a drop in ICP when patient changes from _____ to _____ position.

   supine to erect

25.6.6

19. **Slit ventricles can be diagnosed by frontal-occipital horn ratio of less than _____.**

0.2

25.6.6

20. **Name categories of patients with slit ventricles.**
(Hint: pahms)

a.	p_____	pseudotumor cerebri
b.	a_____	asymptomatic slit ventricles
c.	h_____	intracranial hypotension
d.	m_____	migraine
e.	s_____	slit ventricle syndrome

25.6.6

25

21. **Complete the following concerning hydrocephalus and subdural hematomas (SDs):**
   a. A cause of SD in patients with shunts is _____ of the brain and _____ _____ _____ _____ _____.

   collapse; tearing of the bridging veins

   b. Risk factors
      i.   b_____ a_____
      ii. l_____-s_____ h_____
      iii. n_____ v_____ p_____

   brain atrophy
   long-standing hydrocephalus
   negative ventricular pressure

   25.6.8

22. **If subdural hematoma develops as a shunt complication the subdural is located on**
   a. the same side as the shunt _____%.
   b. opposite side of the shunt _____%.
   c. bilaterally _____%.

   32%
   21%
   47%

   25.6.8

23. **Treatment for subdural hematoma that occurs due to shunting for hydrocephalus could include**
   (Hint: bcdht)
   a. b_____
   b. c_____
   c. d_____

   d. h_____
   e. t_____

   burr holes
   craniotomy
   drainage–subdural peritoneal shunt
   higher pressure shunt
   tie off shunt

   25.6.8

■ Instructions to Patients

24. **True or False. In VP shunt and laparoscopic surgery, abdominal insufflation can increase ICP.**

   true

   25.9

25. **How often does the patient have to pump the shunt?**

   Patient must not touch the pump unless instructed to do so.

   25.9

25

26

Seizure Classification and Anti-Convulsant Pharmacology

■ Seizure Classification

1. Seizure may be classified by   26.1.1
a. t_____   type
b. e_____   etiology
c. e_____ s_____   epileptic syndrome

2. List the major types of primarily   26.1.1
generalized seizures.
a. m_____   myoclonic
b. a_____   atonic (drop attacks)
c. g_____   generalized (grand-mal)
d. c_____   clonic
e. a_____   absence (petit-mal)
f. t_____   tonic

3. What are the major differences   26.1.1
between primarily generalized and
partial seizures?
a. Primarily generalized
  i. areas involved   bilateral and symmetrical
  ii. percent of seizures   40% of all seizures
  iii. consciousness   loss of consciousness at onset
  iv. significance   does not suggest structural
                       lesion

b. Partial
  i. areas involved   one hemisphere
  ii. percent of seizures   57% of all seizures
  iii. consciousness   no loss of consciousness
  iv. significance   suggests structural lesion

4. **Matching. Match the type of seizure with its listed characteristic(s). More than one may apply.**   26.1.1
    Characteristics:
    ① 3% of seizures; ② 40% of seizures; ③ 57% of seizures; ④ consciousness lost from onset; ⑤ tonic-clonic motor activity; ⑥ involves both hemispheres; ⑦ no postictal confusion; ⑧ spike and wave 3/s; ⑨ represents a structural lesion

    a. generalized   ②, ④, ⑤, ⑥
    b. partial   ③, ⑨
    c. unclassified   ①
    d. absence   ⑦, ⑧

5. **The main difference is that simple partial seizures have**   26.1.1
    a. _____ of _____ and complex   no loss of consciousness
        partial seizures have
    b. _____ of _____.   loss of consciousness

6. **Briefly describe the following characteristics of absence seizures**   26.1.1
    a. motor involvement   absent
    b. postictal state   absent
    c. loss of consciousness   absent
    d. characteristic eeg pattern   3/s spike and wave
    e. effect of hyperventilation   induces seizures

7. **Briefly describe the following characteristics of uncinate seizures:**   26.1.1
    a. Arise from _____-_____.   uncus-hippocampus
    b. Produce hallucinations of _____.   odor
    c. Kakosmia is perception of _____   bad odor
        where none exist.

8. **Complete the following about seizures:**   26.1.1
    a. What is the most common cause of   mesial temporal sclerosis
        intractable temporal lobe epilepsy?
    b. due to _____   cell loss in hippocampus
    c. treated by _____   medication until refractory,
                                                then surgery

9. **True or False. Patients with mesial temporal lobe epilepsy have higher incidence of complicated febrile seizures than in other epilepsy types.**   true   26.1.1

26

10. **Name factors that reduce seizure threshold.**   26.1.3
    (Hint: seizure history)
    a. s_____   stroke
    b. e_____   elevated temperature, fever
    c. i_____   infection, intoxication
    d. z_____   "zzzs" lost (sleep deprivation)
    e. u_____   uremia
    f. r_____   repeated seizures (kindling)
    g. e_____   electrolyte imbalance pH,
                                          Mg++, low Na, high Ca++
    h. h_____   hyperventilation,
                                          hyponatremia, hypoglycemia,
                                          hypercalcemia
    i. i_____   ischemia
    j. s_____   stimulation (photic)
    k. t_____   trauma, tumor
    l. o_____   opioids
    m. r_____   removal or withdrawal of
                                          alcohol or AEDs suddenly
    n. y_____   youth (birth asphyxia,
                                          congenital central nervous
                                          system abnormalities)

11. **Juvenile myoclonic epilepsy is**   3   26.1.3
    characterized by _____ seizure types:
    a. m_____ j_____ predominantly after   myoclonic jerks after waking
       _____
    b. g_____ t_____-c_____   generalized tonic-clonic
    c. a_____   absence
    d. Patients with JME are most responsive to   Depakote
       _____.

12. **Infantile spasms in West syndrome**   ACTH or corticosteroids   26.1.3
    usually have a dramatic response to
    _____ or _____.

13. **Complete the following about Lennox-**   26.1.3
    Gastaut syndrome:
    a. Usually begins in childhood as   atonic seizures (drop attacks)
       a_____ s_____.
    b. Seizures are usually d_____ to _____.   difficult to treat
    c. 50% of cases have reduced seizures with   valproic acid
       _____ _____.
    d. c_____ c_____ may reduce the   corpus callosotomy
       number of atonic seizures.

14. **Describe Todd's paralysis.**   26.1.3
    a. occurs after _____   seizure
    b. causes _____   weakness
    c. resolves with _____   time (1/2 to 36 hours)
    d. another name for it is _____ _____.   postictal paralysis

26

■ Antiepileptic Drugs

15. **What % of patients can achieve control of seizures with medical therapy?**
75%
26.2.1

16. **What AEDs interfere with platelet function and may increase the risk of bleeding complications?**
26.2.2
   a. _____ phenytoin
   b. _____ _____ valproic acid

17. **Indicate the drug of choice for each type of seizure**
26.2.3
   a. Generalized tonic-clonic
      i. _____ _____ valproic acid
      ii. _____ phenytoin
   b. Absence
      i. _____ _____ valproic acid
      ii. _____ ethosuximide
   c. Myoclonic _____ lorazepam
   d. Tonic or atonic _____ lorazepam
   e. Partial
      i. _____ carbamazepine
      ii. _____ phenytoin

18. **True or False. Increase a given medication until seizures are controlled or side effects become intolerable, but do not rely soley on therapeutic levels which are only a range in which most patients have seizure control without side effects.**
true
26.2.4

19. **True or False. 80% of epileptics can be controlled on monotherapy.**
true
26.2.4

20. **True or False. Only 10% of epileptics benefit significantly from the addition of a second drug.**
true
26.2.4

21. **True or False. If more than two AEDs are required, consider whether the patient might have nonepileptic seizures.**
true
26.2.4

22. **If a loading dose is not given, it takes _____ half-lives to reach steady state.**
5 half-lives
26.2.4

23. **Give the characteristics of phenytoin.**
26.2.4
   a. half-life: _____ 24 hours, range 9 to 140 hours
   b. oral loading dose: _____ 300 PO every 4 hours until 17mg/kg
   c. Can we use IM route? no

26

    d. rate by IV: _____   not more than 50 mg/min
    e. permitted solution: _____ _____   normal saline
    f. How many days to reach steady state?   7 to 21 days

24. Side effects of phenytoin
    26.2.4

a.	a	ataxia
b.	b	birth control pills less effective
c.	c	cognitive dysfunction
d.	d	drug intercations, Prozac
e.	e	epidermal necrolysis
f.	g	gingival hyperplasia
g.	h	hirsutism
h.	l	liver granulomas
i.	m	megaloblastic anemia
j.	n	newborn hemorrhage
k.	o	osetomalacia
l.	p	papular rash
m.	r	rickets
n.	s	Steven-Johnson syndrome/SLE
o.	t	teratogenic
p.	v	vitamin D antagonism

25. Describe carbamazepine
    26.2.4

    a. Indication
        i. p_____ s_____   partial seizures
        ii. t_____ n_____   trigeminal neuralgia
    b. Therapeutic levels _____   6 to 12 mcg/mL
    c. Side effects

i.	a	ataxia
ii.	a	aplastic anemia
iii.	a	agranulocytosis
iv.	b	blood dyscrasia
v.	c	cymetidine
vi.	d	drowsiness
vii.	d	diplopia
viii.	D	Darvon
ix.	e	erythromycin
x.	f	fatal hepatitis
xi.	g	GI upset
xii.	i	isoniazid
xiii.	s	Steven-Johnson syndrome
xiv.	s	SIADH

26. Describe carbamazepine.
    26.2.4

    a. Also known as _____   Tegretol
    b. Test for C_____, p_____, i_____   CBC, platelets, iron
    c. Test according to what schedule
        i. _____ time(s) per week for _____ _____   1; 3 months
        ii. _____ time (s) per month for _____ _____   1; 3 years

26

d. Discontinue drug if the levels of the following blood components fall below what level
   i.   wbc   4,000
   ii. rbc   3,000,000
   iii. Hct   32
   iv. platelets   100,000
   v.   reticulocytes   0.3%
   vi. iron rises   higher than 150 mcg%
e. Increase dose as follows: _____ pill per _____ per _____.   1 pill per day per week

27. True or False. When used for treatment of trigeminal neuralgia or partial seizures with or without generalization, carbamazepine has   26.2.4

a. erratic oral absorption although oral suspension is absorbed more readily.   true
b. dramatic elevation levels with cimetidine, isoniazid, erythromycin, and Darvon drug-drug interaction.   true

28. True or False. Regarding oxcarbamazepine.   26.2.4

a. Unlike carbamazepine, there is no auto induction.   true
b. There is liver toxicity.   false
c. There is no hematologic toxicity.   true
d. Dosing is BID.   true

29. Describe valproate.   26.2.4

a. Also known as _____.   Depakote
b. Indication   generalized tonic-clonic
c. Therapeutic level is _____ to _____.   50 to 100 mcg/mL
d. Side effects (list at least 5)   confusion, drowsiness, hair loss, liver failure, neural tube defects, hyperammonemia, platelet dysfunction, teratogenic, tremor, weight gain

30. True or False. Acetylsalicyclic acid displaces valproic acid from serum protein.   true   26.2.4

31. True or False. Valproic acid causes neural tube defects in 1 to 2% of patients.   true   26.2.4

26

32. Describe phenobarbital.   26.2.4
  a. Indication   generalized tonic-clonic
  b. Therapeutic level is _____ to _____.   15 to 30 mcg/mL
  c. Half-life _____, steady state _____   5 days; 30 days
  d. Side effects
      i.   c_____   cognitive impairment
      ii. d_____   drowsiness
      iii. p_____ h_____   paradoxical hyperactivity
      iv. h_____ in n_____   hemorrhage in newborns if
                                          mother is on phenobarbital

33. True or False. Indicate whether the following statements about antiepileptic drugs are true or false: 26.2.4
  a. Phenobarbital is a potent inducer of hepatic enzymes that metabolize other AEDs.   true
  b. Cognitive impairment may be subtle and may outlast administration of the drug at least by several months.   true
  c. They may cause hemorrhage in newborn if mother is on phenobarbital.   true

34. Caution is needed when using felbamate due to an unacceptably high rate of _____ _____ as a serious side effect.   aplastic anemia   26.2.4
  a. Can it be used as a first-line drug?   No

35. Describe levetiracetam   26.2.4
  a. Indication   myoclonic seizure, tonic-clonic, partial onset with secondary generalization
  b. Drug-drug interaction?   none
  c. Side effects   somnolence, dizziness

36. Describe topiramate.   26.2.4
  a. Indication   adjunct for refractory partial onset seizures
  b. Side effects   cognitive impairment, weight loss, paresthesias renal stone oligohidrosis
  c. In children it may cause o_____.

37. What is the mechanism of action of lacosamide?   26.2.4
  a. Enhances slow inactivation of _____.   voltage-gated Na channels

38. True or False. The following are characteristics of Diamox (acetazolamide):   26.2.4
  a. It reduces CSF production.   true
  b. It may have anti-epileptic effect either due to slight central nervous system acidosis or due to its direct inhibition of CNS carbonic anhydrase.   true

26

39. Describe withdrawal of AEDs.   26.2.5
a. Taper by _____.   1 unit every 2 weeks
b. Role of EEG?   if EEG shows epileptiform
                                    discharges, discourage
                                    withdrawal
c. Relapse rate is _____ %.   35%
d. over how long?   8 months

40. True or False. These are important   26.2.5
factors to predict freedom from
recurrence after AED withdrawal:
a. longer seizure-free period   true
b. use of only one AED   true
c. tonic-clonic seizure   false (seizures other than
                                    tonic-clonic)

41. Complete the following about   26.2.6
antiepileptic drugs:
a. What effect do antiepileptic medications   They increase the failure rate
   have on birth control pills?   fourfold
b. Why?
   i. AEDs induce liver _____ _____   microsomal cytochrome P450
       _____,
   ii. which degrades the _____ _____   birth control medication
       _____.

42. True or False. Regarding complications   26.2.6
during pregnancy.
a. Women with epilepsy have more   true
   complications.
b. > 90% pregnancies have favorable true
   outcomes.
c. Status epilepticus poses serious risk to   true
   the mother and to the fetus.

43. Considering seizures, AEDs, and birth   26.2.6
defects, describe the following:
a. Effect of seizure history on incidence of   double 4 to 5%
   fetal malformations.
b. Phenobarbital and malformations   the worst, 9.1% - highest rate
                                     of malformation
c. Teratogenic properties in
   i.   Phenytoin   fetal hydantoin syndrome,
                                     low IQ
   ii. Carbamazepine   neural tube defects – rare
   iii. Valproate   neural tube defects 1-2%
d. Therefore, during pregnancy
   i.   first choice is _____   carbamazepine (lowest dose
                                     possible)
   ii. second choice is _____   valproic acid
   iii. add_____   folate
   iv. use _____   monotherapy

26

27

Special Types of Seizures

■ New Onset Seizures

1. **Incidence of new-onset seizures per 100,000 person years is _____.** 44 27.1.1

2. **Neurologic insults resulting in first time seizure include.** 27.1.2
   a. s_____ stroke
   b. h_____ t_____ head trauma
   c. c_____ i_____ CNS infection
   d. f_____ fever
   e. b_____ a_____ birth asphyxia

3. **In patients with stroke, _____% had a seizure within ____ days of a stroke.** 4.2%; 14 27.1.2

4. **What metabolic disturbances can cause first-time seizure?** 27.1.2
   a. u_____ uremia
   b. _____natremia hypo
   c. _____glycemia hypo

5. **In pediatric patients the most common etiology of first-time seizure is _____.** febrile seizures 27.1.2

6. **In patients with new-onset unprovoked seizure,** 27.1.2
   a. _____% had recurrent seizures during follow-up. 27%
   b. If seizure-free for 3 years, _____ had recurrence. none

7. **For new-onset seizure in an adult what should be done?** 27.1.3
   a. s_____ w_____ systemic work-up
   b. C_____ CT
   c. M_____ MRI
   d. E_____ EEG
      i. If all studies negative, you should repeat study at _____. 6 and 12 (and possibly 24) months
      ii. If two EEGs are normal, the 2 year recurrence rate is _____%. 12%

■ Posttraumatic Seizures

8. What are the two categories of posttraumatic seizure?   27.2.1

a. _____ within _____ days after trauma.   Early, within 7 days after trauma

b. _____beyond_____days after trauma.   Late, beyond 7 days after trauma

9. True or False. Regarding posttraumatic seizures.   27.2.1

a. AEDs may be used to prevent early post-traumatic seizures in high risk patients.   true

b. Prophylactic AEDs reduce the frequency of late posttraumatic seizures.   false

c. AEDs can be discontinued after 1 week.   true

10. Incidence of seizures in early posttrauma period (1 to 7 days) is   27.2.2

a. _____% in severe head injuries   30%

b. _____% in mild to moderate head injuries.   1%

11. Incidence of late seizures (> 7 days) is ___ - ___% over a 2-year period.   10-13%   27.2.3

12. The incidence of posttraumatic seizures is higher in _____ head injuries than with _____ head injuries.   penetrating; closed   27.2.4

a. Occur in _____% of penetrating trauma cases followed for 15 years.   50%

13. True or False. High risk criteria for posttraumatic seizures include: Table 27.1

a. acute SDH, EDH, or ICH   true

b. seizure within 24 hours after injury   true

c. Glasgow coma scale > 10   false (GCS < 10)

d. alcohol abuse   true

e. penetrating injury   true

14. Phenytoin has adverse _____ _____when given long-term as prophylaxis against posttraumatic seizures.   cognitive effects   27.2.5

15. Using AEDs after head trauma can result in _____ % reduction of early posttraumatic seizures.   73%   27.2.5

16. In appropriate patients AEDs should be tapered after _____, except in: 1 week   27.2.5

a. p_____ b_____ i_____   penetrating brain injury

b. l_____ p_____ s_____   late posttraumatic seizure

c. p_____ s_____ h_____   prior seizure history

d. c_____   craniotomy

27

17. **In patients not meeting criteria to discontinue AEDs after 1 week,**   27.2.5
    a. AEDs should be maintained for ___ - ___ months.   6-12 months
    b. _____ should be done before discontinuing.   EEG

■ Alcohol Withdrawal Seizures

18. **True or False. Ethanol withdrawal seizures are seen in ____% of habitual drinkers within ___ to ___ _____ of stopping or reducing ethanol intake.**   33%; 7 to 30 hours   27.3.1

19. **Regarding alcohol withdrawal patients.**   27.3.1
    a. What occurs first: delirium tremens or seizures?   seizures
    b. Risk of onset of seizures lasts for _____.   48 hours
    c. Risk of onset of DTs lasts for _____.   96 hours
    d. Risk persists for ___ to ___ days.   1 to 3 days
    e. Are AEDs recommended:
       i.   For prophylaxis?   yes
       ii. For treatement?   no, (because seizure is usually brief, and self-limited. AEDs are not indicated once seizures have occurred.)

20. **True or False. The following patients should be admitted for observation for additional seizures or DT's:**   27.3.2
    a. Those with their first EtOH withdrawal seizure   true
    b. Those with focal findings   true
    c. Those with more than 6 seizures in 6 hours   true
    d. Those with evidence of trauma   true

21. **True or False. Patients with ethanol withdrawal seizures should receive long-term antiepileptic drugs if they have:**   27.3.3
    a. A history of prior ethanol withdrawal seizures   true
    b. Recurrent seizures   true
    c. History of prior seizure disorder unrelated to ethanol   true
    d. Risk factors for seizures (e.g., subdural hematoma)   true

27

■ Nonepileptic Seizures

22. Answer the following about nonepileptic seizures   27.4.1
a. aka pse_____   pseudoseizures
b. aka psy_____   psychogenic
c. True or False
   i.   They are real events   true
   ii. The may not be under voluntary true
        control
   iii. They are helped by AEDs   false

23. What are features suggestive of nonepileptic seizures?   27.4.2
a. This feature is 90% specific for NES: arching back
   a_____.
b. Another highly specific feature is   weeping
   w_____.
c. Forced eye _____.   closure
d. Bilateral shaking with preserved   awareness

   _____.
e. Variable _____   seizure types
f. Clonic UE or LE movements that are   out of phase

   _____.
g. Pelvic _____.   thrust
h. Altered by _____.   distraction

24. A feature strongly suggestive of epileptic seizure is l_____ t_____ l_____.   lateral tongue laceration   27.4.2

25. True or False. Which serum hormone may be used to confirm a true seizure versus nonepileptic seizures: 27.4.2
a. TSH   false
b. ACTH   false
c. Cortisol   false
d. GH   false
e. Prolactin   true

26. Regarding serum prolactin   27.4.2
a. Transient elevations occur in ____% of   80%
   generalized motor seizures.
b. Peak levels are reached in ___ - ___   15-20
   minutes.

27. Overall accuracy of prolactin levels in predicting true seizures is ____%.   72%   27.4.2

27

■ Febrile Seizures

28. **True or False. The most common type of seizure is**   27.5.2
a. ethanol withdrawal   false
b. tumor induced   false
c. posttraumatic   false
d. febrile   true
e. epileptic   false

29. **Regarding treatment of febrile seizures.**   27.5.3
a. Recurrence rate can be _____ by   reduced
b. administering _____   diazepam (0.33 mg/kg)
c. every ___ hours and   8
d. continuing until _____ hours after the 24
   fever subsides.

■ Status Epilepticus

30. **Status epilepticus is defined as**   27.6.1
a. seizure lasting more than _____,   5 minutes
b. or persistent seizure after _____.   1st and 2nd line AEDs

31. **What is the most common etiology for** low AED levels   27.6.1
status epilepticus?

32. **Complete the following about status epilepticus**   27.6.5
a. The mean duration is _____ hours.   1.5
b. The mortality for SE is _____%.   2%
c. The mortality from underlying acute   10-12%
   event is ___ - ___%.
d. Irreversible changes from repetitive   20 minutes
   electrical discharges begin to appear in
   neurons as early as _____ minutes.
e. Cell death may occur after _____   60 minutes
   minutes.

33. **For a patient in status epilepticus, the work-up includes the following**   27.6.6
a. a_____   airway
b. b_____   blood pressure
c. c_____   CPR
d. e_____   EKG, EEG, electrolytes
e. i_____   IV
f. l_____   lumbar puncture

34. **If a lumbar puncture is done after a seizure,**   27.6.6
a. it may show e_____ w_____ c_____,   elevated white count
b. which may be b_____ p_____   benign postictal pleocytosis
   p_____
c. and should be treated as _____.   infection (until cultures
                                             negative)

35. **What is the first line drug for status?**   benzodiazepine   27.6.6

36. **If seizures persist after first dose of benzodiazepine, load with f_____, or p_____.**   fosphenytoin, phenytoin   27.6.6
   a. Loading dose for fosphenytoin is _____ at _____.   15-20 mg/kg at 150 mg/min
   b. Loading dose for phenytoin is _____ at _____.   15-20 mg/kg at 50 mg/min
   c. If no response to loading dose, an additional _____ can be given after _____ minute.   10 mg/kg; 20 minutes

37. **What medication should be avoided in status epilepticus?**   27.6.6
   a. n_____   narcotics
   b. p_____   phenothiazines
   c. n_____ b_____ a_____   neuromuscular blocking agents

38. **True or False. The drug of choice for myoclonic status is**   27.6.8
   a. Lorazepam   true
   b. Benzodiazepine   false
   c. Dilantin   false
   d. Phenobarbital   false
   e. Diazepam   false

39. **True or False. The drug of choice for absence status is**   27.6.8
   a. Valproic acid   true
   b. Benzodiazepine   false
   c. Dilantin   false
   d. Phenobarbital   false
   e. Diazepam   false

27

28

Pain

■ General Information

1. **Complete the following statements about pain:**
28.1

a. The three types of pain are
- i. n_____   nociceptive
- ii. d_____   deafferentation
- iii. s_____ m_____   sympathetically mediated

b. Two types of nociceptive pain are:
- i. s_____   somatic
- ii. v_____   visceral

■ Neuropathic Pain Syndromes

2. **Answer the following about the use of tricyclics to treat neuropathic pain:**
28.2.2

a. Use is limited by _____ and _____ effects, and by _____.   anticholinergic; central; limited pain relief

b. Which is more effective: serotonin reuptake blockers, or norepinephrine reuptake blockers?   serotonin reuptake blockers

---

■ Craniofacial Pain Syndromes

3. **Complete the following statements about craniofacial pain syndromes:**
28.3.1

a. Tic convulsif is g_____ neuralgia plus h_____ spasm.   geniculate; hemifacial

b. Ramsay Hunt syndrome is p_____ g_____ n_____.   postherpetic geniculate neuralgia

c. Tolosa-Hunt syndrome is s_____ o_____ f_____ i_____.   superior orbital fissure inflammation

d. Raeder neuralgia is p_____ n_____.   paratrigeminal neuralgia

4. **Characterize the craniofacial pain syndrome known as SUNCT**   28.3.1

a. s_____ _____   short lasting
b. u_____   unilateral
c. n_____ _____   neuralgiform headache
d. c_____ _____   conjunctival injection
e. t_____   tearing
f. brief—about _____   2 minutes
g. near the _____   eye
h. occurs _____ _____ per day   multiple times
i. affects _____   males

5. **Complete the following regarding primary otalgia:**   28.3.2

a. It may have its origin from which nerves?   fifth, seventh, ninth, tenth, and occipital nerves
b. Cocainization of the pharynx, producing pain relief, suggests _____ _____ instead of primary otalgia.   glossopharyngeal neuralgia
c. Treatment includes
   i. Medicines: T_____, D_____, and b_____   Tegretol, Dilantin, and baclofen
   ii. Surgical procedures: of m_____ d_____ or sectioning the n_____ i_____, the _____ CN, and the upper two fibers of the _____ CN   microvascular decompression (MVD); nervus intermedius; ninth; tenth

6. **Characterize trigeminal neuralgia (TGN).**   28.3.3

a. The incidence is _____, but higher (2%) in patients with _____.   4/100,000; MS
b. It is pathophysiologically caused by what?   ephaptic transmission from large myelinated A fibers to poorly myelinated A delta and C fibers
c. Pathogenesis may be due to vascular compression from what arteries?   superior cerebellar artery (SCA), persistent primitive trigeminal artery, or dolichoectatic basilar artery
d. The neurologic exam in a patient with trigeminal neuralgia should be _____.   entirely normal, or with very mild sensory loss

7. **Complete the following statements about treatment of trigeminal neuralgia:**   28.3.3

a. Tegretol provides pain relief in ____%.   69%
b. What if Tegretol has no effect?   The diagnosis of trigeminal neuralgia is suspect.
c. What is the second drug of choice for trigeminal neuralgia?   baclofen (Lioresal)
d. The two special precautions needed with the use of this medication are as follows:
   i. It may be _____.   teratogenic
   ii. Don't _____ _____.   stop abruptly

28

8. Medicines for trigeminal neuralgia include the following: 28.3.3

a. a_____ (E_____®)   amitriptyline; Elavil®
b. b_____ (L_____®)   baclofen; Lioresal®
c. b_____ (B_____®)   botulinum toxin; Botox®
d. c_____ (Z_____®)   capsaicin; Zostrix®
e. c_____ (T_____®)   carbamazepine; Tegretol®
f. c_____ (K_____®)   clonazepam; Klonopin®
g. g_____ (N_____®)   gabapentin; Neurontin®
h. l_____ (L_____®)   lamotrigine; Lamictal®
i. p_____ (D_____®)   phenytoin; Dilantin®
j. o_____ (T_____®)   oxcarbazepine; Trileptal®

9. The basis upon which percutaneous trigeminal rhizotomy treats trigeminal neuralgia is the destruction of _____ fibers and while preserving _____ fibers.

nociceptive fibers (A-delta and C fibers); touch fibers (A-alpha and A-beta)   28.3.3

10. When treating trigeminal neuralgia, percutaneous trigeminal rhizotomy (PTR) is recommended for whom?   28.3.3

a. Patients with p_____ r____ for general anesthesia.   poor risk
b. Patients who wish to avoid m_____ s_____,   major surgery
c. have u_____ i_____ t_____,   unresectable intracranial tumors
d. have m_____ s_____,   multiple sclerosis
e. have i_____ h_____ on the other side,   impaired hearing
f. or have l_____ l____ e_____.   limited life expectancy

11. State the considerations when choosing radiofrequency rhizotomy (RFR) versus percutaneous microcompression (PMC) rhizolysis for trigeminal neuralgia.   28.3.3

a. Recurrence rates and incidence of dysesthesias are _____ across the various lesioning techniques.   comparable
b. Occurrences of intraoperative hypertension are _____ with PMC than with radiofrequency.   less
c. Bradycardia occurs regularly with _____.   PMC
d. _____ requires a patient who can cooperate; _____ can be done with the patient asleep.   RFR; PMC
e. Paralysis of the ipsilateral trigeminal motor root is more common with _____.   PMC

12. Answer the following concerning trigeminal neuralgia (TGN) and microvascular decompression (MVD):   28.3.3

a. True or False. It is appropriate for patients with <5 years expected survival.   false

28

b. True or False. It may produce anesthesia dolorosa.   false

c. It has a mortality rate of _____.   <1%

d. It has a major neurologic morbidity of ____ to ____%.   1 to 10%

e. It has a failure rate of ____ to _____%.   20 to 25%

f. True or False. It is the procedure of choice in MS patients.   false (MS patients do not respond to MVD and should be treated with a PTR.)

13. Complete the following about TGN and the benefits of stereotactic radiosurgery: 28.3.3

a. Complete pain relief is achieved in _____%.   65%

b. There is significant pain reduction in an additional ____ to ____%.   15 to 31% (80 to 96% total)

c. Must anticoagulation be reversed to have SRS?   No

14. List some complications with percutaneous radiofrequency trigeminal rhizotomy.   28.3.3

a. a_____ d_____   anesthesia dolorosa
b. b_____   bradycardia
c. d_____   dysesthesias
d. h_____ l____   hearing loss
e. h_____ s_____   herpes simplex
f. h_____   hypotension
g. i_____ b_____   intracranial bleed
h. k_____   keratitis
i. l_____ c_____   lacrimation changes
j. m_____ w_____   masseter weakness
k. m_____   meningitis
l. m_____   mortality
m. o_____ p_____   oculomotor paresis
n. s_____ c_____   salivation changes

15. Describe microvascular decompression (MVD) complications: 28.3.3

a. mortality ____ to ____%   0.22 to 2%
b. meningitis: aseptic ___%, bacterial ___%   aseptic 2%; bacterial 0.9%
c. deafness _____%   1%
d. mild facial sensory loss _____%   25%
e. success rate ____ to ____%   75 to 80%

16. Complete the following about supraorbital and supratrochlear nerves: 28.3.4

a. They arise from the _____ nerve.   frontal
b. The larger of the two is the _____.   supraorbital
c. The supraorbital nerve exits the orbit via the _____ notch, usually located within the _____ third of the orbital roof.   supraorbital; medial
d. Which nerve is most medial?   supratrochlear

28

17. Answer the following about differential diagnosis of SON and STN: 28.3.4

a. What are typical TGN features lacking in SON?   SON lacks characteristic triggers and electric shock-like pain

b. If SON is suspected, but associated autonomic activity is present, what conditions should be considered?   cluster H/A or SUNCT

c. Pain of the medial upper orbit exacerbated by supraduction of the eye and palpation of the trochlea might lead one to suspect _____.   trochleitis

18. Characterize glossopharyngeal neuralgia.   28.3.5

a. Pain is located in
   i.   base of t_____ and   tongue
   ii. t_____   throat

b. Other symptoms besides pain:
   i.   h_____   hypotension
   ii. s_____   syncope
   iii. c_____ a_____   cardiac arrest

19. Describe glossopharyngeal neuralgia.   28.3.5

a. The incidence is _____ as frequent as trigeminal neuralgia.   1/70

b. Pain occurs in t_____, b_____ of t_____, e_____, n_____.   throat, base of tongue, ear, neck

c. Treatment includes
   i.   medicine: _____   cocainization
   ii. surgery: _____ _____   microvascular decompression
   iii. nerve division: section of _____ and upper _____ of _____   ninth and upper third of tenth nerve

20. Complete the following concerning geniculate neuralgia: 28.3.6

a. Pain is located _____.   deep in the ear, eye, cheek

b. If there are herpetic lesions, this is called R_____ H_____ s_____.   Ramsay Hunt syndrome (RHS)

c. If combined with hemifacial spasm, it is called t_____ c_____.   tic convulsif

d. Treatment
   i.   medicine: mild cases may respond to c_____, sometimes in combination with p_____   carbamazepine; phenytoin

   ii. surgery: m_____ d_____ together with division of _____ _____   microvascular decompression; nervus intermedius

   iii. What vessel is most often involved?   AICA—compressing sensory and motor roots of seventh nerve

28

■ Postherpetic Neuralgia

21. Complete the following about herpes zoster: 28.4.1

a. The etiologic agent is h_____   herpes varicella zoster virus
v_____ z_____ v_____.

b. It involves the eye in _____%.   10%

c. Pain usually resolves after ____ to ____.   2 to 4 weeks

d. Postherpetic neuralgia occurs in _____% of HZ cases.   10%

e. Vesicles and pain run in the
     i. distribution of the d_____   dermatome
     ii. not the p_____ n_____.   peripheral nerve

22. Complete the following about postherpetic neuralgia:

a. With an acute attack of herpes zoster, you may treat with e_____ or i_____ i_____.   epidural; intercostal injection   28.4.5

b. For acute treatment use
     i. a_____   acyclovir
     ii. v_____ or   valacyclovir
     iii. f_____   famciclovir

c. Medical treatment of PHN is with   Table 28.5
     i. t_____ a_____   tricyclic antidepressants
     ii. l_____ p_____   lidocaine patch
     iii. i_____ s_____ + l_____   intrathecal steroids + lidocaine
     iv. g_____   gabapentin
     v. o_____   oxycodone
     vi. c_____ also may be used as a topical treatment.   capsaicin

d. Start treatment with l_____ p_____, which is better tolerated in the _____.   lidocaine patches; elderly   28.4.5

■ Complex Regional Pain Syndrome (CRPS)

23. Complete the following statements about complex regional pain syndrome (CRPS):

a. Formerly known as _____   causalgia   28.5.1

b. Triad to diagnose:
     i. a_____ d_____   autonomic dysfunction
     ii. b_____ p_____   burning pain
     iii. t_____ c_____   trophic changes

c. What is the cause of CRPS Type II (AKA major causalgia)?   nerve damage due to high-velocity missile injury or other penetrating trauma

28

d. Signs of CRPS: 28.5.5
    i.   tapered _____   fingers
    ii. v_____ c_____   vascular changes, either
                                          vasodilator or vasoconstrictor
    iii. Touching causes pain induced by allodynia   28.5.4
         non-noxious stimulus, known as

         _____.
    iv. hands are _____ and _____.   cold and moist

24. **Complete the following statements**   28.5.7
    about treatments for CRPS:
    a. True or False. Medical therapy is usually   false
        effective.
    b. Medical treatment for CRPS uses   tricyclic antidepressants

        _____ _____.
    c. A common agent used for intravenous   guanethidine
        injection for causalgia is _____.
    d. Surgical sympathectomy may relieve the   90%
        pain of causalgia in _____%.

28

29

Peripheral Nerves

■ General Information

1. **Answer the following about motor and sensory classification of nerves.**

   29.1.1

   a. Which sensory and motor classification has the greatest conduction velocity?

   A-alpha

   b. All post-ganglionic autonomic nerve fibers are of what type?

   C

   c. What types of sensory information are carried by A-delta fibers?

   fine touch, pressure, pain, and temperature

   d. Where can nerves of type B be found?

   preganglionic autonomic fibers

2. **Answer the following about grading muscle strength and muscle reflexes.**

   29.1.2

   a. A muscle with flicker or trace contraction would score what on the MRC scale?

   1

   b. What does an MRC score of 4- mean?

   active movement against slight resistance

   c. What is a normal score for muscle stretch reflex?

   2+

3. **True or False. Upper motor neuron paralysis includes**

   29.1.3

   a. clonus

   true

   b. hyperactive reflexes

   true

   c. muscle spasms

   true

   d. atrophy

   false

   e. fasciculations

   false (Choices d and e are characteristic of lower motor neuron paralysis.)

29

■ Muscle Innervation

4. **For the 11 muscles of the shoulder, list their nerves, roots, and action.**

   Table 29.5

   a. trapezius

   i. nerve, s_____ a_____

   spinal accessory (CN XI)

   ii. roots, _____

   C3,4

   iii. action, _____

   elevate shoulders, abduct arm >90 degrees

b. serratus anterior
    i.   nerve, l_____ t_____   long thoracic
    ii. roots, _____   C5,6,7
    iii. action, _____   forward shoulder thrust
c. supraspinatus
    i.   nerve, s_____   suprascapular
    ii. roots, _____   C4,5,6
    iii. action, _____   abduct arm 15-30 degrees
d. infraspinatus
    i.   nerve, s_____   suprascapular
    ii. roots, _____   C5,6
    iii. action, _____   exorotation of humerus
                                           (backhand tennis shot)
e. rhomboids
    i.   nerve, d_____ s_____   dorsal scapular
    ii. roots, _____   C4,5
    iii. action, _____   adduct and elevate scapulae
f. pronator teres
    i.   nerve, m_____   median
    ii. roots, _____   C6,7
    iii. action, _____   forearm pronation
g. pectoralis major
    i.   nerve, p_____   lat. anterior thoracic and
                                           med. anterior thoracic (aka
                                           pectoral nerve)
    ii. roots, _____   C5,6,7,8
    iii. action, _____   adduct arm and push arm
                                           forward
h. latissimus dorsi
    i.   nerve, t_____   thoracodorsal
    ii. roots, _____   C5,6,7,8
    iii. action, _____   adduct arm (climb ladder)
i. deltoid
    i.   nerve, a_____   axillary
    ii. roots, _____   C5,6
    iii. action, _____   abduct arm 30-90 degrees
j. brachialis
    i.   nerve, m_____   musculocutaneous
    ii. roots, _____   C5,6
    iii. action, _____   flex forearm
k. biceps brachii
    i.   nerve, m_____   musculocutaneous
    ii. roots, _____   C5,6
    iii. action, _____   flex and supinate forearm

5. **The suprascapular nerve innervates**   infraspinatus and   Table 29.5
    which two of the following muscles?   supraspinatus (teres major
                                                innervated by subscapular
                                                nerve; teres minor innervated
                                                by axillary nerve)

    a. teres major
    b. teres minor
    c. infraspinatus
    d. supraspinatus

29

6. **Describe the latissimus dorsi muscle.**   29.2.1
   a. function: _____   adductor—together with
                                           pectoralis
   b. nerve: _____   thoracodorsal
   c. roots: _____   C5,6,7,8

7. **True or False. The deltoid muscle**   29.2.1
   a. abducts the arm 30 to 90 degrees.   true
   b. abducts arm >90 degrees.   false
   c. is innervated by the axillary nerve. true
   d. rotates the arm out.   false (infraspinatus muscle)

8. **True or False. The abductor pollicis**   29.2.1
   longus
   a. is innervated by the median nerve.   false
   b. is innervated by the posterior   true
      interosseous nerve.
   c. is innervated by the ulnar nerve.   false
   d. is innervated by the radial nerve.   true (The posterior
                                           interosseous nerve is a
                                           continuation of the radial
                                           nerve in the forearm.)

9. **True or False. The median nerve is**   29.2.2
   responsible for the following
   movements of the thumb:
   a. adduction   false (ulnar)
   b. abduction   true
   c. extension   false (radial)
   d. flexion   true
   e. opposition   true

10. **Complete the following about the**   29.2.2
    movements of the thumb:
    a. Plane of movement for the thumb
       i.   extension: _____   plane of palm
       ii. flexion: _____   plane of palm
       iii. adduction: _____   perpendicular to palm
       iv. abduction: _____   perpendicular from palm
       v.   opposition: _____   across the palm
    b. Action of nerves to the thumb
       i.   median nerve, Hint: FAO
            F—action, f_____   flexion;
            muscle, f_____ p_____   flexor pollicis brevis;
            b_____
            root, _____   C8, T1;
            A—action, a_____   abduction;
            muscle, a_____ p_____   abductor pollicis brevis;
            b_____
            root, _____   C8, T1;
            O—action, o_____   opposition;
            muscle, o_____ p_____   opponens pollicis;
            root, _____   C8, T1

29

    ii.   ulnar nerve
        action, a_____   adduction;
        muscle, a_____ p_____   adductor pollicis;
        root, _____   C8, T1
    iii. radial nerve
        action, e_____   extension;
        muscle, e_____ p_____   extensor pollicis brevis and
        b_____ and l_____   longus;
        root, _____   C7, C8

11. Complete this list of the peripheral nerves of the lower extremities: 29.2.3
Hint: fosis pdstp (Follow our sign. It says, "please don't spoil the plants.")

a. f_____   femoral
b. o_____   obturator
c. s_____   superior gluteal
d. i_____   inferior gluteal
e. s_____   sciatic (trunk)
f. p_____   peroneal (trunk)
g. d_____   deep peroneal
h. s_____   superficial peroneal
i. t_____   tibial
j. p_____   pudendal

12. Now name the nerves of the lower extremities along with the roots that form them   29.2.3

a. f_____   femoral, L2,3,4
b. o_____   obturator, L2,3,4
c. s_____   superior gluteal, L4,5, S1
d. i_____   inferior gluteal, L5, S1,2
e. s_____   sciatic, L5, S1,2
f. d_____   deep peroneal, L4,5, S1
g. s_____   superficial peroneal, L5, S1
h. t_____   tibial, L4,5, S1,2,3
i. p_____   pudendal, S2,3,4

13. Finally, name the nerves of the lower extremities along with the muscles and their function.   29.2.3

a. nerve, f_____   femoral
    i. muscle, i_____, q_____   iliopsoas, quadriceps femoris,
        f_____, s_____   sartorius
    ii. function, _____   flex hip and leg extension
                                (quadriceps femoris)

b. nerve, o_____   obturator
    i. muscle, a_____, g_____,   adductor, gracilis, obturator
        o_____ e_____   externus
    ii. function, _____   adduct thigh (all), and lateral
                                rotation (obturator externus)

29

c. nerve, s_____   superior gluteal
   i.   muscle, g_____ m_____,   gluteus medius/minimus,
      t_____ f_____ l_____,   tensor fasciae lata,
      p_____   piriformis
   ii. function, _____   abduct thigh (gluteus), thigh
      flexion (tensor fasciae lata),
      lateral thigh rotation
      (piriformis)

d. nerve, i_____   inferior gluteal
   i.   muscle, g_____ m_____   gluteus maximus
   ii. function, _____   thigh abduction

e. nerve, s_____   sciatic trunk
   i.   muscle, b_____ f_____,   biceps femoris,
      s_____, s_____   semitendinosus,
      semimembranosus
   ii. function, _____   leg flexion (and assist thigh
      extension)

f. nerve, d_____   deep peroneal
   i.   muscle, t_____ a_____,   tibialis anterior, extensor
      e_____ d_____ l_____,   digitorum longus, extensor
      e_____ h_____ l_____,   hallucis longus, extensor
      e_____ d_____ b_____   digitorum brevis
   ii. function, _____   foot dorsiflexion (all but EDB),
      foot supination (TA),
      extension toes 2-5 (EDL,
      EDB), extension great toe
      (EHL, EDB)

g. nerve, s_____   superficial peroneal
   i.   muscle, p_____ l_____ and   peroneus longus and brevis
      b_____
   ii. function, _____   plantarflex pronated foot and
      eversion

h. nerve, t_____   tibial
   i.   muscle, p_____ t_____,   posterior tibialis,
      g_____, p_____, s_____,   gastrocnemius, plantaris,
      f_____ h_____ l_____,   soleus, flexor hallucis longus,
      f_____ d_____ l_____,   flexor digitorum longus,
      f_____ d_____ b_____,   flexor digitorum brevis, flexor
      f_____ h_____ b_____   hallucis brevis
   ii. function, _____   plantarflex supinated foot
      (PA, FDL, FHL), plantarflex
      ankle (gastroc, plantaris,
      soleus), inversion (PA), flex
      terminal phalanx toes 2-5
      (FDL), flex terminal phalanx
      great toe (FHL), flex mid
      phalanx toes 2-5 (FDB), flex
      proximal phalanx great toe
      (FHB), knee flexion (gastroc,
      plantaris)

i. nerve, p_____   pudendal
   i.   muscle, p_____, s_____   perineal, sphincters
   ii. function, _____   voluntary contraction of
      pelvic floor

29

14. **True or False. The gluteus maximus muscle**   29.2.3
    a. abducts thigh — true (abducts thigh in a prone position)
    b. adducts thigh — false (obturator externus and pectineus)
    c. medially rotates thigh — false (gluteus medius and gluteus minimus)
    d. laterally rotates thigh — false (obturator externus)
    e. is innervated by superior gluteal nerve — false (inferior gluteal nerve)

15. **True or False. The tibialis anterior muscle is responsible for foot**   29.2.3
    a. dorsiflexion — true
    b. plantarflexion — false (soleus, gastrocnemius)
    c. eversion — false (peroneus longus and brevis)
    d. supination — true

16. **Complete the following about the function of peripheral nerves:**   29.2.3
    a. The function of extension of the great toe is served by
        i. muscle, e_____ h_____ l_____ and e_____ d_____ b_____ — extensor hallucis longus and extensor digitorum brevis
        ii. root, _____ — L5, S1
    b. The function of foot dorsiflexion is served by
        i. muscle, t_____ a_____, e_____ d_____ l_____, and e_____ h_____ l_____ — tibialis anterior, EDL, and EHL
        ii. root, _____ — L4,5 (TA); L4,5, S1 (EDL and EHL)
    c. Which is the best L5 muscle to test clinically? (Hint: E is the 5th letter of the alphabet) — extensor hallucis longus

17. **True or False. The extensor hallucis longus muscle**   29.2.3
    a. extends great toe — true
    b. dorsiflexes foot — true
    c. is innervated by the deep peroneal nerve — true

■ Peripheral Nerve Injury/Surgery

18. **Complete the following regarding timing of surgical repair of nerves:**   29.3.3
    a. If the nerve must regenerate a long distance, repair should be done _____. — early
    b. After _____ months of denervation, most muscles cannot recover. — 24

29

19. **True or False. The brachial plexus is formed by the dorsal rami of C5-T1.**

false (It is formed by the ventral rami of C5-T1. The dorsal rami innervate the paraspinal muscles.)

29.3.4

20. **Draw a diagram of the brachial plexus.**

29.3.4

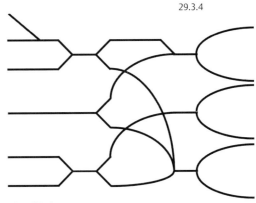

Fig. 29.1

21. **On your diagram of the brachial plexus, label the following:**
① roots C4-T1; ② organization RTDCN (roots, trunks, divisions, cords, nerves); ③ names of trunks—SMI (superior, middle, inferior); ④ add names of cords—LMP (lateral, medial, posterior)

29.3.4

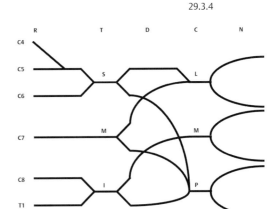

Fig. 29.2

22. **On your outline of the brachial plexus, add the nerves.**
Hint: Donald says somewhat loudly, "Mickey Mouse, you are right to so sincerely love Minnie Mouse madly."

29.3.4

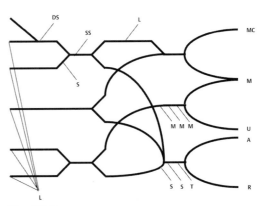

Fig. 29.3

29

23. Draw the left brachial plexus–outline.

29.3.4

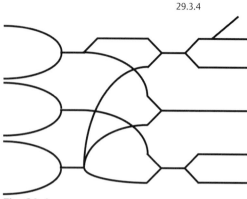

Fig. 29.4

24. Complete the following about the brachial plexus:

29.3.4

a. Name the roots (6).

C4,5,6,7,8, T1

b. Name the segments (5).
(Hint: Run to do Cindy's needs.)

roots, trunks, divisions, cords, nerves

c. Name the nerves (16).
(Hint: Donald says somewhat loudly Mickey Mouse you are right to so sincerely love Minnie Mouse madly)

dorsal scapular;
suprascapular;
subclavius;
lateral pectoral;
musculocutaneous;
median;
ulnar;
axillary;
radial;
thoracodorsal;
subscapular upper;
subscapular lower;
long thoracic;
medial pectoral;
medial brachial cutaneous;
medial antebrachial cutaneous

d. Name the trunks (3).

superior, middle, inferior

e. Name the cords (3).

lateral, medial, posterior

25. Trace, using the brachial plexus diagram, the theoretically possible root contribution to each nerve and then compare with the actual root contribution in each nerve.

(Without rote memorization, this will give accurate answers 83% of the time. Only 8 of 49 theoretical root contributions are not actualized.)

Fig. 29.1

a. nerve, d_____ s_____

dorsal scapular

   i.   theoretical, _____

C4,5

   ii. actual, _____

C4,5

b. nerve, s_____

subscapular

   i.   theoretical, _____

C4,5,6

   ii. actual, _____

C4,5,6

c. nerve, s_____

subclavius

   i.   theoretical, _____

C6

   ii. actual, _____

C6

29

d. nerve, l_____   lateral pectoral
    i.   theoretical, _____   C4,5,6,7
    ii. actual, _____   C4,5,6,7
e. nerve, m_____   musculocutaneous
    i.   theoretical, _____   C5,6,7
    ii. actual, _____   C5,6,7
f. nerve, m_____   median
    i.   theoretical, _____   C5,6,7, T1
    ii. actual, _____   C5,6,7, T1
g. nerve, u_____   ulnar
    i.   theoretical, _____   C8, T1
    ii. actual, _____   C7,8, T1
h. nerve, a_____   axillary
    i.   theoretical, _____   C4,5,6,7,8, T1
    ii. actual, _____   C4,5,6,7,8, T1
i. nerve, r_____   radial
    i.   theoretical, _____   C4,5,6,7,8, T1
    ii. actual, _____   C4,5,6
j. nerve, t_____   thoracodorsal
    i.   theoretical, _____   C5,6,7,8, T1
    ii. actual, _____   C6,7,8
k. nerve, s_____ u_____   subscapular upper
    i.   theoretical, _____   C5,6,7,8, T1
    ii. actual, _____   C5,6,7
l. nerve, s_____ l_____   subscapular lower
    i.   theoretical, _____   C5,6,7,8,T1
    ii. actual, _____   C5,6,7
m. nerve, l_____ t_____   long thoracic
    i.   theoretical, _____   C5,6,7
    ii. actual, _____   C5,6,7
n. nerve, m_____ t_____   medial thoracic (pectoral)
    i.   theoretical, _____   C8, T1
    ii. actual, _____   not listed
o. nerve, m_____ b_____   medial brachial
    i.   theoretical, _____   C8, T1
    ii. actual, _____   not listed
p. nerve, m_____ a_____   medial antebrachial
    i.   theoretical, _____   C8, T1
    ii. actual, _____   not listed

26. **List the brachial plexus nerves (except**   29.3.4
    for median, ulnar, and radial), the
    muscles they serve, and the action of
    the muscles.

    a. nerve, d_____ s_____   dorsal scapular
        i.   muscle 1, l_____ s_____   levator scapulae
        ii. action, _____   elevate scapulae
        iii. muscle 2, r_____   rhomboids
        iv. action, _____   adduct and elevate scapula
    b. nerve, s_____   suprascapular
        i.   muscle 1, s_____   supraspinatus
        ii. action, _____   adduct arm 15 to 30 degrees
        iii. muscle 2, i_____   infraspinatus
        iv. action, _____   exorotation of humerus

29

   c. nerve, m_____   musculocutaneous
       i.   muscle 1, b_____ b_____   biceps brachii
       ii.   action, _____   flex and supinate forearm
       iii. muscle 2, c_____ coracobrachialis
       iv.   action, _____   flex humerus at shoulder
       v.   muscle 3, b_____ brachialis
       vi.   action, _____   flex forearm
   d. nerve, a_____   axillary
       i.   muscle 1, d _____ deltoid
       ii.   action, _____   abduct arm 30 to 90 degrees
       iii. muscle 2, t_____ m_____   teres minor
       iv.   action, _____   exorotate and adduct
                                    humerus
   e. nerve, s_____   subscapular
       i.   muscle 1, _____   teres major
       ii.   action, _____   adduct arm
       iii. muscle 2, _____   subscapularis
       iv.   action, _____   adduct arm
   f. nerve, t_____   thoracodorsal
       i.   muscle, _____   latissimus dorsi
       ii.   action, _____   adduct arm
   g. nerve, l_____ t_____   long thoracic
       i.   muscle, _____   serratus anterior
       ii.   action, _____   forward shoulder thrust

27. **List the branches of the radial nerve**   29.3.4
    cascade in proper sequence.
    (Hint: rest in peace, retbes in peeeeeae)
    a. r_____   radial
    b. e_____   extensor
    c. t_____   triceps
    d. b_____   brachioradialis
    e. e_____   extensor carpi radialis
    f. s_____   supinator
    g. i_____   i
    h. n_____   n posterior interosseous
                           nerve
    i. p_____   p
    j. e_____   extensor carpi ulnaris
    k. e_____   extensor digitorum
                           communis
    l. e_____   extensor digiti minimi
    m. e_____   extensor pollicis brevis
    n. e_____   extensor pollicis longus
    o. a_____   abductor pollicis longus
    p. e_____   extensor indicis

28. **True or False. The radial nerve**   29.3.4
    a. is formed by C5-8.   true
    b. innervates triceps.   true
    c. innervates supinator.   true
    d. innervates brachioradialis.   true
    e. continues into forearm as posterior   true
        interosseous nerve.

29

29. **What muscle is innervated by the axillary nerve?**

teres minor, deltoid

29.3.4

30. **List the branches of the median nerve cascade.**
    (Hint: pfpf³pfaol)

    29.3.4

    a. p_____ t_____   pronator teres
    b. f_____ c_____ r_____   flexor carpi radialis
    c. p_____ l_____   palmaris longus
    d. f_____ d_____ s_____   flexor digitorum superficialis
    e. f_____ d_____ p_____   flexor digitorum profundus I & II
    f. f_____ p_____ l_____   flexor pollicis longus
    g. p_____ q_____   pronator quadratus
    h. f_____ p_____ b_____   flexor pollicis brevis
    i. a_____ p_____ b_____   abductor pollicis brevis
    j. o_____ p_____   opponens pollicis
    k. l_____   lumbricals 1 and 2

31. **Now list the function of the muscles of the median nerve cascade:**
    (Hint: pfpf³pfaol)

    29.3.4

    a. pronator teres: function _____   forearm pronator
    b. flexor carpi radialis: function _____   radial flexion of hand
    c. palmaris longus: function _____   wrist flexion
    d. flexor digitorum superficialis: function _____   flex middle phalanx fingers 2 to 5, flex wrist
    e. flexor digitorum profundus: function _____   flex distal phalanx fingers 2 and 3, flex wrist
    f. flexor pollicis longus: function _____   flex distal phalanx of thumb
    g. flexor pollicis brevis: function _____   flexes proximal phalanx of thumb
    h. abductor pollicis brevis: function _____   abducts thumb metacarpal and radial wrist extension
    i. opponens pollicis: function _____   opposes thumb metacarpal
    j. lumbricals 1 and 2: function _____   flex proximal phalanx and extend 2 distal phalanges Dig 2-3

32. **Which muscles of the hand are innervated by the median nerve?**
    Hint: loaf

    29.3.4

    a. l_____   lumbricals 1 and 2
    b. o_____ p_____   opponens pollicis
    c. a_____ p_____ b_____   abductor pollicis brevis
    d. f_____ p_____ b_____   flexor pollicis brevis

29

33. **List the muscles served by the ulnar nerve cascade in proper order, as well as the function of the muscles.**   29.3.4

    (Hint: "Ffafner I Love Him")

    a.
      i.   f_____ c_____ u_____   flexor carpi ulnaris
      ii. function: _____   ulnar flexion of hand
    b.
      i.   f_____ d_____ p_____   flexor digitorum profundus
      ii. function: _____   flex distal phalanx of fingers 4
                                                    and 5
    c.
      i.   a_____ p_____   adductor pollicis
      ii. function: _____   thumb adductor
    d.
      i.   deep part of f_____ p_____   flexor pollicis brevis
           b_____
      ii. function: _____   flex proximal phalanx thumb
    e.
      i.   i_____   interossei
      ii. function (dorsal): _____   abducts
      iii. function (palmar): _____   adducts, flex proximal
                                                    phalanges at
                                                    metacarpophalangeal joints
    f.
      i.   l_____   lumbricals 3 & 4
      ii. function: _____   extends two distal phalanges
                                                    of fingers 3 and 4 at
                                                    interphalangeal joints
    g.   hypothenar muscles
      i.   a_____ d_____ m_____   abductor digiti minimi
      ii. function: _____   abduction of little finger
      iii. f_____ d_____ m_____   flexor digiti minimi
      iv. function: _____   flex little finger
      v.   o_____ d_____ m_____   opponens digiti minimi
      vi. function: _____   opposition digit 5
    h.   p_____ b_____   palmaris brevis

34. **Complete the following about anatomic variants with Martin-Gruber anastomosis:**   29.3.4

    a.   Connections between the _____ and   median;
         _____ nerves   ulnar
    b.   in the _____   forearm
    c.   found in _____% of cadavers.   23

29

30

Entrapment Neuropathies

■ General Information

1. **List medical etiologies of entrapment neuropathies.**
   a. d_____ m_____
   b. h_____
   c. a_____
   d. a_____

   e. c_____
   f. p_____ r_____
   g. r_____ a_____
   h. g_____

diabetes mellitus
hypothyroidism
acromegaly
amyloidosis (primary or secondary)
carcinomatosis
polymyalgia rheumatica
rheumatoid arthritis
gout

30.1

■ Mechanism of Injury

2. **Does brief compression primarily affect myelinated fibers, unmyelinated fibers, or both?**

myelinated

30.2

■ Occipital Nerve Entrapment

3. **True or False. Occipital nerve entrapment**
   a. is due to compression of a sensory branch of C3.
   b. presents pain in the occiput with a trigger point near the superior nuchal line.
   c. is more common in men.

false (sensory branch of C2)

true

false

30.3.1

4. **Answer the following about non-surgical treatment of occipital nerve entrapment:**
   a. Greater occipital nerve block may provide relief lasting ~_____.
   b. Inject at _____.

1 month

trigger point

30.3.4

30

c. If the case is disabling, and pain doesn't respond to medication, what else may be tried?   surgery, alcohol neurolysis

d. Is a collar indicated?   no

5. **Answer the following about surgical treatment of occipital nerve entrapment:**   30.3.4

a. decompression of _____ nerve root   C2

b. Occipital neurectomy can consist of avulsion of the greater occipital nerve as it exits between the _____ and the _____ _____ muscle.   transverse process of C2 and inferior oblique muscle

c. Another option is release of nerve within the _____ muscle.   trapezius

  i. relief in _____%   46

  ii. improvement in _____%   36

■ Median Nerve Entrapment

6. **Name the two most common syndromes of median nerve entrapment.**   30.4.1

a. c_____ t_____ s_____   carpal tunnel syndrome

b. p_____ t_____ s_____   pronator teres syndrome

7. **Complete the following about the course of the median nerve:**   30.4.2

a. The median nerve passes under the _____ _____ _____.   transverse carpal ligament

b. The motor branch either goes _____ or _____ the ligament   under; pierces

c. and serves the _____ muscles,   LOAF

d. which consist of

  i. _____   lumbricals 1 and 2

  ii. _____   opponens pollicis

  iii. _____   abductor pollicis

  iv. _____   flexor pollicis brevis

8. **Complete the following about the median nerve:**   30.4.2

a. Describe the sensory distribution of the median nerve.

  i. thumb: _____ aspect   palmar

  ii. fingers: _____, _____ , and half of _____   index, middle, and half of ring

  iii. _____ eminence and adjacent   thenar

  iv. _____ palm   radial

b. Palmar cutaneous branch (PCB) crosses _____ transverse carpal ligament.   above

9. **Answer the following about the transverse carpal ligament (TCL):**   30.4.2

a. The TCL extends how far beyond the distal wrist crease?   3 cm

30

b. What is the name of the sensory nerve spared in carpal tunnel syndrome?   palmar cutaneous branch

c. This nerve arises _____cm proximal to the wrist,   5.5

d. passes _____ the transverse carpal ligament   above

e. and serves the _____ _____ sensation.   thenar eminence

10. Describe main trunk median nerve compression.   30.4.3

a. above elbow due to _____   Struther's ligament

b. at elbow

  i. l_____ f_____   lacertus fibrosus (bicipital aponeurosis)

  ii. p_____ t_____   pronator teres

  iii. s_____ b_____   sublimis bridge

c. Honeymoon paralysis is due to _____.   external pressure

d. Benediction hand is due to weakness in what muscle?   flexor digitorum profundus I and II

11. Characterize pronator teres syndrome (PTS).   30.4.3

a. It compresses the _____ nerve   median

b. where it dives between the two heads of the _____ _____.   pronator teres

c. Symptoms:

  i. Pain in _____ distinguishes it from carpal tunnel syndrome   palm

  ii. due to the _____ _____ _____ branch exiting before the TCL.   median palmar cutaneous

  iii. Also presents with weakness in the _____ and   grip

  iv. paresthesias in the _____ and _____.   thumb and index finger

  v. Nocturnal exacerbation is _____.   absent

12. What are the key features of anterior interosseous neuropathy?   30.4.3

a. Presents with

  i. loss of f_____   flexion

  ii. of the d_____ p_____   distal phalanges

  iii. of the _____   thumb

  iv. and _____   index finger

b. due to

  i. weakness of the f_____ d_____ p_____ and the   flexor digitorum profundus

  ii. f_____ p_____ l_____.   flexor pollicis longus

c. No loss of _____.   sensation

d. Patient can't _____.   make "OK" sign

e. treatment

  i. e_____ m_____   expectant management 8-12 weeks

  ii. s_____ e_____   surgical exploration (if no improvement)

30

13. **Describe carpal tunnel syndrome.**   30.4.4
  a. The _____ _____ median nerve   most common
      entrapment neuropathy.
  b. It is due to _____.   compression of the median
                                                     nerve
  c. Where?   distal to wrist crease
  d. Usually occurs in what population?   middle-aged patients
  e. Male/female ratio: _____   4:1
  f. Bilateral in _____% of cases   >50%
  g. Worse in _____   dominant hand
  h. Phalen sign performed by _____ of   forced flexion
      the wrist
  i. and is positive in _____.   80% of cases

14. **Answer the following about carpal**   30.4.4
      tunnel syndrome:
  a. What is the most sensitive   sensory latency nerve
      electrodiagnostics test for carpal tunnel   conduction velocity (NCV)
      syndrome?
  b. Which should be faster, median sensory   median sensory conduction
      conduction velocity or ulnar sensory   velocity
      conduction velocity?
  c. By how much?   4m/s

15. **Complete the following about carpal**   30.4.4
      tunnel syndrome:
  a. Describe treatment.
      i.   sp_____   splint
      ii. st_____   steroids
      iii. su_____   surgery
  b. Incision should be slightly to the   ulnar
      _____ side of the interthenar crease
  c. to avoid
      i.   p_____ c_____ b_____   palmar cutaneous branch
           and/or
      ii. a_____ r_____ t_____   anomalous recurrent thenar
           m_____ b_____.   motor branch

■ Ulnar Nerve Entrapment

16. **Complete the following about the**   30.5.1
      ulnar nerve:
  a. Name the roots.   C7,8, T1
  b. Motor findings of entrapment are:
      i.   wasting of the _____   interossei
      ii. W_____ sign   Wartenberg's
      iii. F_____ sign   Froment's
      iv. _____ deformity of hand   claw
  c.
      i.   disturbance of sensation in   little finger
           _____
      ii. and _____   ulnar half of ring finger

30

17. Describe Wartenberg's sign.   30.5.1
  a. It affects the _____,   little finger
  b. which rests in _____   abduction
  c. due to weakness of the t_____   third palmar interosseous
     p_____ i_____ m_____.   muscle
  d. Which nerve is involved?   ulnar

18. Describe Froment's sign.   30.5.1
  a. Test by having the patient g_____   grasp a piece of paper
  b. using their t_____ and i_____   thumb and index fingers
     f_____.
  c. If the _____ nerve is weak the   ulnar
  d. thumb b_____ b_____   bends backwards
  e. because ulnar-innervated _____   adductor pollicis
     _____ is weak;
  f. therefore, the body substitutes it for the   flexor pollicis longus
     stronger _____ _____ _____,
  g. which is innervated by the _____   anterior interosseous;
     branch of the _____ nerve.   median

19. Describe injury to the ulnar nerve   30.5.2
above the elbow.
  a. Can be due to injury to the _____   medial
     cord of the brachial plexus.
  b. Kinking may be caused by the   arcade of Struthers
     a_____ of S_____,
  c. which is a thin, flat _____ _____.   aponeurotic band

20. Answer the following about ulnar   30.5.3
nerve entrapment at the elbow:
  a. May present as t_____ u_____   tardy ulnar palsy
     p_____.
  b. NCV is less than _____ m/s   50
  c. or there is a drop of more than _____   10
     m/s between the AE and BE segments.
  d. Early symptoms may be purely _____.   motor

21. What are surgical options for   30.5.3
treatment of ulnar compression at the
elbow?
  a. nerve d_____ without t_____   decompression, transposition
  b. nerve d_____ with _____   decompression, transposition
  c. m_____ e_____   medial epicondylectomy
  d. Sometimes e_____ of n_____   excision of neuroma;
     and possibly j_____ g_____ may   jump graft
     be required.
  e. transposition may be to _____   subcutaneous tissue, within
     _____, within the _____ _____   the flexor carpi ulnaris, or a
     _____, or a _____   submuscular position
     _____.

30

22. **Describe the borders of Guyon's canal.**   30.5.5
    a. roof
        i.   p_____ f_____   palmar fascia
        ii. p_____ b_____   palmaris brevis
    b. floor
        i.   f_____ r_____ of the   flexor retinaculum of the
             p_____   palm
        ii. p_____ l_____   pisohamate ligament
    c. Below the floor lies the t_____   transverse carpal ligament
        c_____ l_____.
    d. Contains only the _____ _____ and ulnar nerve and ulnar artery
        _____ _____.

23. **Describe the types of ulnar nerve**   30.5.5
    lesions in Guyon's canal.
    a. Type I
        i.   location of compression   just proximal to or within
                                                Guyon's canal
        ii. weakness   all intrinsic hand muscles
                                                innervated by ulnar n.
        iii. sensory deficit   palmar ulnar distribution
    b. Type II
        i.   location of compression   along deep branch
        ii. weakness   muscles innervated by deep
                                                branch
        iii. sensory deficit   none
    c. Type III
        i.   location of compression   distal end of Guyon's canal
        ii. weakness   none
        iii. sensory deficit   palmar ulnar distribution

■ Radial Nerve Injuries

24. **Complete the following regarding**   30.6.3
    radial nerve injuries:
    a. Sensation loss in the web space of the hand
        thumb indicates injury in the _____.
    b. Pain at the lateral epicondyle indicates supinator tunnel at the elbow
        compression of the _____.
    c. Wrist drop indicates injury to _____-   mid-upper arm;
        _____ _____, where the nerve is in the spiral groove
        _____ _____ of the humerus.
    d. Triceps plus all distal muscle weakness axilla
        indicates injury at the _____.
    e. Weakness of the above, plus the deltoid posterior cord
        and latissimus dorsi indicates injury to
        the _____ _____ .

30

25. **Describe mid-upper or forearm radial nerve compression.** 30.6.3

   a. Radial nerve compression in mid-upper arm produces
      i. w_____ (w_____ d_____) weakness (wrist drop)
      ii. w_____ n_____ wrist numbness
      iii. because it compresses _____ PIN; and _____ _____ _____. superficial radial nerve
   b. Injury to the posterior interosseous nerve (PIN) produces _____ of fingers. weakness
   c. Injury at the supinator tunnel produces _____ but no _____. pain; weakness

26. **Complete the following about radial nerve anatomy.** 30.6.3

   a. PIN refers to the _____ _____ _____, posterior interosseous nerve
   b. a continuation of the _____ nerve, radial
   c. which serves the
      i. _____ of the fingers extensors
      ii. and the a _____ p_____ l_____. abductor pollicis longus

27. **Describe management of radial nerve injury.** 30.6.3

   a. posterior interosseous syndrome
      i. e_____ exploration (if case doesn't respond to 4-8 weeks expectant management)
      ii. l_____ c_____ lyse constrictions (including arcade of Frohse)
   b. supinator tunnel syndrome Surgery rarely required, but responds to nerve decompression.
   c. hand injury
      i. Clinical finding is _____ _____ of _____ loss at the d_____ w_____ s_____ of the thumb small area of sensory loss; dorsal web space of the thumb
      ii. often caused by _____. handcuffs

■ Axillary Nerve Injuries

28. **List possible etiologies of axillary nerve neuropathy.** 30.7

   a. s_____ d_____ shoulder dislocation
   b. sleeping in the _____ position with arms _____ _____ __ _____ prone; abducted above the head
   c. compression from a _____ thoracic harness
   d. i_____ i_____ injection injury
   e. entrapment in the _____ _____ quadrilateral space

30

■ Suprascapular Nerve

29. Describe suprascapular nerve injury.   30.8
   a. Nerve formed from roots _____   C5,6
   b. Entrapped at s_____ n_____   suprascapular notch beneath
       beneath the _____ _____   the transverse scapular
       _____   ligament
   c. Sensory symptoms: _____   deep, poorly localized
                                                  (referred) shoulder pain
   d. Motor symptoms: weakness and atrophy   supraspinatus and
       of _____ and _____   infraspinatus
   e. May be difficult to distinguish from   rotator cuff injury
       _____ _____ injury.
   f. Differentiate from C5 cervical
       radiculopathy and upper brachial plexus   rhomboid and deltoid
       lesion by testing _____ and
       _____.

■ Meralgia Paresthetica

30. Define meralgia paresthetica.   30.9.2
   a. Also known as _____, or   Bernhardt-Roth syndrome
   b. _____.   "swashbuckler's disease"
   c. Hyperpathia located at the l_____   lateral upper thigh (burning
       u_____ t_____.   pain)
   d. Entrapment of the l_____ f_____   lateral femoral cutaneous
       c_____ nerve.
   e. True or False. Involves both motor and   false (sensory only)
       sensory fibers.

31. Answer the following regarding   30.9.4
    differential diagnosis of meralgia
    paresthetica:
   a. Femoral neuropathy sensory changes   anteromedial
       tend to be more _____.
   b. L2 or L3 radiculopathy: look for _____   motor weakness (thigh
       _____.   flexion or knee extension)
   c. Nerve compression by abdominal or   concomitant GI or GU
       pelvic tumor suspected if _____.   symptoms

32. Describe treatment options for   30.9.5
    meralgia paresthetica.
   a. Nonsurgical measures achieve relief in   91
       ~_____% of cases.
   b. True or False. Centrally acting pain   false
       medications are often effective.
   c. Neurectomy may be _____   more;
       (more/less) effective than   denervation pain
       decompression, but risks _____
       _____.
   d. If neurectomy instead of neurolysis is   electrical stimulation to rule
       elected, what should be done prior to   out a motor component
       sectioning?

30

■ Common Peroneal Nerve Palsy

33. Complete the following about common peroneal nerve palsy: 30.12.1

a. True or False. The peroneal nerve is the most common nerve to develop acute compression palsy. — true

b. At what location? — fibular head

34. Describe the clinical findings in peroneal nerve palsy.   30.12.3

a. True or False. The anterior tibialis is the most commonly involved muscle in peroneal nerve palsy. — false (EHL)

b. Results in impairment of
  i. motor function: _____ — foot drop, weak foot eversion
  ii. sensory loss in _____ — dorsum of foot and lateral calf

c. The peroneus longus and brevis are innervated by the _____ _____ branch of the common peroneal nerve. — superficial peroneal

d. The deep peroneal branch innervates the _____, _____ _____, and _____ muscles. — EHL, anterior tibialis, and EDL (extensor digitorum longus)

35. If EMG stimulation is absent, both above and below fibular head, prognosis is _____. — poor   30.12.4

■ Tarsal Tunnel

36. True or False. The posterior tibial nerve may be   30.13.1

a. found in the tarsal tunnel. — true

b. found posterior and inferior to the medial malleolus. — true

c. trapped at the retinacular ligament. — true

d. classically responsible for nocturnal pain and paresthesia at the heel. — false (heel is spared)

37. Answer the following about clinical findings of posterior tibial nerve entrapment: 30.13.2

a. Percussion of the nerve at _____ _____ produces paresthesias that radiate _____. — medial malleolus; distally

b. Exacerbated by _____. — maximal inversion and eversion of foot

c. Dorsiflexion-eversion test: Examiner maximally everts and dorsiflexes the ankle while _____ for 5-10 seconds. — dorsiflexing the toes at MTP joints

30

31

Non-Entrapment Peripheral Neuropathies

■ Definitions

1. Define:
31.1

a. peripheral neuropathy — diffuse lesions of peripheral nerves producing weakness, sensory disturbance, and/or reflex changes

b. mononeuropathy — disorder of a single nerve, often due to trauma or entrapment

c. mononeuropathy multiplex — involvement of 2 or more nerves, usually due to a systemic abnormality

---

■ Etiologies of Peripheral Neuropathy

2. List the etiologies of non-entrapment peripheral neuropathies.
(Hint: Grand Therapist)
31.2

a.	G_____	Guillain-Barré
b.	R_____	Renal (uremic neuropathy)
c.	A_____	Alcoholism
d.	N_____	Nutritional
e.	D_____	Diabetes
f.	T_____	Traumatic
g.	H_____	Hereditary
h.	E_____	Endocrine or Entrapment
i.	R_____	Radiation
j.	A_____ or A_____	Amyloid or AIDS
k.	P_____ or P_____ or P_____	Psychiatric or Paraneoplastic or Pseudoneuropathy
l.	I_____	Infectious
m.	S_____	Sarcoidosis
n.	T_____	Toxins

■ Classification

3. **Complete the following regarding peripheral neuropathy:**   31.3
   a. The most common peripheral neuropathy that is an inherited disorder is C_____-M_____-T_____.   Charcot-Marie-Tooth
   b. Psychogenic somatoform disorders or malingering with symptoms of pains, paresthesias, hyperalgesia, weakness, an even objective changes in temperature are associated with p_____.   pseudoneuropathy

■ Clinical

4. **Regarding peripheral neuropathy.**
   a. Symptoms of peripheral neuropathies include: 31.4.1
      i.   l_____ of s_____   loss of sensation
      ii. p_____   pain
      iii. w_____   weakness
      iv. i_____   incoordination
      v.   d_____ a_____   difficulty ambulating
   b. Work-up includes: 31.4.2
      i.   H___-A___   Hgb-A1C
      ii. T____   TSH
      iii. E____   ESR
      iv. V_____ B___   Vitamin B12
      v.   E____   EMG

■ Syndromes of Peripheral Neuropathy

5. **True or False. Regarding critical illness polyneuropathy (CIP).**   31.5.1
   a. Most often affects proximal muscles.   false (distal muscles)
   b. Occurs in the presence of sepsis or multi-organ failure.   true
   c. Abnormal EMG is seen.   true
   d. Serum CPK may be normal.   true
   e. Treatment is supportive.   true
   f. Complete recovery rarely occurs.   false (occurs in 50% of patients)

6. **Which syndrome is associated with a pure sensory neuropathy?**   paraneoplastic syndrome (also associated with pyridoxine therapy)   31.5.2

7. **True or False. Alcohol neuropathy includes:**   31.5.3
   a. motor neuropathy   false
   b. sensory neuropathy   true
   c. absent Achilles reflex   true
   d. intense pain   false

31

8. **Brachial neuritis:**   31.5.4
    a. aka P_____-T_____ syndrome   Parsonage-Turner
    b. aka i_____ brachial plexus   idiopathic
        neuropathy
    c. Etiology: _____   unclear
    d. Prognosis: _____   good
    e. Predominant symptom: _____   pain
    f. Followed by: _____ in ____%   weakness in 96%
    g. Confined to shoulder girdle in   50%
        _____%

9. **True or False. The most important   31.5.5
    study in the diagnosis of lumbosacral
    plexus neuropathy is**
    a. MRI   false
    b. CT   false
    c. EMG   true (EMG in lumbosacral
                                               neuropathy – rule out
                                               diabetic neuropathy)
    d. ESR   false

10. **EMG in lumbosacral neuropathy shows   31.5.5
    what in regards to:**
    a. Fibrillation potentials in number   decreased
        _____.
    b. Motor unit potentials in number   decreased
        _____.
    c. Motor unit potentials in amplitude   increased
        _____.
    d. Motor unit potentials in duration   increased
        _____.
    e. Motor unit potentials that are   polyphasic
        _____.
    f. Have changes involving at least   2
        _____ segments.
    g. _____ the paraspinal muscles is highly   Sparing;
        _____.   diagnostic

11. **Complete the following about diabetic   31.5.6
    neuropathy:**
    a. Diabetic patients show neuropathy or   50%
        EMG changes __%.
    b. The first symptom of diabetes may be   neuropathy
        _____.
    c. Neuropathy might be reduced by control sugar
        of blood _____.

12. **Complete the following about drug-   31.5.7
    induced neuropathy:**
    Hint: CDEF
    a. C_____   Chemotherapy drugs
    b. D_____   Dilantin (Phenytoin)
    c. E_____   Elavil (Amitriptyline)
    d. F_____   Flagyl (Metronidazole)

31

13. **True or False. Femoral neuropathy includes:**   31.5.8
    a. weakness of the quadriceps and iliopsoas   true
    b. patellar reflex – reduced   true
    c. femoral stretch – positive   true
    d. sensation over lateral calf reduced   false (femoral neuropathy includes ↓ sensation over anterior thigh and medial calf.)

14. **Answer the following regarding femoral neuropathy:**   31.5.8
    a. Name the muscle responsible for
       i.   knee extension   quadriceps femoris
       ii. hip flexion   iliopsoas
    b. To distinguish L4 radiculopathy from   iliopsoas
       femoral neuropathy, L4 radiculopathy
       would not involve the _____.
    c. Femoral neuropathy is caused by
       i.   d_____   diabetes
       ii. c_____   compression

15. **True or False. The most frequent cause of femoral neuropathy is**   31.5.8
    a. intrabdominal tumor   false
    b. retroperitoneal hematoma   false
    c. diabetes   true (All other options can cause femoral neuropathy.)
    d. entrapment due to inguinal hernia   false
    e. trauma   false

16. **True or False. Regarding AIDS neuropathy.**   31.5.9
    a. It usually presents as proximal symmetric   false (distal, symmetric
       polyneuropathy.   polyneuropathy)
    b. HIV+ only patients do not develop it.   true
    c. It never includes sensory elements.   false (usually includes numbness and tingling)
    d. It has an infectious etiology.   true
    e. It may be caused by lymphomatous   true
       invasion of the meninges or nerves.
    f. Drugs used to treat HIV can also cause   true
       neuropathies, most commonly NRTIs
       and protease inhibitors.

31

17. Complete the following about monoclonal gammopathy: 31.5.10
a. Included entities such as
    i.   m_____   myeloma
    ii. Waldenstrom _____   macroglobulinemia
    iii. M_____   MGUS
b. Responsible for _____% of neuropathies. 10%
c. Patient risk factors for anesthesia-related ulnar neuropathy include:
    i.   m_____ g_____   male gender
    ii. o_____   obesity (BMI > 38)
    iii. prolonged post-op b_____ r_____ bed rest

18. Complete the following about perioperative ulnar neuropathies: 31.5.11
a. Avoid elbow flexion of greater than _____ degrees. 110
b. It tightens the _____ _____ cubital tunnel
    retinaculum.

19. Complete the following about lower extremity neuropathy: 31.5.11
a.
    i.   common peroneal in _____%   81%
    ii. risk is _____ position   lithotomy
b. Femoral neuropathy where there is hemorrhage in the _____ muscle. psoas
c. Meralgia paresthetica
    i.   tends to occur _____   bilaterally
    ii. in young slender _____   males
    iii. positioned _____   prone
    iv. in operations lasting _____ hours 6 to 10
    v.   recovers in approximately _____ _____ 6 months

20. What is the management of lower extremity neuropathy?   31.5.11
a. Call neurologist if not better in _____ days. 5
b. Do EMG not earlier than _____ weeks.   3

21. Complete the following about amyloid neuropathy and uremic neuropathy: 31.5.12
a. Amyloid neuropathy
    i.   Amyloid can be deposited in   peripheral nerves
         _____ _____.
    ii. It produces a _____   sensory
         neuropathy.
    iii. It can produce pressure on nerves, carpal tunnel
         i.e., _____ _____.
b. Uremic neuropathy
    i.   occurs in _____ _____   chronic renal failure
         _____ patients.
    ii. symptoms include _____ _____   "Charlie horses" and "restless
         and _____ _____.   legs"
    iii. can be relieved by _____.   dialysis

31

22. **Complete the following about post-cardiac catheterization neuropathy:**
       31.5.12
    a. It involves the _____ nerve.   femoral
    b. It usually involves _____.   hematomas

■ Peripheral Nerve Injuries

23. **Describe the anatomy of the peripheral nerve.**
       31.6.1
    a. The connective tissue membrane that surrounds individual axons is the _____.   endoneurium

    b. _____ surrounds groups of axons (i.e. fascicles).   Perineurium

    c. _____ surrounds groups of fascicles (i.e. nerves).   Epineurium

24. **Complete the following regarding injury and regeneration of nerve:**
       31.6.1
    a. The regeneration rate = _____   1 mm/day (i.e. 1 inch/month)
    b. Sunderland system
       i. first degree: anatomy   preserved; conduction block, compression, or ischemia

       ii. second degree: axon _____ connective tissue is _____   injuried; endo-, peri-, epineurium intact (endoneurium provided tube for regeneration)

       iii. third-degree: axon and endoneurium d_____   disrupted (grossly normal appearance, recovery related to the extent of intrafascicular fibrosis)

25. **Complete the following about peripheral neuropathies:**
       31.6.1
    a. Fourth-degree axon injury involves _____ of all the elements but _____ is intact.   interruption of all elements but epineurium is intact (nerve is indurated and enlarged)

    b. Fifth-degree axon injury: endo-, peri-, and epineurium is completely t_____.   transected

    c. Sixth-degree axon injury: mixed _____ through _____ degree injuries   first through fourth

26. **Describe injury classification of peripheral nerves and regeneration prognosis.**   Two classifications: Seddon and Sunderland   31.6.1
    a. Axon compressed   First degree = Seddon neuropraxia; conduction block from compression or ischemia, anatomy preserved

31

b.   Axon injured

Second-degree = Seddon axonotmesis; injury to axon and Wallerian degeneration; endo-, peri-, epineurium intact; endoneurium provides "tube" to optimize successful reinnervation of target muscle

c.   Axon and endoneurium disrupted

Third degree = axon and endoneurium disrupted; recovery inversely related to interfascicular fibrosis; gross normal appearance

d.   Axon, endoneurium and perineurium disrupted

Fourth-degree = interruption of axon, endo- and per-neurium; gross reveals indurated enlarged nerve

e.   Axon endo-, peri-, and epineurium disrupted

Fifth-degree = Seddon neurotmesis; complete transection of axon, endo-, peri-, and epineurium

27.   **What are the etiologies of brachial plexus injuries?**
      Hint: CPT

      a.   C_____   compression
      b.   P_____   penetration
      c.   T_____   traction

31.6.2

28.   **Complete the following about traction (stretch) injuries of the brachial plexus selectively:**

      a.   Spare the
           i.   _____ _____   medial cord
           ii. _____ _____   median nerve
      b.   Injure the
           i.   _____ _____   posterior cord
           ii. _____ _____   lateral cord

31.6.2

29.   **Complete the following about the pre- and post-ganglionic injuries:**

      a.   What nerve injury cannot be repaired?   proximal to the dorsal root ganglion (i.e. preganglionic)

      b.   What is the evidence for such an injury? (Hint: prEHms)
           i.   p_____   pain
           ii.   r_____   rhomboids
           iii. E_____   EMG
           iv.   H_____   Horner's syndrome
           v.   m_____   meningocele
           vi.   s_____   scapula

31.6.2

31

30. **Describe upper and lower brachial plexus injury.**   31.6.2
    a. Upper brachial plexus injury
        i.   E____-D_____ palsy   Erb-Duchenne palsy
        ii. C__-C__   C5-C6
        iii. f_____ s_____ of h_____ h_____   forceful separation of
             from s_____   humeral head from shoulder
        iv. i_____ r_____ a___ with   internally rotated arm with
             e_____ e_____   extended elbow
        v.   Commonly shoulder d_____ or   dystocia or motorcycle crash
             m_____ c_____
        vi. B_____ t_____   Bellhop's tip, hand not
                                                      affected
    b. Lower brachial plexus injury:
        i.   aka K_____ palsy   Klumpke's palsy
        ii. C__-T__   C8-T1
        iii. s_____ p____ of a_____ a_____ in   sudden pull of abducted arm
        iv. f____ or P_____ t_____   fall or Pancoast tumor
        v.   c____ h___ with w_____ of s_____   claw hand with weakness of
             h___ m_____   small hand muscles
        vi. s_____ h_____   Simian hand

31. **Complete the following about brachial plexus birth injuries:**   31.6.2
    a.
        i.   most common is _____   upper
        ii. consisting of C5-C6 _____% and   50%
        iii. C5, C6-C7 _____%   25%
        iv. lower C8-T1 _____%   2%
    b. Combined is _____%   20%
    c. Bilateral _____%   4%
    d. Spontaneous recovery is _____%   90%

32. **Characterize upper brachial plexus injury – Erb's palsy.**   31.6.2
    a. Roots involved: _____   C5 (ABCDE) fifth letter of
                                                      alphabet, Erb palsy mainly C5
                                                      and also C6, C7

    b. Position of upper extremity (Hint: erp)
        i.   e_____   extended
        ii. r_____   rotated
        iii. p_____   pronated
        iv. looks like _____ _____ _____   Bellhop's tip position

31

c. Weak muscles and their roots.
   i. d_____   deltoid;
       roots, _____   C5, C6
   ii. b_____   biceps;
       roots, _____   C5, C6
   iii. r_____   rhomboids;
       roots, _____   C4, C5
   iv. b_____   brachioradialis;
       roots, _____   C5, C6
   v. s_____   supraspinatus;
       roots, _____   C4, C5, C6
   vi. i_____   infraspinatus;
       roots, _____   C5, C6
d. Mechanism: _____ _____   shoulder separation
e. From:
   i. b_____ i_____   birth injuries
   ii. m_____ a_____   motorcycle accidents

33. Characterize lower brachial plexus   31.6.2
    injury – Klumke's palsy.
a. Roots involved: _____   C7, C8, T1
b. Position of upper extremity (Hint: klump)
   i. kl_____   claw hand (Simian hand)
   ii. u_____   ulnar claw
   iii. m_____   median claw
   iv. p_____   paralysis
c. Weak muscles
   i. upper extremity: _____   small muscles of hand
   ii. face: _____   Horner's syndrome if T1
                                       involved
d. Mechanism: traction on _____ arm   abducted
e. From:
   i. f_____   falls
   ii. b_____   birth
   iii. P_____ t____   Pancoast tumors

34. Complete the following regarding   31.6.2
    birth injury of brachial plexus:
a. Incidence is _____   0.3 to 2/1000 births
   i. upper: ___%   50% (C5, C6)
   ii. upper plus C7: ___%   25% (C5, C6, C7)
b. mixed   20%
c. lower   2% C7, C8, T1
d. bilateral   4%

35. True or False. The following are   31.6.2
    indications for early surgical
    exploration of the brachial plexus:
a. any injury needs repair   false (most injuries will have
                                      maximal deficit at onset then
                                      improve)
b. progressive deficit   true (progressive deficit likely
                                      vascular injury, explore
                                      immediately)

31

| c. | clean sharp injury | true (clean, sharp, fresh lacerating injuries → explore acutely and repair end-to-end) |
| d. | gunshot wound (GSW) to brachial plexus | false (surgery is of little benefit) |

■ Missile Injuries of Peripheral Nerves

36. Regarding gunshot wounds: 31.7

a. Most injuries are the result of s____ and c_____ and not d_____ n_____ t_____.   shock and cavitation; direct nerve transection

b. Approximately ____% will recover with expectant management.   70%

c. However, if there is lack of improvement on EMG, intervention should occur about ___ - ___ months after the injury to avoid further nerve fibrosis and muscle atrophy.   5-6 months

■ Thoracic Outlet Syndrome

37. True or False. Clinical presentation of thoracic outlet syndrome may include   31.8.1

a. pallor and ischemia of hand and fingers.   true

b. arm swelling and edema.   true

c. brachial plexus lower trunk dysfunction.   true

d. brachial plexus median cord dysfunction.   true

38. List the differential diagnosis for thoracic outlet syndrome.   31.8.2

a. h_____ _____ _____   herniated cervical disc

b. c____ ____   cervical arthrosis

c. l____ ____   lung cancer (Pancoast tumor)

d. t_____ _____ _____ ____   tardy ulnar nerve palsy

e. c____ ____ ____   carpal tunnel syndrome

f. o_____   orthopedic shoulder problems

g. c_____ _____ _____ syndrome   complex regional pain syndrome (CPRS)

39. True of False. Regarding thoracic outlet syndrome, conservative treatment may be as effective as the surgical treatment.   true   31.8.3

40. True or False. Scalenus syndrome is a well characterized and accepted cause of thoracic outlet syndrome.   false   31.8.4

31

32

Neurophthalmology

■ Nystagmus

1. Complete the following about nystagmus: 32.1.1

a. What is nystagmus? i_____ r_____   involuntary rhythmic
    o_____ of the eyes   oscillation

b. What is the most common form?   jerk nystagmus

c. How is it directionality defined?   fast component

d. What is the abnormal component?   slow component

e. What is vertical nystagmus indicative of?

    i.   p_____ f_____ p_____   posterior fossa pathology

    ii.   s_____   sedatives

    iii.   a_____ d_____   antiepileptic drugs

2. Seesaw nystagmus occurs with a lesion in the _____.   diencephalon   32.1.2

3. Nystagmus retractorius occurs with a lesion in the _____ _____ _____; for example p_____.   upper midbrain tegmentum; pinealoma   32.1.2

4. Ocular bobbing occurs with a lesion in the _____ _____.   pontine tegmentum   32.1.2

5. Matching. Match the form of nystagmus and the location of the lesion.   32.1.2

Form:
① seesaw nytagmus; ② convergence nystagmus; ③ nystagmus retractorius; ④ downbeat nystagmus; ⑤ upbeat nystagmus; ⑥ abducting nystagmus; ⑦ ocular bobbing

Location: (a-f) below

a. diencephalon   ①

b. upper midbrain tegmentum   ②

c. midbrain tectum   ③

d. pons medial longitudinal fasciculus (MLF)   ⑥, ⑦

e. medulla   ⑤

f. posterior-fossa – cervicomedullary junction   ④

6. **Name the location of the lesion for the following forms of nystagmus:**   32.1.2

   a. seesaw nystagmus   diencephalon
   b. nystagmus retractorius   upper midbrain
                                          tegmentum/pineal region
   c. downbeat nystagmus   cervicomedullary junction
                                          (foramen magnum)
   d. upbeat nystagmus   medulla
   e. ocular bobbing   pons

■ Papilledema

7. **Complete the following about papilledema:**   32.2.1

   a. What is papilledema caused by?   Thought to be caused by
                                          axoplasmic stasis. Theory: 1.
                                          Increased intracranial
                                          pressure (ICP) transmitted to
                                          the optic disk via
                                          subarachnoid (SA) space.
                                          Retinal venous pulsations
                                          obliterated. 2. Retinal arterial:
                                          venous pressure < 1.5:1.
   b. How long does it take to develop?   24 to 48 hours
   c. What is the earliest it is seen?   6 hours
   d. Does it cause visual blurring?   no (unless severe and
                                          prolonged)
   e. Does it cause visual field distortion?   no (unless severe and
                                          prolonged)
   f. Differentiate from optic neuritis.
      i. funduscopy _____ _____   may look alike
         _____
      ii. visual loss more with _____ optic neuritis
          _____
      iii. pain on palpation more with _____   optic neuritis
           _____

8. **What is the differential diagnosis for unilateral papilledema?**   32.2.2
   (Hint: FIOM)

   a. F_____-_____ _____   Foster-Kennedy syndrome
   b. I_____   Inflammation
   c. O_____ _____   Optic glioma
   d. M_____ _____   Multiple Sclerosis

32

■ Visual Fields

9. **Complete the following concerning visual fields:**   32.3.1
   a. Normal visual field extends approximately from:
      i.   ____° nasally in each eye   35
      ii. ____° temporally in each eye   90
      iii. ____° above and below the horizontal meridian in each eye   50
   b. The normal blind spot is due to _____ and is located to the _____ side of the macular visual area in each eye.   absence of light receptors in the optic disc where the retina is penetrated by the optic nerve; temporal
   c. Macular splitting occurs with lesions _____ or _____ to the lateral geniculate body (LGB).   anterior or posterior   32.3.2
   d. Macular sparing tends to occur with lesions _____ to the LGB.   posterior

■ Visual Field Deficits

10. **Regarding visual field deficits:**   32.4
    a. Can be tested either at the _____ or with _____ _____.   bedside; formal perimetry
    b. Visual field deficits depend on the location of the injury, for example:
       i.   right optic nerve: _____ _____ _____   right monocular blindness
       ii. optic chiasm: _____ _____   biltemporal hemianopsia
       iii. right Meyer's loop: _____ _____ _____ with ____ _____   left superior quadrantanopsia with macular sparing
       iv. right occipital (visual cortex): _____ _____ _____ with ____ _____   left homonymous hemianopsia with macular sparing

■ Pupillary Diameter

11. **Complete the following concerning the pupillodilator nerve fibers:**   32.5.1
    a. First-order sympathetic nerve fibers
       i.   origin: p_____ h_____   posterolateral hypothalamus
       ii. destination: i____ cell column (_____ to _____)   intermediolateral (C8 to T2)
       iii. neurotransmitter: a_____   Acetylcholine (ACh)
    b. Second-order sympathetic nerve fibers
       i.   origin: i____ cell column   intermediolateral
       ii. destination: s_____ c_____ g_____   superior cervical ganglion

32

c. Third-order sympathetic nerve fibers
  i. origin: s_____ c_____
     g_____   superior cervical ganglion
  ii. destination: p_____ m_____ of   pupillodilator muscle (long
     the eye, l_____ g_____,   ciliary nerves); lacrimal gland,
     M_____ m_____   Müller's muscle
  iii. neurotransmitter: n_____   norepinephrine

12. How are pupillodilator muscles   radially   32.5.1
   arranged?

13. Describe the anatomy of sympathetic   32.5.1
   outflow to the eye.
   (Hint: hilsc)
   a. h_____   hypothalamus
   b. i_____ _____ _____   intermediolateral cell column
   c. l_____ _____ _____   lateral horn cells;
      c_____ _____   ciliary ganglion
                                                    Sympathetic summary: first
                                                    order: posterolateral (a)
                                                    hypothalamus → descend in
                                                    midbrain tegmentum
                                                    uncrossed to pons, medulla,
                                                    spinal cord (SC) to the (b)
                                                    intermediolateral cell
                                                    columns, C8-T2 (ciliospinal
                                                    center of Budge) → synapse
                                                    with (c) lateral horn cells
                                                    acetylcholine and give off
                                                    second-order neurons (a)
                                                    (preganglionics). Second
                                                    order: enter sympathetic
                                                    chain → (b) superior cervical
                                                    ganglion. Third order: (a)
                                                    (postganglionics): go up with
                                                    common carotid artery (CCA)
                                                    (b), those that mediate sweat
                                                    to face go up external carotid
                                                    artery (ECA), the rest go up
                                                    internal carotid artery (ICA).
                                                    Some pass: = (d) V1 → ciliary
                                                    ganglion → (e) pupillodilator
                                                    norepinephrine = ICA → (f)
                                                    ophthalmic artery → (g)
                                                    lacrimal gland and the Muller
                                                    muscle.

14. The pupilloconstrictor   concentric as a sphincter   32.5.2
   (parasympathetic) are muscles
   arranged c_____ as a
   s_____.

32

15. **Describe the parasympathetic outflow to the eyes.**   32.5.2
    (Hint: Ect)
    a. E_____-_____   Edinger-Westphal
    b. c_____ _____   ciliary ganglion
    c. t_____ _____   third nerve
    Parasympathetics summary: Preganglionics arise in the Edinger-Westphal nucleus at the level of the superior colliculus synapse in the ciliary ganglion. Postganglionics travel on the third nerve to (e) innervate sphincter pupillae and ciliary muscle (thickens lens causing accommodation via relaxation).

16. **Describe the pupillary light reflex.**   32.5.3
    (Hint: ropEtcs)
    a. r_____   retina
    b. o_____   optic nerve
    c. p_____   pretectal
    d. E_____   Edinger-Westphal
    e. t_____   third nerve
    f. c_____   ciliary ganglion
    g. s_____   sphincter light reflex
    Summary: Mediated by (a) rods and cones of retina. Transmit via axons to (b) optic nerve. Bypass lateral geniculate body (unlike vision) synapse in (c) pretectal nuclear complex. Connect to both (d) Edinger-Westphal nuclei. Preganglionics travel in (e) third nerve to (f) ciliary gangion, etc. Postganglionics via third nerve to pupillary sphincter. Ciliary muscles thicken (relax) causing accommodation.

17. **Complete the following about Argyll Roberston pupil:**   32.5.4
    (Hint: ALRP = Argyll Robertson pupil = absent light response pupil)
    a. Key feature is _____ _____   absent light response pupil
       _____ _____ or ALRP.
    b. It occurs in _____.   syphilis
    c. Light-near dissociation means the pupil   near (i.e. convergence)
       constricts when focusing on an object
       _____

    d. but the pupil does not react to _____.   light

18. **Does afferent pupillary defect cause anisocoria?**   no   32.5.5

19. **Complete the following about anisocoria:**   32.5.5
    a. unequal pupils with an afferent pupillary   two lesions
       defect (Marcus-Gunn) means there are

       ____ _____
    b. Physiologic anisocoria occurs in _____%   20%
       of people.
    c. The difference is usually _____ mm.   0.4
    d. Sudden onset of anisocoria is usually due   drugs
       to _____.
    e. Sympathomimetics cause _____ to   1 to 2
       _____ mm of dilation and
    f.
       i.   parasympatholytics cause _____   8
            mm of dilation and the
       ii. eye _____ _____ react to light.   does not

20. **What is the differential diagnosis of anisocoria?**   32.5.5
    Hint: u tAp Hat
    a. u_____   uncal herniation (also has
                                                             mental status changes)
    b. t_____   trauma (traumatic iridoplegia
                                                             mydriasis or miosis)
    c. A_____   Adie's pupil (iris palsy –
                                                             impaired postganglionic
                                                             parasympathetics)
    d. p_____   physiologic (less than 1 mm
                                                             difference – 20% of
                                                             population)
    e. H_____   Horner's syndrome (impaired
                                                             sympathetics to pupillodilator
                                                             muscle)
    f. a_____   aneurysm (posterior
                                                             communicating, basilar)
    g. t_____   third nerve palsy (pupil
                                                             sparing-diabetes mellitus
                                                             [DM 1], EtOH, cavernous
                                                             aneurysm)

32

21. **What is the differential diagnosis for Marcus-Gunn pupil?**   32.5.5
    a. Location of lesion: _____   ipsilateral to impaired direct reflex anterior to chiasm
        i.   r_____ - d_____   retina – detachment, infarction
             i_____
        ii. n_____ - n_____ (m_____   nerve – neuritis (multiple sclerosis, viral) or trauma
             s_____, v_____), or t_____
    b. In Marcus Gunn is/are the
        i.   third nerve intact?   Yes
        ii. parasympathetic nerves intact?   Yes

22. **Complete the following about Adie's pupil:**   32.5.5
    a. Dilated or constricted pupil?   dilated
    b. Due to impaired preganglionic or   postganglionic
        postganglionic fibers?
    c. Thought to be caused by a _____   viral infection
        _____
    d. of the _____ _____.   ciliary ganglion

23. **Complete the following about third nerve compression:**   32.5.5
    a. example is _____   aneurysm
    b. most common is _____   P-comm
    c. occasionally _____ _____   basilar bifurcation
        aneurysm
    d. usually _____ _____ _____ the pupil   does not spare

24. **Complete the following about Horner's syndrome:**   32.5.6
    a. The abnormal pupil is _____.   smaller
    b. Ptosis is on the side of the _____   small
        pupil.

25. **The ptosis is due to paralysis of the**   superior and inferior tarsal   32.5.6
    _____ and _____ _____ muscles.

26. **Is the ptosis complete or partial?**   partial   32.5.6

27. **Enophthalmos is due to paralysis of**   Müller's muscle; is involved   32.5.6
    M_____ muscle, which is or is not
    involved in Horner's syndrome?

28. **Horner's syndrome is caused by**   32.5.6
    interruption of sympathetics to the
    eye and face anywhere along their
    path. Name specific causes that affect
    the following:
    a. first-order neurons (three causes)
        i.   i_____ from v_____   infarction from vascular occlusion (usually PICA)
             o_____
        ii. s_____   syringobulbia
        iii. i_____ n_____   intraparenchymal neoplasm

32

   b. second-order neurons (three causes)

      i.   l_____ s_____   lateral sympathectomies

      ii. s_____ c_____ t_____   significant chest trauma

      iii. a_____ p_____ n_____   apical pulmonary neoplasms

          (P_____ t_____)   (Pancoast tumors)

   c. third-order neurons (five causes)

      i.   n_____ t_____   neck trauma (e.g. carotid dissections)

      ii. c_____ v_____ d_____   carotid vascular disease

      iii. c_____ b_____ a_____   cervical bony abnormalities

      iv. m_____   migraine

29. **Trace the third-order neuron in the pupillodilation/sympathetic path.**   32.5.6

   a. neurons from the s_____ c_____ g_____   superior cervical ganglion

   b. to the p_____ m_____   pupillodilator muscle

   c. and M_____ m_____   Müller's muscle

30. **True or False. Answer the following regarding Horner's syndrome:**   32.5.6

   a. In a patient with Horner's syndrome and preserved sweating of the face, the lesion is located

      i.   in the first-order neuron   false

      ii. in the second-order neuron   false

      iii. in the third-order neuron   true (injured fibers on ICA produce Horner, intact sweat fibers to face on ECA).

   b. this is compatible with a Pancoast tumor.   false (Pancoast tumor would affect the sympathetics between the spinal cord and superior cervical ganglion [i.e., second-order neurons]. The fibers to sweat glands would be damaged because they had not yet separated to travel with the ECA.)

31. **Complete the following about Horner's syndrome:**   32.5.6

   a. What medication is used if diagnosis of Horner's syndrome is in doubt?   cocaine

   b. How does it work?   cocaine blocks norepinephrine (NE) reuptake

   c. Therefore in Horner's syndrome the pupil will _____ _____ with _____.   not dilate with cocaine (no NE release)

   d. In a normal patient the pupil will _____ _____.   dilate normally

32

■ Extraocular Muscle (EOM) System

32. Matching. From the list below identify the cranial nerve that innervates the muscle: 32.6.1
Nerve:
① CN III; ② CN IV; ③ CN VI
Hint: L6 SO4
Muscle: (a-f) below

a. medial rectus   ①
b. inferior rectus   ①
c. inferior oblique   ①
d. superior rectus   ①
e. superior oblique   ②
f. lateral rectus   ③

33. Complete the following regarding the frontal eye field: 32.6.1

a. True or False. It moves eyes laterally to the opposite side.   true
b. It is located in the Brodmann area _____.   8
c. Its fibers go through the _____ of the _____ _____.   genu of the internal capsule
d. It sends fibers to the ipsilateral _____ _____ _____ _____ nucleus.   paramedian pontine reticular formation (PPRF)
e. It sends fibers to the ipsilateral _____ nucleus   sixth
f. and the contralateral _____ nucleus   third
g. via the _____ _____ _____.   medial longitudinal fasciculus (MLF)
h. The right paramedian pontine reticular formation (PPRF) controls lateral eye movements to the _____.   right

34. Complete the following about the extraocular motor system: 32.6.2

a. Injury to the medial longitudinal fasciculus (MLF) is called _____ _____.   internuclear ophthalmoplegia (INO)
b. Convergence is _____ _____.   not impaired
c. If the right MLF is injured the right eye will not _____ _____.   move medially (adduct)
d. The left eye when looking laterally shows
   i.   w_____ on a_____   weakness on abduction
   ii. n_____ on a_____   nystagmus on adduction
e. The most common cause of MLF malfunction is _____ _____.   multiple sclerosis (MS)

35. With third nerve palsy, if there is ptosis it will be on the side of the _____ pupil.   large   32.6.3

32

36. **Complete the following about oculomotor neuropathy:**   32.6.3
   a. Example is _____.   diabetes
   b. Usually _____ the pupil.   spares
   c. Usually resolved in _____ _____.   8 weeks

37. **Name three causes of non-pupil-sparing oculomotor palsy.**   32.6.3
   (Hint: tau)
   a. t_____   tumor
   b. a_____   aneurysm (PComm, Basilar tip)
   c. u_____ _____   uncal herniation

38. **Name seven causes of pupil-sparing oculomotor palsy.**   32.6.3
   (Hint: mEtDacc)
   a. m_____   myasthenia gravis
   b. E_____   EtOH
   c. t_____   temporal arteritis
   d. D_____   DM
   e. a_____   atherosclerosis
   f. c_____ _____ _____   chronic progressive ophthalmoplegia
   g. c_____ _____ _____   cavernous sinus lesions

39. **Complete the following about trochlear nerve palsy (CN IV):**   32.6.4
   a.
     i. In relation to the aqueduct the trochlear nucleus lies _____   ventral
     ii. at the level of the _____ _____.   inferior colliculi
   b.
     i. The axons pass _____ and   dorsally
     ii. decussate _____.   internally
   c. It innervates the _____ _____ muscle   superior oblique
   d. Superior oblique muscle
     i. Primarily depresses the _____ eye.   adducted
     ii. In primary gaze it moves the eye _____ and ___.   down and out

40. **Complete the following about the unique features of the trochlear nerve:**   32.6.4
   a. Nucleus is on the _____ side of the   opposite
   b. muscle it goes to: _____ _____ _____   superior oblique muscle
   c. It is the only nerve to decussate _____.   internally
   d. It is the only nerve to exit _____ to the brainstem.   posterior
   e. True or False. It passes through the annulus of Zinn.   false
   f. Palsy results in eye deviation "_____ and ___."   "up and in"

32

g. Head is tilted to the _____ _____ the   side opposite
    CN IV palsy.
h. Diplopia is exacerbated with looking   down; stairs
    _____ (i.e., _____).

41. Name the causes of abducens palsy.   32.6.5
    Hint: abducens
a. a_____   arteritis, aneurysms
b. b_____   sixth nerve palsy
c. d_____   diabetes, Dorello canal
                                      (Gradenigo's syndrome)
d. u_____   uncontrolled ICP,
                                      pseudotumor, trauma, tumor
e. c_____   cavernous sinus lesions,
                                      clivus, chordoma, or fracture
f. e_____   eye disease, thyroid,
                                      myasthenia gravis
g. n_____   neoplasms
h. s_____   sphenoid sinusitis
                                      (Gradenigo's syndrome)

42. Matching. Match the syndrome with   32.6.6
    the nerves involved in multiple
    extraocular motor involvement
    disorders.
    Syndrome:
    ① cavernous sinus; ② superior orbital
    fissure; ③ orbital apex
    Nerves involved: (a-g) below
a. II   ③
b. III   ①, ②, ③
c. IV   ①, ②, ③
d. V1   ①, ②, ③
e. V2   ①
f. V3
g. VI   ①, ②, ③

■ Neurophthalmologic Syndromes

43. Regarding Tolosa-Hunt Syndrome: 32.7.2
a. Is the ophthalmoplegia painful or   painful
    painless?
b. Which nerve(s) is/are involved?   any nerve traversing the
                                         cavernous sinus
c. The pupil is usually _____.   spared
d. How long do symptoms last?   days to weeks
e. Can there be spontaneous remission? yes
f. Can there be recurrent attacks?   yes
g. Is there systemic involvement?   no
h. How is it treated?   systemic steroids = 60 to 80
                                         mg of prednisone by mouth
                                         daily (slow taper)

32

i. The disease is thought to be a   nonspecific inflammation
_____ _____.
j. The inflammation is located at the   superior orbital fissure
_____ _____ _____.

44. Complete the following about   32.7.3
Raeder's paratrigeminal neuralgia:
a. Name two components.
   i. u_____ o_____ p_____   unilateral oculosympathetic
paresis (think Horner's
syndrome – anhidrosis ±
ptosis)
   ii. h_____ t_____ n_____   homolateral trigeminal nerve
     i_____   involvement (Horner's
syndrome and tic-like pain)
b. The pupil is _____.   small
c. True or False. The pain is continuous.   false (intermittent, tic-like)
d. The pain is located at the _____.   trigeminal nerve V1
(ophthalmic division) and
sympathetics

45. Complete the following regarding   32.7.4
Gradenigo's syndrome:
a. What is Gradenigo's syndrome?   Apical petrositis
b. Involves _____ canal.   Dorello's canal
c. Name the classic triad.
   i. p_____ of _____   palsy; abducens
   ii. p_____ where? _____   pain; retro-orbital
   iii. d_____ e_____   draining ear
d. Pain is located at the p_____   petrous apex
     a_____.
e. Features
(Hint: Gradenigo)
   i. G_____   Gradenigo
   ii. r_____ _____   retro-orbital pain
   iii. a_____ _____   apical petrositis – abducens
palsy
   iv. d_____ _____   draining ear – Dorello's canal
   v. e_____ _____   ear draining
   vi. n_____ _____ _____   neuropathy of VI
   vii. i_____   inflammation
   viii. p_____   petrositis
   ix. o_____ p_____   orbital pain

■ Miscellaneous Neurophthalmologic Signs

46. Complete the following about ocular   32.8
bobbing:
a. The eyes move _____.   downward
b. How many times per minute?   2 to 12
c. Ocular bobbing is associated with   horizontal gaze
bilateral paralysis of _____ _____.
d. It is seen with destruction of the _____   pontine tegmentum
_____.

32

47. **Optic atrophy is due to a _____ lesion.**   compressive   32.8

48. **Opsoclonus is _____, _____, _____, ___-_____ eye movement.**   rapid, conjugate, irregular, non-rhythmic   32.8

49. **Oscillopsia is the visual sensation that stationary objects are _____ or _____ side-to-side.**   vibrating or swaying   32.8

32

33

Neurotology

■ Dizziness and Vertigo

1. The differential diagnosis for dizziness includes: 33.1.1
a. n_____ s_____   near syncope
b. d_____   disequilibrium
c. v_____   vertigo
d. l_____   lightheadedness

2. What is the definition of vertigo?   33.1.1
a. Sensation of _____   movement (usually spinning)
b. from
    i.   i_____ e_____ d_____   internal ear dysfunction
      or
    ii.   v_____ n_____ d_____   vestibular nerve dysfunction

3. True or False. Inner ear dysfunction presenting with vertigo includes the following: 33.1.1
a. labyrinthitis   true
b. trauma, i.e. e_____ l____   true (i.e. endolymphatic leak)
c. drugs, i.e. a_____   true (i.e. aminoglycosides)
d. acoustic neuroma   false (acoustic neuroma does not cause inner ear dysfunction but may cause vertigo from compression of the vestibular nerve)
e. vertebrobasilar insufficiency   true (other causes of vertigo include inner causes: Meniere disease, benign/paroxysmal positional vertigo, syphilis)

4. Complete the following regarding cupulolithiasis: 33.1.1
a. What is cupulolithiasis? c_____
    c_____ in s_____ c_____   Calcium concentrations in semicircular canal
b. It is also known as b_____
    p_____ p_____ v_____.   benign paroxysmal positional vertigo
c. Symptoms are made manifest by
    _____ _____.   head turning
d. Patient is usually in _____.   bed

33

e. Is it self-limiting?	yes
f. For how long?	usually not for > 1 year
Is hearing affected?	no hearing loss

5. Describe indications and complications of selective vestibular neurectomy (SVN).   33.1.2

a. Indications
   i.   M_____ d_____   Meniere's disease
   ii. p_____ v_____ i_____   partial vestibular injury

b. Rationale?   In disabling cases of vertigo, refractory to medical/nondestructive surgical treatment. SVN preserves hearing; is 90% (Meniere disease) and 80% (vertiginous spells) effective.

c. Complications
   i.   h_____ l_____   hearing loss (unusual)
   ii. o_____   oscillopsia (Dandy's syndrome)
   iii. l_____ of b_____ in the d_____ with bilateral SVN   loss of balance in the dark with bilateral SVN (loss of vestibule-ocular reflex)

6. Answer the following about the vestibular nerve: 33.1.2

a. In which half of the eighth nerve complex?   superior

b. What color relative to the cochlear nerve?   more gray

c. To preserve hearing what vessel must be preserved?   artery of the auditory canal

7. True or False. CN VII can be differentiated from CN VIII at the internal auditory canal (IAC) by all of the following: 33.1.2

a. direct stimulation/recording   true
b. lies anterior/superior to VIII   true
c. transverse crest and Bill bar   true
d. darker color c/w CN VIII   false (CN VII is paler/whiter)
e. Electromyographic (EMG) monitoring of CN VII during manipulation   true

---

■ Meniere's Disease

8. Meniere's disease is also known as e_____ h_____.   endolymphatic hydrops   33.2.1

9. What is the clinical triad of Meniere's disease?   33.2.3

a. v_____ v_____ a_____   violent vertigo attacks
b. t_____   tinnitus "escaping steam"
c. h_____ l_____   hearing loss (fluctuating, low-frequency)

10. **Diagnostic studies for patients with Meniere's disease include:**   33.2.3
   a. E____ with b_____ c_____   ENG with bithermal caloric
      s_____   stimulation
   b. a_____   audiogram
   c. B_____   BAER
   d. No findings on r_____ i_____ radiographic imaging

11. **True or False. Treatment of Meniere's disease includes:**   33.2.3
   a. middle ear perfusion with gentamicin   true
   b. bilateral vestibular neurectomy   false (bilateral ablative
                                              procedure is to be avoided)
   c. salt restriction   true
   d. vestibular suppressants (e.g. Valium,   true
      meclizine)
   e. endolymphatic shunting   true
   f. diuretics (e.g. Diamox)   true

■ Facial Nerve Palsy

12. **Answer the following about supranuclear facial palsy:**   33.3.2
   a. Which part of the face is involved?   lower only
   b. Emotional facial expression (e.g. smiling) intact
      is _____.
   c. The lesion is the lowest part of the   precentral gyrus
      _____ _____.
   d. Part of the face is spared paralysis   upper face; bilateral
      because the _____ _____ has _____ representation
      _____.

13. **Complete the following regarding nuclear facial palsy:**   33.3.2
   a. It causes paralysis of all _____   ipsilateral CN VII innervated
      _____ _____ muscles.
   b. Plus sixth nerve palsy constitutes the Millard-Gubler
      _____-_____ syndrome.
   c. It can be caused by a particular tumor medulloblastoma
      called _____.
   d. Especially when it _____ the _____ of invades the floor of the fourth
      the _____ _____.   ventricle
   e. True or False. Nuclear facial palsy is due true
      to damage to the motor nucleus at the
      pontomedullary junction.

14. **True or False. Regarding CN VII anatomy:**   33.3.2
   a. Enters superior-anterior portion of IAC. true
   b. External genu is geniculate ganglion.   true
   c. GSPN is first branch after the ganglion. true
   d. Exits at stylomastoid foramen.   true

33

15. Complete the following about the seventh nerve: 33.3.2

a. It exits the brainstem at the _____ _____.   pontomedullary junction

b. It enters the IAC at the _____.   superoanterior portion

c. The geniculate ganglion is located in the _____ bone.   temporal

d. The first branch is the _____ _____ _____ _____,   greater superficial petrosal nerve

e. which goes to the _____ _____   pterygopalatine ganglion

f. and innervates the _____ _____ and _____ _____.   lacrimal gland and nasal muscosa– dry eye and nasal mucosa if injured

g. The next branch goes to the _____ _____.   stapedius muscle – to ear – hyperacusis

h. The next branch is the _____ _____.   chorda tympani – taste

i. It then exits the s_____ f_____   stylomastoid foramen

j. and sends branches to the _____.   face

16. Name the facial nerve branches within the temporal bone and their function.   33.3.2

a. g_____   greater superficial petrosal nerve (GSPN) to pterygopalatine ganglion, innervates nasal and palatine mucosa and lacrimal gland

b. s_____   branch to stapedius muscle, volume regulation

c. c_____   chorda tympani, taste sensation from anterior two thirds of the tongue

d. fibers to s_____ g_____   salivary glands, submandibular, sublingual

e. the nerve travels on to _____ _____   facial muscles

17. Name the facial nerve branches to the facial muscles cranial to caudal.   33.3.2

a. t_____   temporal

b. z_____   zygomatic

c. b_____   buccal

d. m_____   mandibular

e. c_____   cervical

18. Name the three most common causes of facial nerve palsy.   33.3.3

a. B_____   Bell's palsy

b. h_____   herpes zoster oticus

c. t_____   trauma/basal skull fracture

33

19. **Provide the differential diagnosis for facial nerve palsy.**

acoustic tumor
Bell's palsy
congenital
diabetes
fracture
Guillain-Barré
herpes zoster
Klippel-Feil
lyme disease
meningioma
neoplasm
otitis media
parotid surgery
sarcoid
trauma

33.3.3

20. **Describe seventh nerve palsy.**
    a. The most common cause of facial palsy is _____ _____.
    b. Etiology: _____
    c. Probable etiology: v_____ i_____
       d_____ p_____
    d. Usually proceeded by a _____ _____.
    e. It is caused by the _____ _____ virus.
    f. It progresses _____ to _____.
    g. Meaning
       i. first
       ii. then
       iii. and then
       iv. and then
    h. Percent that recover completely is ____%; partially _____%
    i. Manage with _____ and _____.
       S_____ d_____ is rarely used.
    j. If herpetic vesicles are present and VZV antibody titers rise, these patients are diagnosed with h_____ z_____ o_____ f_____ p_____ and there is a higher chance of f_____ n_____ d_____.

Bell's palsy

unknown
viral inflammatory
demyelinating polyneuritis
viral syndrome

herpes simplex

distally to proximally

facial movements weak
loss of taste and salivation
hyperacusis
decreased tearing
75 to 80%; 10%

EMG and steroids;
Surgical decompression
herpes zoster oticus facial
paralysis;
facial nerve degeneration

33.3.4

33.3.5

21. **What are the considerations for facial nerve injury surgical repair?**
    a. If known to be interrupted, _____ _____.
    b. Options for anastomosis include:
       i. h_____, which creates some t_____ morbidity
       ii. s_____ a_____, which sacrifices some s_____ m_____
    c. If known to be in continuity, _____.
    d. Role of electrical testing?

reanastomose early

hypoglossal; tongue

spinal accessory; shoulder
movement
several months of observation
serial electrical testing after 1
week

33.3.6

■ Hearing Loss

33

22. **Describe the following about hearing loss:**   33.4.1
    a. Conductive
        i.   patient speech   Normal or low volume voice
        ii. Rinne   Air < bone = negative (i.e. abnormal)
        iii. Weber lateralizes to _____ _____ side.   poor hearing
    b. Sensorineural   33.4.2
        i.   patient speech   loud voice
        ii. Rinne   Air > bone = positive (i.e. normal)
        iii. Weber lateralizes to _____ _____ side.   good hearing

34

General Information, Classification and Tumor Markers

■ Classification of Nervous System Tumors

1. **True or False. The following tumor is considered to be a World Health Organization (WHO) grade IV:**

   Table 34.2

   a. anaplastic astrocytoma — false, anaplastic astrocytoma is grade III

   b. gliosarcoma — true

   c. fibrillary astrocytoma — false, fibrillary astrocytoma is grade II

   d. subependymal giant cell astrocytoma — false, SEGA is grade II

2. **True or False. Tumors of mixed neuronal-glial origin include the following:**

   Table 34.2

   a. ganglioglioma — true

   b. central neurocytoma — true

   c. primitive neuroectodermal tumor (PNET) — false, PNET is listed under embryonal tumors

   d. desmoplastic infantile ganglioglioma (DIG) — true

   e. pineoblastoma — false, listed under pinealocyte tumor

3. **Complete the following about medulloblastoma:**

   Table 34.2

   a. Medulloblastoma is considered to be an _____ type of tumor. — embryonal

   b. It is also known as _____. — PNET

4. **Name the two types of craniopharyngiomas:**

   Table 34.2

   a. a_____ — adamantinomatous

   b. p_____ — papillary

5. **The following primary cancers commonly metastasize to the brain:**

   Table 34.2

   a. l_____ (especially s_____ c___) — lung, small cell

   b. b_____ — breast

   c. m_____ — melanoma

   d. r_____ c____ c_____ — renal cell carcinoma

   e. l_____ — lymphoma

   f. g_____ — gastrointestinal

■ Brain Tumors – General Clinical Aspects

6. List the four most common presentations of brain tumors and their frequency.

   34.2.1

   a. p_____ n_____ d_____: ___%

   b. h_____: ___%

   c. m_____ w_____: ___%

   d. s_____: ___%

   progressive neurologic deficit: 68%

   headache: 54%

   motor weakness: 45%

   seizure: 26%

7. When encountering a first-time seizure in a patient older than 20 years of age, think _____ until proven otherwise.

   tumor

   34.2.1

8. Describe the characteristic "syndromes" of the following:

   34.2.2

   a. Frontal lobe: a_____, d_____, p_____ changes

   abulia, dementia, personality changes

   b. Temporal lobe: a_____ or o_____ hallucinations, m_____ impairment, c_____ s_____ q_____

   auditory or olfactory; memory impairment, contralateral superior quadrantanopsia

   c. Parietal lobe: contralateral m_____ or s_____ impairment, h_____ h_____

   motor or sensory; homonymous hemianopsia

   d. Occipital lobe: contralateral v_____ f_____ deficits, a_____

   visual field deficits; alexia

9. What are 5 common etiologies of headache in the setting of an intracranial tumor?

   34.2.3

   1. Increased ICP due to mass effect or hydrocephalus
   2. Invasion of pain sensitive structures including dura, blood vessels, or periosteum
   3. Secondary to difficulty with vision
   4. Hypertension secondary to increased ICP
   5. Psychogenic due to stress from loss of functional capacity

10. Complete the following concerning a > 20-year-old patient presenting with a headache:

    34.2.3

    a. The classical headache associated with a brain tumor is characterized by:

    i. worsening in the _____ (A.M. vs. P.M.)

    AM

    ii. _____ (Increased vs. Decreased) with cough

    increased

    iii. _____ (Increased vs. Decreased) with bending forward

    increased

    iv. associated with n_____ and/or v_____

    nausea; vomiting

b. What percentage of patients have these "classic" headaches?

8% (77% had headache similar to tension headache, 9% were similar to migraine, only 8% showed classic brain tumor headache; two thirds of these had high ICP)

11. The _____ _____ is the so-called vomiting center.

area postrema

34.2.5

12. Cranial nerve ___ has the longest intracranial course.

CN VI (abducens nerve)

34.2.5

13. Match the area of cerebellum/brainstem with symptoms
① cerebeller hemisphere; ② vermis;
③ brainstem
Symptoms: (a-g) below

34.2.5

a. ataxia of extremities   ①
b. broad-based gait   ②
c. truncal ataxia   ②
d. dysmetria   ①
e. intention tremor   ①
f. nystagmus   ③
g. cranial nerve dysfunction   ③

14. What are the pros and cons of placing a shunt or external ventricular drain (EVD) into a pediatric patient with a posterior fossa tumor and hydrocephalus?

34.2.5

a. Pros:
   i. may possibly lower o_____
     m_____   operative mortality
b. Cons:
   i. l___-____ shunt   life-long
   ii. s_____ of peritoneum   seeding
   iii. u____ _____ herniation   upward transtentorial
   iv. i_____ of shunt   infection
   v. d_____ in definitive treatment   delay

■ Pediatric Brain Tumors

15. Common pediatric brain tumors include:

34.3.2

a. g_____   gliomas
b. p_____ tumors   pineal tumors
c. c_____   craniopharyngiomas
d. t_____   teratomas
e. g_____   granulomas
f. P_____ tumors including   PNET;
   m_____   medulloblastoma

34

16. **Complete the following about infra-**   Table 34.3
    vs. supra-tentorial pediatric tumors:
    a. Age vs. % Infratentorial:
        i.   0-6 mos: _____%   27%
        ii. 6-12 mos: _____%   53%
        iii. 12-24 mos: ___%   74%
        iv. 2-16 years: ___%   42%
    b. _____ are the most common   Astrocytomas   34.3.3
        supratentorial tumor in pediatrics as a
        whole.
    c. True or False?   34.3.1
        i.   Brain tumors are the second most   true
             common cancer in childhood.
        ii. They are the most common solid   true
             tumors in childhood.
    d. In neonates, 90% of brain tumors are of neuroectodermal;   34.3.4
        n_____ origin with _____   teratomas
        being the most common.

17. **Common presentations for pediatric**   34.3.4
    tumors include:
    a. v_____   vomiting
    b. a_____ of d_____   arrest of development
    c. f_____ to t_____   failure to thrive
    d. s_____   seizures

■ Medications for Brain Tumors

18. **The beneficial effects of steroids are**   metastatic tumors   34.4.1
    greater for _____ (metastatic vs.
    primary) tumors.

19. **In terms of prophylactic**   34.4.2
    anticonvulsants with brain tumors:
    a. There is Level ____ evidence that AEDs   Level I;
        _____ (should/should not) be used should not
        routinely in patients with newly
        diagnosed brain tumors.
    b. There is Level ____ evidence that in   Level II;
        patients undergoing craniotomy for a   can
        brain tumors, prophylactic AEDs
        _____ (can or cannot) be used.

■ Chemotherapy for Brain Tumors

20. **Match the chemotherapeutic agent with its mechanism of action:**
① DNA crosslinking; ② DNA alkylation; ③ Microtubule function inhibitor; ④ Topoisomerase II inhibitor; ⑤ Topoisomerase I inhibitor; ⑥ PKC inhibitor; ⑦ Anti-VEGF antibody

Table 34.5

a. Bevacizumab: _____   ⑦
b. Vincristine: _____   ③
c. Irinotecan (CPT-11): _____   ⑤
d. Temozolomide: _____   ②
e. BCNU: _____   ①

21. **Complete the following about Temozolomide:**

34.5.2

a. It is an _____ (oral vs. IV) medication that works through DNA _____.   oral; alkylation
b. It functions as a p_____ and undergoes rapid non-enzymatic conversion at physiologic pH to _____.   prodrug; MITC (monomethyltriazenoimidazo lecarboxamide)
c. MITC alkylation occurs primarily at the __ and ___ positions on _____ but some tumors can repair this damage with _____ that is coded by the _____ gene.   O6; N7; guanine; AGT; MGMT

22. **The following are tactics that can be used to circumvent the blood-brain barrier (BBB):**

34.5.4

a. l_____ agent   lipophilic agent
b. h___ d_____   higher doses (of medication)
c. d_____ of BBB   disruption of BBB (e.g. with mannitol)
d. b_____ BBB   bypass BBB (e.g. intrathecal methotrexate for primary lymphoma)
e. d_____ i_____ polymers   directly implantable polymers

23. **Complete the following about tumor imaging:**

34.5.5

a. The proper time to obtain post-op imaging to check for bleeding is typically within __ - __ hours.   6-12 hours
b. The proper time to obtain post-op imaging to check for residual tumor is either within __ - __ days or after about ___ days.   2-3 days; 30 days
c. An exception to this timing rule of thumb is for _____ tumors.   pituitary

34

■ Select Commonly Utilized Stains in Neuropathology

24. True or False. This tumor marker usually indicates astroglial origin.   34.7.2, 34.7.3

a. glial fibrillary acid protein (GFAP)   true (GFAP is rarely found outside the CNS. Thus, the presence of GFAP in a tumor found in the CNS is usually taken as good evidence for glial origin of the tumor)

b. S-100 protein   false

c. cytokeratin   false

d. neuron specific enolase (NSE)   false

e. human chorionic gonadotropin (hCG)   false

25. True or False. This tumor marker may be helpful in differentiating metastatic tumor from primary CNS tumors.   34.7.2, 34.7.3

a. GFAP   true (Indicates astroglial origin; unusual for metastatic lesion to stain positive)

b. S-100 protein   true (Associated with metastatic melanomas)

c. cytokeratin   true (Associated with metastatic tumors as it stains epithelial cells)

d. NSE   true (Associated with metastatic small cell lung cancer)

e. hCG   true (Associated with cerebral metastases from uterine or testicular choriocarcinoma)

f. α-fetoprotein   true (Associated with cancers of ovary, stomach, lung, colon, and pancreas)

g. carcinoembryonic antigen (CEA)   true

h. CSF-CEA   true (Associated with leptomeningeal spread of several cancer types)

26. Complete the following about tumor marker MIB-I: 34.7.2

a. Detects _____ antigen.   Ki-67

b. A high number indicates m_____ a_____.   mitotic activity

c. It correlates with degree of m_____.   malignancy

d. It is used for a_____, m_____, l_____, and e_____ tumors   astrocytomas, meningiomas, lymphomas, and endocrine tumors

27. **β-hCG is elevated in the following tumors:**   34.7.3
    a. metastatic u_____ or t_____   uterine, testicular
       choriocarcinoma
    b. primary c_____ or e_____   choriocarcinoma, embryonal
       c_____ c_____ of pineal or suprasellar   cell carcinoma
       region

28. **The tumor marker _____ may rise**   S-100   34.7.3
    after head trauma and may be
    elevated in Creutzfeldt-Jakob disease.

34

35

Syndromes Involving Tumors

■ Neurocutaneous Tumors

1. **Most neurocutaneous disorders demonstrate an _____ _____ inheritance pattern.**

   autosomal dominant

   35.1.1

2. **True or False. The following are neurocutaneous disorders:**

   35.1.1

   a. Sturge-Weber syndrome — true
   b. Neurofibromatosis — true
   c. Tuberous sclerosis — true
   d. Von Hippel-Lindau disease — true
   e. Foix-Alajouanine syndrome — false (Foix-Alajouanine syndrome, acute or subacute neurologic deterioration in a patient with a spinal arteriovenous malformation without evidence of hemorrhage)

3. **Schwannomas tend to _____ nerve fibers whereas neurofibromas tend to _____ a nerve of origin.**

   displace; encapsulate

   35.1.2

4. **True or False. The following is correct about differences between NF-1 and NF-2:**

   Table 35.1

   a. Alternate name for NF-1 is von Recklinghausen's syndrome. — true
   b. NF-2 has a greater incidence and prevalence than NF-1. — false (NF-1 represents >90% of cases of neurofibromatosis)
   c. The inheritance pattern of both NF-1 and NF-2 is autosomal dominant. — true
   d. Bilateral vestibular schwannomas are commonly seen in NF-2 but not NF-1. — true
   e. Lisch nodules are associated with NF-2. — false (associated with NF-1)
   f. Skeletal anomalies are common with NF-1. — true
   g. Cataracts are common with NF-2. — true

h. Gene product of NF-2 is neurofibromin.

false (NF-1 gene product is neurofibromin, NF-2 gene product is schwannomin (merlin).)

i. An increased frequency of malignant tumors are seen in both NF-1 and NF-2.

true

5. Diagnostic criteria for NF-1 include 2 or more of the following:

Table 35.2

a. six or more c___ a_ l___ spots

café au lait

b. p_____ n_____

peripheral neurofibromatosis

c. h_____ in the axillary or inguinal areas

hyperpigmentation

d. o_____ g_____

optic gliomas

e. Two or more L_____ n_____

Lisch nodules

f. Distinctive o_____ abnormality

osseous (e.g. sphenoid dysplasia)

g. __ first degree relative with NF-1

One

6. Complete the following about genetics of NF-1:

35.1.2

a. generally _____ _____ inheritance pattern

autosomal dominant

b. __ - __% of cases are due to new somatic mutations.

30-50%

c. After age 5, it has _____% penetrance.

100%

d. It is on chromosome _____.

17q11.2

e. Gene product is _____.

neurofibromin

7. Diagnostic criteria for NF-2 include:

Table 35.3

a. Definite diagnosis if b_____ v_____ s_____ on imaging

bilateral vestibular schwannomas

b. Definite diagnosis if first degree relative with NF-2 AND either u_____ v_____ s_____ at age less than ____ or any two of the following:

unilateral vestibular schwannoma; 30

   i. m_____

meningioma

   ii. s_____

schwannoma

   iii. g_____

glioma

   iv. p_____ s_____ l__ o_____

posterior subcapsular lens opacity

8. What are clinical features of NF-2?

35.1.2

a. multiple i_____ s_____ t_____ are common

intradural spinal tumors

b. Most NF-2 patients will become _____.

deaf

c. R_____ h_____

retinal hamartomas

d. Pregnancy may _____ the growth of eight nerve tumors.

accelerate

35

9. **Complete the following about genetics of NF-2:**   35.1.2
   a. Generally _____ _____   autosomal dominant
      inheritance pattern
   b. It is on chromosome _____.   22q12.2
   c. Mutation leads to inactivation of   schwannomin (merlin), a
      _____.   tumor suppression peptide

10. **List the key clinical features of tuberous sclerosis:**   35.1.3
    a. s_____   seizures
    b. a_____ s_____   adenoma sebaceum
    c. m_____ r_____   mental retardation
    d. This triad is seen in less than _____ of   1/3
       cases.

11. **Complete the following about tuberous sclerosis:**   35.1.3
    a. Typical CNS finding: s_____   subependymal nodules
       n_____
    b. Common associated neoplasm is a   giant cell astrocytoma
       g_____ c___ a_____.
    c. CT shows i_____ c_____.   intracerebral calcifications

12. **Complete the following about genetics of tuberous sclerosis complex:**   35.1.3
    a. The majority of cases are due to   spontaneous mutation
       s_____ m_____.
    b. The two distinct tumor suppressor genes   TSC1;
       that may be involved are _____ which   hamartin;
       codes for h_____ and _____   TSC2;
       which codes for t_____.   tuberlin
    c. If one affected child, __ - __% chance of   1-2%
       recurrence.

13. **Complete the following about the major diagnostic criteria for tuberous sclerosis:**   35.1.3
    a. Cutaneous manifestations:
       i.   f_____ a_____   facial angiofibroma
       ii. u_____ f_____   ungual fibroma
       iii. >3 h_____ m_____   hypomelanotic macules
       iv. s_____ p _____   shagreen patch
    b. Brain and eye lesions:
       i.   c_____ t_____   cortical tubers
       ii. s_____ n_____   subependymal nodules
       iii. s_____ g____ c___ a_____ subependymal giant cell
                                            astrocytoma
       iv. r_____ n_____ h_____ retinal nodular hamartomas
    c. Tumors in other organs:
       i.   c_____   cardiac
       ii. r_____   rhabdomyoma
       iii. l_____   lymphangioleiomyomatosis
       iv. r_____ _____   renal angiomyolipoma

14. Complete the following about tuberous sclerosis: 35.1.3

a. In infants, the earliest findings are a____ l_____ m_____ which can be observed with a w____ l_____ examination.   ash leaf macules; wood's lamp

b. M_____ found in children is often replaced by s_____ in adults.   Myoclonus; seizures

c. F_____ a_____ appear by 4 years.   Facial adenomas

d. R_____ h_____ are present in 50% of patients.   Retinal hamartomas

e. CT demonstrates c_____ in 97% of cases along l_____ v_____ or near f_____ of M_____.   calcifications; lateral ventricles; foramina of Monro

f. Enhancing subependymal lesions on MRI are usually g_____ c_____ a_____.   giant cell astrocytomas

15. List the key features of Sturge-Weber syndrome.   35.1.4

a. a_____   atrophy: localized cerebral cortical atrophy and calcification

b. b____ m____   birth mark: ipsilateral port-wine facial nevus (usually in distribution of trigeminal nerve)

c. c_____   calcification: plain skull films classically show "tram tracking"

16. Complete the following about neurocutaneous melanosis: 35.1.5

a. Presence of benign or malignant m_____ t_____ of the l_____.   melanocytic tumors of the leptomeninges

b. Sometimes associated with S_____-W_____ syndrome and n_____.   Sturge-Weber syndrome; neurofibromatosis 1

c. >__% of patients die within 3 years after first neurologic manifestation.   >50%

■ Familial Tumor Syndromes

17. Match the familial syndrome and associated CNS tumor: Table 35.5
① von Hippel-Lindau; ② Tuberous sclerosis; ③ NF-1; ④ NF-2; ⑤ Turcot syndrome; ⑥ Li-Fraumeni; ⑦ Cowden

a. Hemangioblastoma   ①

b. Bilateral vestibular schwannomas   ④

c. Colorectal neoplasms and neuroepithelial tumors of the CNS (e.g. medulloblastoma, pineoblastoma)   ⑤

d. Subependymal giant cell astrocytoma   ②

e. Optic glioma   ③

35

36

Astrocytomas

■ Classification and Grading of Astrocytic Tumors

1. For the following astrocytomas, the respective WHO grading are:

a. Anaplastic astrocytoma: _____   WHO III

b. Glioblastoma: ____   WHO IV

c. Diffuse astrocytoma: ____   WHO II

d. Juvenile pilocytic astrocytoma: _____   WHO I

e. Subependymal giant cell astrocytoma: WHO I

    ____

f. Pilomyxoid astrocytoma: ____   WHO II

g. Gliosarcoma: ___   WHO IV

36.2.1

2. Complete the following about astrocytoma:

a. grade I

   i. frequency _____%   0.7%   *36.2.2*

   ii. median survival _____ years   8-10   *Table 36.10*

b. grade II

   i. frequency _____%   16%   *36.2.2*

   ii. median survival _____ years   7-8   *Table 36.10*

c. grade III

   i. frequency _____%   17%   *36.2.2*

   ii. median survival _____ years   2-3   *Table 36.10*

d. grade IV

   i. frequency _____%   65%   *36.2.2*

   ii. median survival _____ year   <1   *Table 36.10*

3. Complete the following on low-grade astrocytomas:

a. Y_____ a____ is a favorable prognosticator.   Young age

b. Mean time to dedifferentiation for patients diagnosed <45 years is about ___ months whereas for patients diagnosed ≥45 years it is about ___.   44.2 months; 7.5 months

c. Once dedifferentiation occurs, median survival is __ - __ years after.   2-3 years

36.2.2

4. **Histologic features of GBM include:** 36.2.2

a. c_____   cellular
b. g_____ a_____   gemistocytic astrocytes
c. m_____   mitosis
d. p_____   pleomorphism
e. n_____   neovascularization
f. areas of n_____   necrosis
g. p_____   pseudopalisading

■ Molecular Genetics and Epigenetics

36

5. **What are three major genetic** 36.3.1
   pathways in the development of GBM?

a. Inactivation of the _____ and _____ tumor   p53; Rb
   suppressor pathways.
b. Activation of P_____, A_____, and   PI3K, AKT; mTOR
   m_____, an intracellular signaling
   pathway.
c. Amplification and mutational activation   EGF, VEGF, and PDGF
   of RTK genes including _____, _____,
   and _____.

6. **In terms of the genetics underlying**
   GBMs:

a. Loss of _____ expression makes   MGMT; temozolomide   36.3.2
   alkylating agents such as t_____
   more effective.
b. Mutant IDH1 and IDH2 demonstrate the α-KG; 2-hydroxyglutarate   36.3.3
   capacity to convert _____ into
   _____.
c. These mutations are associated with   lower-grade,
   l_____-g_____, o_____,   oligodendrogliomas, and
   and s_____ g_____ with   secondary gliomas
   better overall survival than glioblastomas
   that are wild type for both genes.

7. **True or False. The following are** 36.3.4
   associated with secondary
   glioblastomas rather than primary
   glioblastomas:

a. EGFR amplification   false, associated with primary
     GBMs
b. TP53 mutations   true, seen in 60% of
     secondary GBMs
c. IDH1/IDH2 mutations   true, seen in the majority of
     secondary gliomas
d. PTEN mutations   false, more associated with
     primary GBMs

8. **The four subclassifications of GBM** 36.3.5
   based on gene expression analysis are:

a. I - _____   Classical
b. II - _____   Mesenchymal
c. III - _____   Proneural
d. IV - _____   Neural

36

■ Neuroradiological Grading and Findings. Spread. Multiple Gliomas

9. **Describe the following features of low-grade gliomas on imaging:**   36.5
    a. Usually are _____(hypo vs. hyper dense) on CT.   hypodense
    b. Most are _____ (hypo vs. hyper intense) on T1WI MRI but _____ (hypo vs. hyper intense) on T2WI.   hypointense; hyperintense
    c. Most _____ (do vs. do not) enhance on CT or MRI.   do not
    d. Low-grade astrocytomas usually appear as _____ (hypo vs. hyper metabolic) areas on fluorodeoxyglucose PET scans.   hypometabolic

10. **Describe the following features of high-grade malignant gliomas:**
    a. About ____% of highly anaplastic astrocytomas do not enhance on CT.   31%   36.5
    b. The non-enhancing center of ring enhancement seen with GBM represents _____ while the rim is c_____ t_____.   necrosis; cellular tumor
    c. Gliomas can spread by the following mechanisms: T_____ through w_____ m_____ or spread through the C_____ p_____.   Track through white matter; CSF pathway   36.6
    d. G_____ c_____ is used to describe a diffuse, infiltrating astrocytoma that invades almost all of the cerebral hemispheres.   Gliomatosis cerebri   36.7
    e. Meningeal gliomatosis occurs in ___% of high-grade gliomas at autopsy.   20%

■ Treatment

11. **Describe what should prompt consideration for surgical resection of a low-grade astrocytoma:**   36.8.1
    a. e_____ a d_____   establish a diagnosis
    b. presence of p_____ a_____   pilocytic astrocytoma
    c. evidence of h_____   herniation
    d. evidence of o_____ C___ f_____   obstructed CSF flow
    e. prevention of m_____ t_____   malignant transformation

12. **The standard of care for treatment of high-grade gliomas includes c_____ s_____ followed by e_____ b_____ r_____ and t_____. Median survival with this regimen is ____ months.**

cytoreductive surgery; external beam radiation (60 Gy); temozolomide; 14.6 months

36.8.2

13. **Use of 5-ALA for tumor resection leads to _____ (less/equal/more) resection which translates into _____ (decreased/increased/no effect on) 6-month progression free survival and _____ (decreased/increased/no effect on) on overall survival.**

more; increased; no effect on

36.8.2

14. **Complete the following regarding stereotactic biopsy:**

36.8.2

a. It underestimates the occurrence of GBM by _____%. 25%

b. Some CNS _____ mimic GBM radiographically. lymphomas

c. Yield of biopsy is highest when the following are sampled:

i. low density _____ center

ii. enhancing_____ rim

d. If Karnofsky rating is higher than _____. 70

15. **Complete the following about radiation therapy for malignant gliomas:**

36.8.4

a. ___ - __Gy 50-60 Gy

b. Is whole brain x-ray treatment (XRT) valuable? No, it does not increase survival

16. **Complete the following about pseudoprogression:**

36.8.3

a. Occurs in up to __ - __% of patients after XRT and temozolomide. 28-60%

b. Typically seen ≤__ months after treatment. 3 months

c. Histologically resembles r_____ n_____. radiation necrosis

17. **Complete the following about recurrent GBM:**

36.8.4

a. B_____ is approved for progressive GBM following prior treatment. Bevacizumab

b. S_____ is the mainstay of treatment and is usually recommended on for patients with KPS ≥ ___. Surgery; 70

■ Outcome

18. **The following are prognostic indicators for malignant astrocytomas:**   36.9

    a. a____   age, found to be the most
                                                 significant prognosticator
    b. h_____ features   histological features
    c. p_____ s_____   performance status
    d. M____ m_____ status   MGMT methylation status

19. **How does MGMT methylation status affect median overall survival in malignant gliomas?**   Unmethylated – median OS 12.2 months; Methylated – median OS 18.2 months   36.9

36

37

Other Astrocytic Tumors

■ Pilocytic Astrocytomas

1. Pilocytic astrocytomas can be found in the following locations: 37.1.2
- a. o_____ n_____   optic nerve
- b. h_____   hypothamus
- c. c_____ h_____   cerebral hemispheres
- d. b_____   brainstem
- e. c_____   cerebellum
- f. s_____ c_____   spinal cord

2. Characteristic histologic findings in pilocytic astrocytomas are 37.1.3
- a. R_____ f_____   Rosenthal fibers
- b. f_____ cells   fibrillated cells
- c. m_____   microcysts
- d. e_____ g_____ b_____   eosinophilic granular bodies
- e. typically grossly w___-d_____   well-demarcated

3. Complete the following about the radiographic appearance of PCAs: 37.1.4
- a. Over 66% are c_____ with m_____ n_____.   cystic with mural nodules
- b. ____% enhance with contrast.   94%
- c. ___% are periventricular.   82%
- d. Are these tumors typically surrounded by edema?   no
- e. Cyst wall enhancement indicates _____.   tumor

4. Pilocytic astrocytomas typically occur within the ____ decade of life.   2nd (75% occur before age 20) 37.1.5

5. Complete the following about the treatment of PCAs: 37.1.5
- a. The main treatment of PCAs is _____.   surgery
- b. In tumors composed of a nodule with a true cyst, excision of the _____ is sufficient   nodule
- c. If the cyst wall enhances, it _____ (should vs. should not) be removed.   should
- d. Generally, radiation therapy _____ (is vs. is not) recommended as an additional treatment.   is not

37

6. **According to Collins' law, a patient's tumor is considered cured if it does not recur after a post-op period equal to the patient's _____ plus _____.**

age; 9 months

37.1.6

7. **Complete the following about optic gliomas:**

37.1.7

   a. Gliomas in both optic nerves are usually only seen in _____.

   neurofibromatosis

   b. Often occur in conjunction with a _____ glioma.

   hypothalamic

   c. P_____ p_____ is an early sign of an optic nerve tumor, whereas a tumor of the chiasm may cause p_____ d_____ or h_____.

   Painless proptosis; pituitary dysfunction; hydrocephalus

8. **Complete the following about the treatments for optic gliomas:**

37.1.7

   a. If the tumor involves a single optic nerve, spares the chiasm, and produces proptosis as well as visual loss, then _____ of the ____ _____ should be performed.

   excision of the optic nerve (from globe back to the chiasm)

   b. More posterior lesions with nonspecific visual defects and no proptosis, hypothalamic dysfunction, pituitary dysfunction, or hydrocephalus, it is likely a _____ _____. This usually undergoes b_____ and _____.

   chiasmal lesion; biopsy; XRT

9. **Describe the features of diencephalic syndrome:**

37.1.8

   a. c_____

   cachexia

   b. h_____

   hyperactivity

   c. o_____-a_____

   over-alertness

   d. e_____

   euphoria

   e. f_____ __ t_____

   failure to thrive

   f. h_____

   hypoglycemia

   g. m_____

   macrocephaly

   h. Is usually associated with glioma in _____ _____.

   anterior hypothalamus

   i. Usually affects _____.

   children

10. **Characterize brainstem gliomas:**

37.1.10

   a. Lower-grade tumors tend to occur in the _____ brainstem.

   upper

   b. Higher-grade tumors tend to occur in the _____ brainstem.

   lower

   c. Can present with multiple _____ _____ _____.

   cranial nerve palsies

   d. Most _____ (are vs. are not) surgical candidates.

   are not

11. **Upper brainstem gliomas present with:**   37.1.10
  a. _____ signs   cerebellar
  b. _____   hydrocephalus

12. **Lower brainstem gliomas present with**   37.1.10
  a. l_____ c_____ n____ deficits   lower cranial nerve
  b. l_____ t_____ signs   long tract

13. **Characterize four MRI growth patterns of brainstem gliomas:** 37.1.10
  a. Diffuse
     i.   Location: _____, _____, _____ _____   pons, medulla, spinal cord
     ii. Grade (high vs low): _____   high (100%)
     iii. Surgical Resection? _____   no
  b. Cervicomedullary
     i.   Location: _____   cervicomedullary
     ii. Grade (high vs low): _____   low (72% are low-grade astrocytomas)
     iii. Surgical Resection? _____   yes if exophitic
  c. Focal
     i.   Location: _____   medulla
     ii. Grade (high vs low): _____   low (66% are low-grade astrocytomas)
     iii. Surgical Resection? _____   yes if exophitic
  d. Dorsally Exophytic
     i.   Location: _____, _____ _____   medulla, spinal cord
     ii. Grade (high vs low): _____   low (60% are low-grade astrocytomas)
     iii. Surgical Resection? _____   yes if accessible

14. **On MRI, brainstem gliomas appear:**   37.1.10
  a. T1: _____, _____   hypointense, homogeneous
  b. T2: _____, _____   hyperintense, homogeneous
  c. Enhancement? _____ _____   highly variable

15. **Surgery may be indicated in the treatment of brainstem gliomas in the following circumstances:**   37.1.10
  a. tumors with _____ _____ component   dorsally exophytic
  b. some success with resecting ___-_____ astrocytomas   non-malignant
  c. if s_____ needed for h_____   shunting; hydrocephalus

16. **Complete the following about the prognosis of brainstem gliomas:**   37.1.10
  a. Prognosis of most patients is __ - __ months.   6 to 12 months
  b. Subgroup of dorsally exophytic pilocytic astrocytomas have a longer survival of up to _____ years.   5 years

37

17. **These neurological findings are possible with a tectal glioma:**   37.1.11

a. P_____ s_____   Parinaud's syndrome
b. a_____   ataxia
c. n_____   nystagmus
d. d_____   diplopia
e. s_____   seizures
f. More commonly presents with signs of   hydrocephalus
_____.

18. **Characterize tectal gliomas:**   37.1.11

a. Present primarily in _____ with a   childhood; 6-14 years
median age of symptom onset of __ - __
years.
b. Pathology is usually ___-_____ _____.   low-grade glioma (diffuse
astrocytoma, pilocytic
astrocytoma, ependymoma,
etc)
c. Diagnostic study of choice is _____.   MRI
d. Symptoms resolve with treatment of the   hydrocephalus
_____.

e. MRI appearance
  i.   mass arising from the q_____   quadrigeminal plate
  _____
  ii. on T1: _____   isointense
  iii. on T2: _____   iso- or hyperintense
  iv. with gadolinium: _____% enhance   18%

19. **Complete the following about the treatment of tectal gliomas:**   37.1.11

a. A _____-_____ _____ may lead to good   ventriculo-peritoneal shunt
long-term symptom control.
b. An alternative is _____ _____.   endoscopic third
ventriculostomy

■ Pleomorphic Xanthoastrocytoma (PXA)

20. **Complete the following about pleomorphic xanthoastrocytomas:**

a. Grade (low vs. high): _____   low (typically WHO II)   37.2.1
b. Location: >90% _____ (supra- vs.   supratentorial;
infratentorial) and typically s_____.   superficial;
Meninges involved in >__% of cases.   67%
c. Most have a _____ component.   cystic
d. Treatment: _____, _____ or _____   surgery (maximal safe
usually only considered for grade III.   resection), XRT or chemo
e. 5-year survival with gross or subtotal   80%   37.2.8
resection, with or without radiation and
chemo is ___%.

37

38

Oligodendroglial Tumors and Tumors of the Ependyma, Choroid Plexus, and Other Neuroepithelial Tumors

---

■ Oligodendroglial Tumors

1. Characterize oligodendrogliomas (ODGs).

a.	Frequent presenting symptom is _____ in __ - __%.	seizure; 50-80%
b.	>__% are _____ (supra- vs. infratentorial).	>90%; supratentorial
c.	They have a predilection for which part of the CNS?	frontal lobe
d.	Calcified on __ - __% of skull x-rays and __% of CT scan.	30-60%; 90%
e.	Oligodendroglioma cells in a tumor suggest what sort of prognosis for the patient?	a better prognosis

Reference column:
- a. 38.1.3
- b. Table 38.1
- c. 38.1.1
- d. 38.1.4

2. Complete the following about the histologic findings of oligodendrogliomas (ODGs): — 38.1.5

a.	The classic description of the cytoplasm of ODG cells is a ____ ____ appearance.	fried egg appearance (perinuclear halos)
b.	A "_____ _____" characteristic vascular pattern can be seen.	"chicken-wire"
c.	The above (a & b) are felt to be unreliable findings. What are more consistent findings?	cells with monotonous round nuclei with an eccentric rim of eosinophilic cytoplasm lacking obvious cell processes

3. Which of the following features are associated with low-grade vs. high-grade oligodendrogliomas? (e.g. WHO II (low-grade) vs. WHO III (high-grade)) — Table 38.3

a.	Contrast enhancement: _____	WHO III
b.	Absence of astrocytic component: _____	WHO II

38

c. Endothelial proliferation on histology: _____ — WHO III

d. Large variability in nuclear and cytoplasmic size and shape: _____ — WHO III

4. Complete the following about the treatment of oligodendrogliomas: 38.1.6

a. Following surgical resection, what general adjuvant therapy is preferred in the treatment of these lesions? — chemotherapy

b. P_____, C_____, v_____, and t_____ are chemotherapy agents used for oligodendrogliomas. — PCV (procarbazine, CCNU, vincristine) and temozolomide

c. Indications for surgery include:
    i. Tumors with significant m_____ e_____ regardless of grade. — mass effect
    ii. If ____-grade, surgery is recommended for _____ lesions but not at the expense of neurological functions. — low; accessible
    iii. Benefit of surgery less clear with ____-grade tumors — high

5. Arrange the following from best to worst prognosis: 38.1.7

a. mixed oligodendroglioma
b. pure astrocytoma
c. pure oligodendroglioma
— c, a, b

6. Complete the following about the prognosis of oligodendrogliomas (ODGs):   38.1.7

a. Chromosomal 1p/19q loss is associated with _____ (shorter vs. longer) survival. — longer

b. What is the 10-year survival of tumors that are predominantly ODGs? — 10-30%

c. Post-op median survival is __ months. — 35

d. Calcification is thought to convey a _____ (better vs. worse) prognosis. — better

■ Ependymal Tumors

7. Complete the following about ependymomas: 38.3.1

a. Arise along the v_____ and c_____ c____ of the s_____ c____. — ventricles, central canal, spinal cord

b. 69% of ependymomas occur in _____ (adults vs. children). — children

c. Account for __% of spinal cord gliomas — 60% (most common primary intramedullary spinal cord glioma below the mid-thoracic region)

d. In adults, tend to be _____. In   intraspinal, posterior fossa
    children, frequently found in the
    _____ _____.

e. Have the potential to spread via _____   CSF;
    forming "_____ _____"   "drop mets"

8. **Complete the following about**   38.3.1
    histological findings in ependymomas:
a. WHO II grade variants include c_____,   cellular, papillary ("classic
    p_____, c_____ c_____, and   lesion"), clear cell; tanycytic
    t_____.
b. Myxopapillary ependymomas are WHO   WHO I
    grade ___.
c. Subependymomas are WHO grade ___.   WHO I
d. Anaplastic ependymomas are WHO   WHO III
    grade ___.
e. The m_____ subtype occurs in the   myxopapillary
    filum terminale.

9. **Complete the following about**   38.3.1
    ependymomas:
a. Incidence among intracranial tumors in   5-6%
    adults is __ - __%.
b. Incidence among pediatric brain tumors   9%
    is __%.
c. It occurs in children __% of the time.   70%
d. Incidence among spinal cord gliomas is   60%
    __%.
e. Drop metastases occur in __% of   11%
    patients.

10. **When evaluating a patient with an**   38.3.1
    intracranial ependymoma:
a. Which parts of the neuraxis should be   usually MRI of the brain as
    imaged?   well as cervical, thoracic, and
                                                   lumbar spine to check for
                                                   potential seeding
b. An alternative to MRI for detecting drop   myelography (with water-
    mets is _____.   soluble contrast)
c. Commonly occur in the floor of the   fourth ventricle;
    _____ _____ so may present with   hydrocephalus; CN VI
    h_____ as well as cranial nerve ___   (involvement of nucleus) & VII
    and ____ palsies.   (involvement of genu)

11. **Complete the following about the**   38.3.1
    treatment of ependymomas:
a. 2 weeks post-op, should perform a ____   lumbar puncture; drop mets
    _____ to look for _____ _____.
b. Ependymomas _____ (are vs. are   are (rank 2nd only to
    not) radiosensitive.   medulloblastomas in
                                                   radiosensitivity)
c. Role of chemo is _____ (important vs.   limited
    limited) in the treatment of these
    lesions.

d. With surgery and _____, 5-year survival is estimated at ___ - ___% in adults. But in pediatric group, 5-year survival is estimated at ___ - ___%.

XRT; 40-80% (adults); 20-30% (pediatrics)

e. Difficult to surgically resect because they can invade the _____.

obex

f. Current operative mortality estimated at __ - __%

5-8%

g. Is mortality higher in adults or in children?

children

12. **If CSF after ependymoma resection demonstrates positive cytology, what should be done?**

Usually provide low dose XRT to entire spinal axis with an increased dose to any visible drop mets.

38.3.1

13. **True or False. Regarding medulloblastomas and ependymomas:**

38.3.1

a. Although uncommon in medulloblastomas, calcifications may be seen ~20% of the time.

false (<10%)

b. The "banana sign" in the fourth ventricle refers to medulloblastomas rather than to ependymomas.

true

c. Ependymomas rank second only to medulloblastomas in radiosensitivity.

true

d. Medulloblastomas arise from the roof of the fourth ventricle, the fastigium.

true

e. Ependymomas arise from the floor of the fourth ventricle, the obex.

true

f. Ependymomas are the most common glioma of the spinal cord below the midthoracic region

true

■ Neuronal and Mixed Glial Tumors

14. **Complete the following about central neurocytomas:**

38.4.2

a. Grade: _____

WHO grade II

b. Location: usually within the _____ _____ attached to s_____ p_____ or within the _____ _____.

lateral ventricles; septum pellucidum; third ventricle

c. Histologically, can mimic oligodendrogliomas as cells may have a "_____ ____" appearance.

"fried egg"

d. Imaging findings:

  i.   On CT, 25-50% show _____.

calcifications

  ii. MRI T1: _____

isointense

  iii. MRI T2: _____

hyperintense

  iv. Enhancement? _____

yes

e. Surgery _____ (is vs. is not) potentially curative.

is

15. **Complete the following about dysembryoplastic neuroepithelial tumors (DNET):**   38.4.4
   a. Most common locations are the _____ and _____ lobes.   frontal; temporal
   b. Grade: _____   WHO Grade I
   c. Age: Usually presents in _____ or _____ _____ with s_____.   children; young adults; seizures
   d. Imaging findings:
      i. Edema?   typically no surrounding edema
      ii. On CT: _____   hypodense
      iii. MRI T1: _____   hypointense
      iv. MRI T2: _____   hyperintense
      v. PET: _____   hypometabolic (with 18-FDG and negative 11C-methionine uptake)
   e. What therapy is recommended for this tumor type?   Surgical resection – adjuvant therapies with XRT or chemo do not benefit these patients.

16. **Lhermitte-Duclos disease is a g_____ of the c_____.**   gangliocytoma of the cerebellum   38.4.5

38

■ Choroid Plexus Tumors

17. **True or False. Regarding choroid plexus tumors:**
   a. The majority of choroid plexus tumors occur in patients less than 2 years old.   true   38.5.2
   b. Choroid plexus tumors do not grow rapidly.   false (they may grow rapidly)   38.5.1
   c. They do not produce drop mets.   false, they can produce drop mets (WHO III grade do so more commonly)
   d. They are usually located infratentorially in adults.   true   38.5.2
   e. They are usually located infratentorially in children.   false, usually supratentorially
   f. Hydrocephalus with choroid plexus tumors may result from overproduction of CSF although tumor removal does not always cure the problem.   true   38.5.3

18. **Imaging findings associated with choroid plexus tumors include:**   38.5.4
   a. Location: _____   intraventricular
   b. Enhancement? _____ _____   densely enhancing
   c. Shape: _____   multi-lobulated with projecting "fronds"
   d. Usually seen associated with _____.   hydrocephalus

39

Neuronal and Mixed Neuronal-Glial Tumors

■ Ganglioglioma

1. **Answer the following about gangliogliomas:**
   a. Peak incidence occurs around _____ years.   11   39.1.2
   b. Characterized by _____ growth.   slow   39.1.1
   c. Have a tendency to c_____.   calcify
   d. Two major classifications include: _____ and _____   ganglioneuromas and gangliogliomas   39.1.4
   e. Most common presenting symptom is s_____.   seizures   39.1.5

■ Paraganglioma

2. **Provide the name of paragangliomas based on location:**   Table 39.1
   a. Carotid bifurcation: _____ _____   carotid body tumors
   b. Auricular branch of vagus: _____   glomus tympanicum
   c. Superior vagal ganglion: _____   glomus jugulare
   d. Inferior vagal ganglion: _____   glomus intravagale
   e. Adrenal medulla & sympathetic chain: _____   pheochromocytoma

3. **Paragangliomas may secrete:**   39.2.1
   a. e_____   epinephrine
   b. n_____   norepinephrine
   c. c_____   catecholamines

4. **Familial syndromes associated with pheochromocytomas include:**   39.2.2
   a. v____ H_____-L_____ disease   von Hippel-Lindau disease
   b. M_____ ___ & ____   MEN 2A & 2B
   c. n_____   neurofibromatosis

5. **Resection of carotid body tumor has a:**   39.2.3
   a. stroke risk of __ - __%.   8-20%
   b. cranial nerve injury risk of __ - __ %.   33-44%
   c. mortality of __ - __%.   5-13%

6. **The most common neoplasm of the**   glomus tympanicum   39.2.4
   middle ear is _____ _____.

7. **Complete the following about glomus**   39.2.4
   jugulare tumors:
   a. They arise from _____ _____.   glomus bodies
   b. Are they vascular or avascular?   very vascular
   c. Receive vascular supply from e_____   external carotid artery
      c_____ a_____ branches including:
      i.   a_____ p_____   ascending pharyngeal
      ii.   p_____ a_____   posterior auricular
      iii. o_____   occipital
      iv.   i_____ m_____   internal maxillary
   d. Receives vascular supply from _____   petrous; internal carotid
      portion of the _____ _____   artery
      _____.

8. **Characterization of glomus tumors**   39.2.4
   include:
   a. Female-to-male ratio:_____   6:1
   b. Does it typically occur bilaterally?   no, almost non-existent
   c. Typical presenting symptoms:
      i.   h_____ l_____   hearing loss
      ii.   p_____ t_____   pulsatile tinnitus
   d. Other clinical exam abnormalities:
      i.   V_____ due to CN VIII   Vertigo
            involvement
      ii.   Loss of t_____ of p_____   taste of posterior third of
            t_____ of t_____ from CN IX   tongue
            involvement
      iii. V_____ c_____ paralysis from   Vocal cord
            CNX involvement
      iv.   T_____ and s_____   Trapezius and
            weakness from CN XI involvement   sternocleidomastoid
      v.   Ipsilateral t_____ a_____ from tongue atrophy
            CN XII involvement

9. **True or False. During surgical excision**   39.2.4
   of a paraganglioma, the patient is
   noted to have abrupt onset of
   hypotension and respiratory distress.
   Is this most related to:
   a. intracranial pressure (ICP) changes   false
   b. vasovagal response   false
   c. inadvertent compression of airway   false
   d. tumor manipulation   true
   e. due to r_____ of h_____ or   release of histamine or
      b_____   bradykinin

39

10. **What is the major differential diagnosis for potential glomus tumors at the CPA?**

   vestibular schwannoma   39.2.4

11. **Complete the following about glomus jugulare:**   39.2.4

   a. Testing for v_____ _____ should be done.

   vanillyl mandelic acid (VMA)

   b. If elevated, indicative of secretion of _____,

   catecholamines

   c. which is similar to _____.

   pheochromocytoma

   d. New clinical marker is _____.

   normetanephrine (NMN)

12. **Complete the following about treatment of glomus jugulare:**   39.2.4

   a. Treat medically with _____ and _____ prior to surgery.

   alpha and beta blockers

   b. S_____ can be used to inhibit release of serotonin, bradykinin, and histamines.

   Somatostatin

   c. E_____ can lead to tumor swelling, which can compress brainstem or cerebellum but can be used to reduce vascularity.

   Embolization

   d. Recurrence after surgical resection may be as high as _____ of cases.

   1/3

39

40

Pineal Region and Embryonal Tumors

■ Pineal Region Tumors

1. True or False. Regarding pineal region tumors.
40.1.1

a. The absence of the BBB in the pineal gland makes this area susceptible to hematogenous metastasis. — true

b. Nongerminomas include:
   i. embryonal carcinoma — true
   ii. choriocarcinoma — true
   iii. teratoma — true
   iv. medulloblastoma — false

c. Germ cell tumors rarely give rise to tumor markers. — false

d. CSF tumor markers are more useful for following response to treatment than they are for diagnosis. — true

e. Obtaining a tissue diagnosis prior to treatment with a test dose of XRT is a growing trend. — true

2. True or False. Regarding pineal cysts.
40.1.2

a. Pineal cysts are a common incidental finding either on MRI or at autopsy. — true

b. Surgery should be performed for all pineal cysts to obtain a diagnosis. — false

c. Surgery can be performed to relieve symptoms should the cyst lead to hydrocephalus. — true

3. Pineocytoma and pineoblastoma are both_____ tumors that are _____. — malignant; radiosensitive
40.1.3

4. Complete the following about germ cell tumors.
40.1.3

a. In the CNS they arise in the _____. — midline

b. In males they are most likely in the _____ region. — pineal

c. In females they are most likely in the _____ region. — suprasellar

40

d. Are germ cell tumors benign or malignant?   malignant

e. They spread via the _____.   CSF

5. **True or False. Regarding germ cell tumors.**   40.1.3

a. Germ cell tumors and pineal cell tumors occur primarily in childhood and young adults (< 40 years old).   true

b. Clinical features of pineal region tumors may include hydrocephalus and Parinaud's syndrome.   true

c. Optimal management strategy for pineal region tumors has yet to be determined.   true

6. **True or False. Germinomas are very sensitive to radiation but not to chemotherapy.**   false – they are sensitive to both   40.1.3

7. **Complete the following about surgery for pineal tumors:**   40.1.3

a.

   i. The most common approach is the _____ _____.   infratentorial supracerebellar

   ii. This cannot be used if the _____ is steep.   tentorium

b.

   i. Another common approach is the _____ _____,   occipital transtentorial

   ii. which is best for lesions _____ at   centered

   iii. or _____ to the tentorial edge   superior

   iv. or _____ the vein of Galen.   above

c. Anatomically,

   i. the base of the pineal gland is the _____ wall of the _____ ventricle.   posterior; 3rd

   ii. the _____ surrounds both sides of the pineal gland.   thalamus

   iii. d_____ c_____ v____ are a major obstacle to operations in this region.   deep cerebral veins

■ Embryonal Tumors

8. **Complete the following about embryonal tumors:**   40.2.1

a. PNET stands for _____ _____ _____   primitive neuroectodermal tumors

b. These tumors include:

   i. p_____   pineoblastoma

   ii. n_____   neuroblastoma

   iii. e_____   esthesioneuroblastoma

   iv. r_____   retinoblastoma

   v. m_____   medulloblastoma

c.

   i. They are _____ indistinguishable   histologically

   ii. but genetically _____.   distinct

9.   Regarding embryonal tumors.   40.2.1

a.   The term primitive neuroectodermal   embryonal
     tumor (PNET) is entrenched, but the
     recommendation is to call them
     _____ tumors.

b.   A medulloblastoma (MB) is more than   beta-catenin;
     just a PNET of the posterior fossa   APC
     because mutations such as ____-_____
     and ____ seen in MB are absent in other
     PNETs.

c.   The most common location for an   cerebellar vermis
     embryonal tumor is the _____ _____
     (hint: think about MB).

d.   Embryonal tumors spread via the ____.   CSF

e.   _____ law for children with treated   Collins
     embryonal tumors states that the period
     of risk of recurrence is equal to the age
     at diagnosis plus 9 months.

f.   Require entire _____ _____   spinal axis
     evaluation.

g.
     i.   Cranial radiotherapy is avoided   3
          before ___ years of age
     ii. to avoid i_____ impairment   intellectual
     iii. and growth r_____.   retardation

10. Complete the following about   40.2.1
**   supratentorial PNET (sPNETs):**

a.   They occur in children under _____   5
     years of age.

b.   They occur _____ in adults.   rarely

c.   Histologically, they are _____ to   identical
     medulloblastoma.

d.
     i.   They are ____ aggressive than   more
          medullobastomas.
     ii. Survival is _____ and they   worse
     iii. respond _____ to therapy.   poorly

11. True or False. Regarding   40.2.2
**   medulloblastoma.**

a.   It accounts for 15 to 20% of all   true
     intracranial tumors in children.

b.   It is the most common malignant   true
     pediatric brain tumors.

c.   There is a standardized chemotherapy,   false (There is no
     including lomulstine (CCNU) and   standardized regimen; CCNU
     vincristine.   and vincristine are usually
                                                used for recurrences.)

d.   Patients with residual medulloblastoma   true
     post-resection and dissemination are a
     poor risk, with only a 35 – 40% chance of
     being disease free at 5 years.

e.   MB are WHO grade ___.   IV

40

40

12. **Complete the following about medulloblastoma:**   40.2.2
    a. The clinical history is _____,   brief
    b. typically only ____ to ____ weeks.   6 to 12
    c. Their location of orgin predisposes   hydrocephalus
       patients to _____.
    d. Patients present with:
       i.   h_____   headache
       ii. n_____   nausea
       iii. a_____ and   ataxia
       iv. seeding of the axis in ____ to ____ %   10 to 35

13. **True or False. Radiologically, medulloblastomas are**   40.2.2
    a. cystic   false
    b. solid   true
    c. enhancing   true
    d. on non-contrast CT they are hyperdense   true

14. **Complete the following about medulloblastoma location:**   40.2.2
    a. Most are in the _____.   midline
    b. Laterally situated tumors are more   adults
       common in _____.

15. **Complete the following about drop mets to the spine with medulloblastoma:**   40.2.2
    a. The test that should be is a _____ _____   MRI w/ contrast
       _____.
    b. Staging should be done _____ or   pre-op;
       within ____ to _____ weeks post-op.   2 to 3

16. **Regarding the molecular biology of**   17p   40.2.2
    medulloblastoma, in 35 to 40% there
    is a deletion of _____.

17. **Poor prognosticators for patients with MB include:**   40.2.2
    a. y_____ a_____   younger age
    b. m_____ d_____   metastatic disease
    c. i_____ to p_____ g____-t_____   inability to perform gross-
       r_____   total removal
    d. histological differentiation along g_____,   glial, ependymal, or neuronal
       e_____, or n_____ lines   lines

18. **Regarding atypical teratoid/rhabdoid tumors:**   40.2.4
    a. Occur primarily in i_____ and   infants and children
       c_____.
    b. Most patients die with ____ year of   1
       diagnosis.
    c. Have a deletion or monosomy of   22
       chromosome __.

19. **Complete the following about esthesioneuroblastoma:**

40.2.5

a. Are a rare _____ _____.   nasal neoplasm
b. Are believed to arise from the   olfactory neural crest
   _____ _____ _____.
c. The _____ grading system should be   Hyams
   used to characterize the disease course.
d. Median survival is typically _____ years.   approx. 7 years
e. Primary treatment is controversial but   chemoradiotherapy;
   typically involves _____ and   craniofacial resection
   _____ _____.

40

41

Tumors of Cranial, Spinal and Peripheral Nerves

■ Vestibular Schwannoma

1. True or False. Vestibular Schwannaoms (VS) usually arise from which nerve? 41.1.1

a. facial nerve — false
b. cochlear nerve — false
c. nervus intermedius — false
d. vestibular nerve, inferior division — true
e. vestibular nerve, superior division — true

2. Vestibular schwannomas arise from the junction 41.1.1

a. of the _____ and _____ myelin called — central and peripheral
b. the _____-_____ zone — Obersteiner-Redlich

3. Complete the following about vestibular schwannomas: 41.1.1

a. What is the Obersteiner-Redlich zone? — site of junction of central and peripheral myelin
b. Where is it located? — 8 to 12 mm from brain stem
c. From what cells do acoustic tumors arise? — the neurilemmal sheath
d. On what structure do they arise? — superior division of vestibular nerve
e. Therefore, are they schwannomas or neuromas? — schwannomas
f. They are the result of a chromosomal defect that leads to
   i. loss of t_____ s_____ gene on the — tumor suppressor
   ii. l_____ arm of c_____ #____. — long arm of chromosome 22
   iii. If this defect is inherited the patient has_____ _____ ___. — neurofibromatosis Type 2

4. **Pathologically, what fibers constitute vestibular schwannomas?**   41.1.3

a. A_____ ____ n_____   Antoni A narrow elongated
   e_____ b_____   bipolar fibers
   f_____

b. A_____ ___ l_____   Antoni B loose reticulated
   r_____ f_____   fibers

5. **List the common triad of symptoms seen with vestibular schwannomas.**   41.1.4

a. h_____ l_____ - ____%   hearing loss – 98%
b. t_____ - ____%   tinnitus – 70%
c. d_____ - ____%   disequilibrium – 70%
                                        (insidious, progressive, 70%
                                        have high-frequency loss,
                                        word discrimination
                                        difficulties)

6. **A patient with good hearing has an MRI study that shows a cerebellopontine angle mass.**   41.1.4

a. Is this compatible with a vestibular   no (at the time of diagnosis
   schwannoma?   virtually all VS have otological
                                                 symptoms)

b. When hearing is involved in VS, what is
   lost?
   i.   low frequencies?   no
   ii. high frequencies?   yes (70% have a high-
                                  frequency loss pattern)
   iii. word discrimination?   yes (e.g. telephone
                                  conversation)

7. **What cranial nerve deficits, other than CN VIII, occur with VS?**   41.1.4

a. CN ____; o_____, f_____   CN V; otalgia, facial
   n_____, and t_____ c_____   numbness, and taste changes
b. CN ____; f_____   CN VII, facial weakness
   w_____
c. CN ____,_____,____; h_____   CN IX, X, XII; horseness and
   and d_____   dysphagia

8. **Answer the following about VS:**   41.1.4

a. As tumor increases in size the following
   occur in what sequence?
   i.   facial weakness   iii, ii, i (facial numbness
   ii. facial numbness   occurs earlier than
   iii. impaired hearing   weakness even though CN V
                                 is only slightly compressed
                                 and CN VII is severely
                                 compressed – a paradox
                                 because of differential
                                 resilience of motor nerves
                                 relative to sensory nerves.)

b. What size of tumor causes CN V and CN   > 2 cm
   VII compression?

41

9. **Complete the following about vestibular schwannomas:**   41.1.4

a. What percentage have no abnormal physical findings except for hearing loss?   66%

b. The Weber test lateralizes to the _____ side.   uninvolved (hearing loss is sensorineural)

c. Is the Rinne test positive or negative if hearing is preserved?   positive

d. What is normal for the Rinne test?   air conduction > bone conduction = positive means normal (Note: An A is better than a B.)

10. **Regarding vestibular schwannomas.**   41.1.4

a. What causes nystagmus?   vestibular involvement

b. Vestibular involvement also causes an abnormal _____ with   electronystagmography (ENG);

c_____ s_____   caloric stimulation

c. What is the growth rate for VS?   1 to 10 mm/year

d. What is the proper follow-up protocol, if no surgery is done?   repeat scan at 6 month intervals for 2 years then once each year

e. Recommend surgery if:

i. size changes by _____   > 2 mm/year

ii. or symptoms _____   progress

11. **Answer the following about the House and Brackmann scale?**   41.1.4

a. What does the House-Brackmann scale measure?   facial nerve function

b. What are the categories?   normal, mild, moderate, moderate-severe, severe, total paralysis

c. Synkinesis is defined as i_____ m_____ accompanying a v_____ m_____   involuntary movement; voluntary movement

12. **What is the major differential diagnosis for a CPA lesion?**   meningioma vs. vestibular schwannoma vs. neuroma of adjacent cranial nerve (e.g. CN V).   41.1.4

13. **Describe the audiometric findings for "useful" hearing in vestibular schwannomas.**   41.1.5

a. pure-tone audiogram threshold: _____   < 50 dB

b. speech discrimination of: _____   ≥ 50%

41

14. Complete the following regarding the modified Gardener-Robertson system:

41.1.5

a. System is used to grade h_____ p_____.

hearing preservation

b. It consists of testing patient with _____ _____ of increasing loudness.

pure tones (decibels [dB]) (if patient hears dB 0 to 30 – excellent hearing; 31 to 50 dB – serviceable; 50 to 90 dB – nonserviceable; 90 dB max-poor; not testable – none)

c. Evaluating patient ability to understand spoken words is called _____ _____.

speech discrimination (understands words spoken correctly 100 to 80% - excellent; 70 to 50% - serviceable; 50 to 5% - nonserviceable)

d. Useful hearing is judged to be present up to a cutoff point of _____.

50/50–patient can hear at 50 dB or less and understands at least 50% of words spoken to him/her

15. Name the findings for the following tests in vestibular schwannomas:

41.1.5

a. pure-tone audiogram

hearing difference between each ear > 10 to 15 dB

b. speech discrimination

4 to 8% score (normal is 92 to 100%)

c. brainstem auditory evoked response (BSAER) or auditory brainstem response (ABR)

prolonged I-III and I-V interpeak latencies (not used for diagnostic purposes but good for prognostication)

d. electronystagmography (ENG)

abnormal if there is >20% difference between the two sides (normally, 50% of response is from each ear.)

e. vestibular evoked myogenic potential (VEMP)

assess inferior vestibular nerve independent of hearing (can be used even with deafness present).

f. MRI

diagnostic procedure of choice; round, enhancing tumor centered on IAC

41

16. Complete the following concerning vestibular schwannoma:

41.1.5

a. It causes what kind of hearing loss?

sensorineural loss of high tones

b. This is the same as the loss from
   i. o_____ a_____
   ii. l_____ n_____ e_____

old age
loud noise exposure

c. Think tumor if the difference between the ears on audiogram is more than _____ dB.

10 to 15

17. **True or False. A 55 year old male is referred for evaluation of a 4.0 cm right cerebellopontine angle (CPA) mass. You conclude it is a vestibular schwannoma. Which of the following is least likely to be a factor in your treatment? Give a rationale for each.**   41.1.6

a. pure-tone audiogram score of 95 dB

false – audiogram with hearing threshold < 50 dB may allow consideration of hearing-sparing procedure, but with a score of 95 dB hearing-saving procedure is not an option

b. effacement of the fourth ventricle with modest ventriculomegaly

false – evidence of hydrocephalus warrants CSF diversion – needs a shunt

c. stereotactic surgery 2 years previously

true – stereotactic radiosurgery 2 years previously is long enough for SRS effect to be over. Surgery should be avoided during the interval 6 to 18 months after SRS because this is the time of maximum damage from radiation

d. contralateral (left) vestibular schwannoma, 1.0 cm in diameter

false – bilateral VS unable to preserve right hearing [95 dB], will need to plan for second procedure to address left-sided lesion. Chance of preserving left hearing is 35 – 71% for a 1 cm tumor

e. angiogram showing absence of right transverse sinus

false – atretic/obstructed right transverse sinus allows consideration of translabyrinthine and suboccipital approach as a combined procedure

18. **True or False. Possible treatments for vestibular schwannomas include:**   41.1.6

a. expectant observation, following symptoms, hearing testing, serial CT or MRI   true

b. radiation therapy, external beam radiation therapy (EBRT)   true

c. radiation therapy, stereotactic radiosurgery (SRS), single dose   true

d. radiation therapy, stereotactic radiotherapy, fractionated (SRT)   true

e. retrosigmoid (suboccipital) resection   true

f. translabyrinthine resection   true

g. extradural subtemporal (middle fossa approach) resection   true

41

19. **Answer the following about vestibular schwannomas:**   41.1.6
   a. What is the growth rate of VSs?   slow (1 to 10 mm/year)
   b. Do some shrink?   yes (6%)
   c. Can they remain stable?   yes
   d. Can they grow faster?   yes (2 to 3 cm/year)
   e. If followed most will show _____ in 3   enlargement
      years.

20. **Complete the following about vestibular schwannoma treatment:**   41.1.6
   a. Under 25 mm with perfect hearing can   observed
      be _____.
   b. Protocol is to retest at 6, 12, 18, 24, 36,   months
      48, 60, 84, 108, and 168 _____.
   c. Growth of more than _____ mm   2
      between studies deserves treatment.
   d. Tumors larger than 15 to 20 mm should   treated
      be _____.
   e. Tumors with cysts can _____   grow dramatically
      _____.

21. **Comparing microsurgery and SRS:**   41.1.6
   a. Better outcome for hearing?   SRS
   b. Better outcome for trigeminal   microsurgery
      neuropathy and tumor control?
   c. No difference for preservation of   facial nerve function
      f_____ n_____ f_____.
   d. Quicker improvement of vertigo?   microsurgery

22. **Classically, vestibular schwannomas**   forward and superiorly in 75%   41.1.7
    push the facial nerve in which   of cases
    direction?

23. **Complete the following about vestibular schwannomas:**   41.1.7
   a. Small, laterally located intracanalicular   subtemporal extradural (also
      VSs can be removed by what surgical   known an middle fossa
      approach?   approach)
   b. A disadvantage is that the seventh nerve   injured at the geniculate
      may be _____ at the _____ ganglion.
   c. An advantage is that hearing function   preserved
      may be _____.

24. **What is the size vestibular**   < 2 to 2.5 cm   41.1.7
    schwannomas should be considered
    for hearing and CN VII preservation
    procedures?

41

25. What are the advantages of translabyrinthine approach for resecting vestibular schwannomas? 41.1.7

a. early identification of the _____ _____   facial nerve
b. less risk to _____ and   cerebellum; lower cranial
_____ _____ _____   nerves
c. patients do not get "ill" from _____   blood in cisterna magna
in _____ _____
d. best for VS that are located   intra-canalicular
_____

26. What are the disadvantages of the translabyrinthine approach for resecting vestibular schwannomas? 41.1.7

a. Hearing is _____.   sacrificed
b. Exposure is _____.   limited
c. May take _____.   longer
d. CSF leak is ____ _____.   more common

27. Complete the following about vestibular schwannomas: 41.1.7

a. what are the disadvantages of suboccipital approach (also known as retrosigmoid) for VSs?
　　i.　Higher _____ when compared   morbidity (H/A more
　　　　with the translabyrinthine approach.   common)
　　ii.　Small tumors are _____.   difficult to remove in lateral
　　　　　 recess of internal auditory
　　　　　 canal (IAC)
　　iii.　Facial nerve is located   on blind side deep to the
　　　　_____   tumor
b. the advantage is the possibility of   hearing preservation
h_____ p_____.

28. Complete the following about localizing the CN VII origin: 41.1.7

a. The seventh nerve originates in the   pontomedullary
_____ sulcus.
b. Is anterior to the eighth nerve by ____   1-2
mm.
c. It lies just anterior to the foramen of   Luschka
_____
d. and anterior to a tuft of _____.   choroid
e. It originates _____ mm cephalad to the   4
IX nerve.

29. How do you treat posteroperative facial nerve weakness after a vestibular schwannoma resection? 41.1.7

a. n_____ t_____   natural tears (2 drops in each
　　　 eye every 2 hours as needed)
b. l_____   lacrilube (to eye and tape eye
　　　 at bedtime)
c. t_____   tarsorrhaphy within a few
　　　 days if there is a complete CN
　　　 VII palsy

41

d. Anastomose by attaching a portion of the _____ nerve to the _____ nerve.

hypoglossal; facial (facial re-animation)

e. When there is no CN VII function and
   i. nerve is known to be divided, you may anastomose in _____.

2 months

   ii. nerve is known to be intact, you may anastomose in _____.

1 year

30. True or False. The following symptoms of brainstem compression from a vestibular schwannoma if present post-op is not likely to improve

41.1.7

a. nausea

false (resolves with time)

b. vomiting

false (resolves with time)

c. balance difficulties

false (clear rapidly)

d. ataxia

true (may be permanent)

31. True or False. The routes of CSF leakage after vestibular schwannoma resection can be via the

41.1.7

a. apical cells

true (to tympanic cavities or Eustachian tube – most common)

b. vestibule

true (posterior SCC is usually entered by drilling – via the oval window)

c. perilabyrinthine cells

true (and tracks to mastoid antrum)

d. mastoid air cells

true (at craniotomy site)

32. With vestibular schwannoma, postoperative routes for rhinorrhea are:
Hint: avpam

41.1.7

a. a_____

apical cells to tympanic cavity and down the Eustachian tube

b. v_____

vestibule of the horizontal SCC

c. p_____

posterior SCC (most common area entered with drilling)

d. a_____

to antrum of mastoid via the perilabyrinthine cells

e. m_____

mastoid air cells at site of craniotomy

41

33. **What are treatment strategies for CSF leakage after vestibular schwannoma resection?**   41.1.7
   a. What percentage stop spontaneously?   25 – 35%
   b. Do what with the head of the bed?   elevate
   c. Place a drain where?   lumbar
   d. if hydrocephalus is present place a ____
       _____.   CSF shunt

   e. If leak persists _____
       _____.   re-explore surgical site to pack with tissue or apply bone wax

34. **What are common complications of vestibular schwannoma surgery?**   41.1.7
   a. CSF leak in ____ – ____%   4 – 27%
   b. infection in _____%   5.7%
   c. stroke in _____%   0.7%
   d. CN VII palsy in ____ – ____%   0 – 50%
   e. hearing loss in ___ – ___%   34 – 43%
   f. death in _____%   1%

35. **Complete the following concerning hearing loss and CN VII weakness after suboccipital removal of VS?**   41.1.7
   a. Tumor < 1 cm
       i.   CN VII preserved, ___ – ___%   95 – 100%
       ii. CN VIII preserved, _____%   57%
   b. Tumor 1 to 2 cm
       i.   CN VII preserved, ___ – ___%   80 – 92%
       ii. CN VIII preserved, _____%   33%
   c. Tumor > 2cm
       i.   CN VII preserved, ___ – ___%   50 – 76%
       ii. CN VIII preserved, _____%   6%

36. **Complete the following concerning hearing loss after suboccipital removal of VS:**   41.1.7
   a. hearing preserved ___ – ____% with tumors < 1.5 cm   35 to 71%
   b. after SRS hearing preserved _____% with tumors < 3 cm   26%

37. **Concerning acoustic neuroma, recurrence following microsurgery is**   41.1.7
   a. ___ – ___% after   7-11%
   b. ___ – ___ years follow-up   3-16
   c. with a subtotal resection of about _____%   20%

38. **Complete the following concerning SRS for vestibular schwannoma:**   41.1.7
   a. Dose recommended is _____.   14 Gy
   b. Local control achieved is _____%.   94%

41

39. **For vestibular schwannoma, what are short-term local control rates for?**   41.1.7
   a. microsurgery   97%
   b. SRS   94%

40. **When is the time of maximal damage (possible tumor enlargement) from radiation to vestibular schwannomas?**   41.1.7
   a. from _____ to _____ months   6 to 18 months
   b. This is important to know because it can produce a false appearance of tumor _____.   enlargement (Surgery should be avoided during the interval 6 to 18 months after SRS because of damage from radiation and the appearance of tumor enlargement.)

■ Tumors of Peripheral Nerves: Perineurioma

41. **Regarding tumors of peripheral nerves:**   41.2
   a. Intraneural perineurioma:
      i.   Lesion is usually found in _____ or _____ _____.   adolescents; young adults
      ii. Mitotic activity is _____.   rare
      iii. MIB-1 labeling is _____.   low
      iv. Treatment is _____.   conservative sampling of lesion (not resection)

   b. Soft tissue perineurioma:
      i.   almost exclusively _____   benign
      ii. more common in _____   females
      iii. is ___ encapsulated   not
      iv. Treatment is _____.   gross total resection

41

42

Meningiomas

■ General information. Common Locations

1. **Characterize meningiomas:**
   a. They arise from what cell of origin? · Arachnoid cap cells · 42.1
   b. What percentage of meningiomas occur at the falx (includes parasagittal)? · 60 to 70% · 42.3.1
   c. With contralateral foot drop plus hyperreflexia, think _____ _____. · parasagittal meningioma · 42.3.3
   d. Olfactory groove meningiomas · · 42.3.4
      i. can produce what syndrome? · Foster Kennedy syndrome
      ii. Consisting of a_____, i_____ o_____ a_____, and c_____ p_____ · anosmia, ipsilateral optic atrophy, and contralateral papilledema
      iii. What other syndrome? · frontal lobe
      iv. Consisting of a_____, i_____ · apathy, incontinence

2. **List the most common locations for adult meningiomas.** · Parasagittal (20.8%) – grouped as either anterior, middle, or posterior; up to 50% invade the superior sagittal sinus (SSS); Convexity (15.8%); Tuberculum sellae (12.8%); Sphenoidal ridge (11.9%) – three basic categories: lateral spenoid wing, middle third, and medial; Olfactory groove (9.8%); Falx (8%); Lateral ventricle (4.2%) · Table 42.1

3. **Abulia** · · 42.3.4
   a. is l_____ o_____ w_____. · lack of willpower
   b. is characteristic of damage to f_____ l_____. · frontal lobes
   c. can occur with a meningioma of the o_____ g_____. · olfactory groove

■ Pathology

4. **Regarding the pathology of meningiomas.**   42.4
   a. List the four histopathological variables.   Grade, histological subtype, proliferation indices, and brain invasion
   b. There are _____ WHO grades.   3 (I, II, III)
   c. As the WHO grade increases, there is increased risk of _____ and an increase in the _____ _____ (i.e. K__-6___).   recurrence; proliferative index; Ki-67

5. **The presence of brain invasion increases the likelihood of _____ to levels similar to atypical meningiomas, but it is not an indicator of _____ _____.**   recurrence; malignant grade   42.4.1

6. **True or False. Regarding meningiomas.**   42.4.2
   a. They commonly metastasize outside of the CNS.   false
   b. The most common site of metastatis is the adrenal gland.   false – most common sites include the liver, lung, LNs and heart
   c. The angioblastic and malignant subtypes most commonly metastasize.   true

7. **Complete the following regarding meningiomas:**   42.4.3
   a. If you see multiple meningiomas, it suggests _____.   NF2
   b. _____ _____ can mimic menigiomas since they may have a dural tail.   Pleomorphic xanthoastrocytoma (PXA)
   c. Massive painless lymphadenopathy with sinus histiocytosis that has MRI signal characteristics similar to a meningioma is typical of _____-_____ _____.   Rosai-Dorfman disease

■ Presentation

8. **Give a description of asymptomatic meningiomas.**   42.5
   a. The most common primary intracranial tumor is _____   meningioma
   b. Percent of primary brain tumors that are meningiomas: _____%   32%
   c. Percent that are stable in size over 2.5 years: _____%   66%
   d. Percent that increase in size when observed for 2.5 years: _____   33%

42

e. What does calcification tell us about rate of growth?   slower

f. Operative morbidity in patients under 70 is _____% and   3.5%

g. above 70 it is _____%   23%

h. classic histological finding is the p_____ b_____.   psammoma body

---

■ Evaluation

9. Complete the following about MRI and meningioma: 42.6.1

a. Meningioma on T1W1 and T2W1 may be _____.   isointense

b. With contrast most will _____.   enhance

c. Accurately predicts sinus involvement in _____%.   90%

d. A common finding is a d_____ t_____.   dural tail

10. What metastatic cancer can mimic meningioma in the bone of MRI?   prostate cancer   42.6.2

11. Olfactory groove meningiomas tend to be fed by the   42.6.3

a. _____ arteries,   ethmoidal

b. which are branches of the _____ artery;   ophthalmic

c. compared to other meningiomas, which are supplied by feeders from the _____ _____ _____.   external carotid artery

d. Classically, meningiomas "_____ _____, _____ _____" on angiography.   "comes early, stays late"

12. The artery of B_____ and C_____ is enlarged in lesions involving the tentorium (i.e. tentorial meningiomas).   Bernasconi and Cassinari (a branch of the meningohypophyseal trunk, the "Italian artery")   42.6.3

13. True or False. The artery most likely to be enlarged on an angiogram depicting a tentorial meningioma is the   42.6.3

a. superificial temporal artery   false

b. artery of Bernasconi and Cassinari   true

c. occipital artery   false

d. posterior inferior cerebellar artery   false

e. anterior choroidal artery   false

42

14. **Regarding meningiomas and plain x-rays, the plain x-rays may show**   42.6.4
   a. b_____ _____ _____   blistering of bone
   b. c_____ _____ _____   calcification in tumor 10%
   c. d_____ _____ – _____   density changes –
                                                  hyperostosis
   d. e_____ _____ _____   enlarged vascular grooves
   e. f_____ _____ _____   frontal fossa hyperostosis

■ Treatment

15. **Complete the following regarding sinus involvement.**   42.7.2
   a. Occlusion of the middle third of the SSS   treacherous
       is _____
   b. Morbidity/mortality rate is   8/3%
       _____/_____%
   c. due to v_____ i_____   venous infarction
   d. The sinus may be divided safely anterior   coronal suture
       to the _____ _____.
   e. Posterior to this site the sinus _____   must not
       _____ be divided.
   f. If tumor is attached, it is best to leave   residual tumor
       _____ _____.
   g. True or False. It is safe to occlude the   false
       dominant transverse sinus.

16. **Complete the following about removal of meningiomas:**   42.7.2
   a. The Simpson grading system grades the   meningiomas
       degree of removal of _____.
   b. It is important because it correlates with recurrence rate
       _____ _____.
   c. What is the most important factor?   extent of tumor removal;
                                                   in order of complexity, from
                                                   minimal surgery to complete
                                                   removal
   d. Components of the system are
       i.   s_____ r_____, b_____   small removal, biopsy
       ii. p_____ r_____   partial removal
       iii. c_____ r_____   complete removal
       iv. c_____ d_____   coagulate dura
       v.   r_____ d_____ and   remove dura and bone and
            b_____ and s_____   sinus
   e. correlates with grade
       i.   _____   V
       ii. _____   IV
       iii. _____   III
       iv. _____   II
       v.   _____   I

42

17. **True or False. Complete the following about radiation therapy (XRT) for meningiomas:**   42.7.3
    a. XRT is effective as a primary modality for treatment.   false
    b. XRT is often used for "benign" lesions.   false
    c. XRT can be used for invasive, aggressive, recurrent, or non-resectable meningiomas.   true
    d. XRT may be beneficial in preventing recurrence for meningiomas that are partially resected.   true

■ Outcome

18. **Five year survival for patients with meningioma is _____%.**   91.3%   42.8

19. **The most important factor in for preventing recurrence is the _____.**   extent of surgical removal   42.8

42

43

Other Tumors Related to the Meninges

■ Mesenchymal, Non-meningothelial Tumors

1. **True or False. Complete the following about hemangiopericytoma:**   43.1.1
   a. Sarcoma that arises from _____.   pericytes
   b. May mimic _____ on CT or MRI.   meningioma (MRS demonstrating a high inositol peak may help distinguish)
   c. Primary treatment is _____.   surgery

■ Primary Melanocytic Lesions

2. **Where does primary CNS melanoma arise?**   probably from melanocytes in the leptomeninges   43.2

3. **In what decade of life does primary CNS melanoma peak?**   4th decade (compared to the 7th decade for primary cutaneous melanoma)   43.2

■ Hemangioblastoma

4. **Characterize hemangioblastoma (HGB).**   43.3.2
   a.
      i. It can be associated with _____ _____-_____   von Hippel-Landau
      ii. in _____%.   20%
   b. Surgically treat it like an _____.   AVM

5. **Answer the following about hemangioblastoma:**   43.3.2
   a. What is the most common primary intraaxial tumor in the adult posterior fossa?   hemangioblastoma
   b. Can also be located in the r_____.   retina
   c. What blood paraneoplastic syndrome is associated?
      i. p_____ due to   polycythemia
      ii. e_____   erythropoietin
   d. Histologically, they are _____ tumors.   benign

43

6. Regarding hemangioblastoma: 43.3.2
a. They present with typical p-fossa mass symptoms:
  i.   h_____   headache
  ii. n_____/v_____   nausea/vomiting
  iii. c_____ f_____   cerebellar findings
b. Cardinal pathological feature?   numerous capillary channels
c. Most common cyst pattern seen?   peritumoral cyst alone
d. p-fossa HGB should be evaluated with   MRI of entire neuroaxis
   _____.   (possibility of spinal HGB)
e. Vertebral angiography usually   intense vascularity
   demonstrates ____ _____.
f. Check a ____ to identify polycythemia.   CBC

7. Complete the following about surgery on a solitary HGB: 43.3.2
a. It may be _____ in sporadic HGB   curative
b. but not in _____.   VHL
c. _____ _____ may help reduce   Pre-op embolization
   vascularity.

8. Complete the following about surgery on HGB: 43.3.2
a. Avoid _____ removal,   piecemeal
b. work along the _____   margin
c. and _____ the blood supply   devascularize
d. using the same technique as for an   AVM
   _____.

9. Complete the following about von Hippel-Landau (VHL) disease: 43.3.3
a. Has hemangioblastoma tumors or cyst in the following sites
  i.   c_____   cerebellum
  ii. r_____   retina
  iii. b_____ s____   brainstem
  iv. s_____ c____   spinal cord
  v.   p_____   phemochromocytoma
  vi. c____ in the k_____   cysts in the kidney
b. Most common location is the _____.   cerebellum
c. Second most common location is the _____.   retina
d. Always manifests before age ____.   60
e. Incidence is 1 in every ____ persons.   35,000
f. The mode of inheritance is _____   autosomal dominant
   _____.
g. The VHL gene is on chromosome ___.   3

10. What is the diagnostic criteria for VHL?   43.3.3
a.
  i.   One lesion of VHL is necessary if there is a _____ _____.   family history
  ii. It will be present in ____%.   80%
b. Two lesions of VHL are required to make it a ___ _____ mutation.   de novo

11. **Complete the following about tumors associated with VHL?**   43.3.3
    a. Occur in younger persons if patient has _____.   VHL
    b. True or False. Cysts are associated with HGBs.   true
    c. Cerebellar HGBs are located in the
       i.   s_____   superficial
       ii. p_____   posterior
       iii. s_____ half of the hemisphere   superior
    d. _____% of cerebellar HGBs were found in the _____.   7%; vermis

12. **Complete the following about spinal cord hemangioblastoma:**   43.3.3
    a. ____% are in the cervical and thoracic cord.   90%
    b. ____% are located in the posterior cord.   96%
    c. ____% of spinal HGBs are associated with VHL.   90%
    d. ____% symptoms are associated with syringomyelia.   95%

13. **The only disease with bilateral endolympathic sac tumors is ____.**   VHL   43.3.3

14. **Complete the following about VHL:**   43.3.3
    a. Retinal hemangioblastomas occur in ____%.   50%
    b. Typically located in the _____.   periphery
    c. Frequently there are _____.   multiple
    d. Treat with laser _____.   photocoagulation

15. **Complete the following about renal cell carcinoma (RCC):**   43.3.3
    a. Which is the most common malignant tumor in VHL?   RCC
    b. Usually it is a _____ _____ _____.   clear cell carcinoma
    c. It is the cause of death in __ to __% of VHL patients.   15 to 50%

16. **Complete the following about surgical treatment of HGB:**   43.3.3
    a. reserved until _____   symptomatic
    b. treatment of choice for _____ _____ HGBs   accessible cystic
    c. True or False. The wall must be removed.   false
    d. The _____ _____ must be removed.   mural nodule

17. **Regarding renal cysts in VHL:**   43.3.3
    a. True or False. They usually cause significant renal impairment.   false
    b. True or False. They are more problematic than polycystic kidney disease. false

43

18. **Complete the following regarding pancreatic lesions in patients with VHL:**   43.3.3

   a.   ____ to ____% of patients with VHL develop a pancreatic endocrine tumor or cyst.   35 to 70%

   b.   Pancreatic cysts are often _____ and _____.   multiple and asymptomatic

   c.   Most neuroendocrine tumors are _____ and only ___% are malignant.   nonfunctional; 8%

43

44

Lymphomas and Hematopoietic Neoplasms

■ CNS Lymphoma

1. **Complete the following about CNS lymphoma:**
   a. Associated with an eye condition called _____. — uveitis — 44.1.1
   b. How frequently does it occur? — 1 to 2% of all brain tumors — 44.1.3
   c. What relationship does CNS lymphoma have with the ventricles? — up close to ventricles — 44.1.5
   d. What form of radiation therapy is given? — whole brain — 44.1.9

2. **Regarding secondary CNS lymphoma.** — 44.1.2
   a. It is pathologically _____ to primary CNS lymphoma. — identical
   b. Systemic lymphoma spread to the cerebral parenchyma occurs in _____% of cases at autopsy. — 1 to 7%

3. **The incidence of primary CNS lymphoma is _____ relative to other brain lesions.** — rising — 44.1.3

4. **The following increase the risk of primary CNS lymphoma:** — 44.1.4
   a. c_____ v_____ d_____ — collagen vascular disease
   b. i_____ — immunosuppression
   c. E_____ B_____ v_____ — Epstein-Barr virus

5. **True or False. Regarding primary CNS lymphoma.** — 44.1.5
   a. B-cell lymphomas are more common than T-cell. — true
   b. Painful skin nodules/plaques occur in approx. 10% of patients. — true
   c. Intravascular lymphomatosis rarely involves the CNS. — false

44

6. **Regarding the presentation of CNS lymphoma.**   44.1.6
   a. The two most common manifestations   spinal cord compression;
       are s_____ c_____ c_____ and   carcinomatous meningitis
       c_____ m_____.
   b. Most patients present with n__-f_____   non-focal neurological
       n_____ symptoms.

7. **Regarding diagnosis of CNS lymphoma.**   44.1.8
   a. CT characteristics
       i.   plain CT tumor is _____   hyperdense to brain
       ii. contrast CT tumor _____   enhances homogenously
       iii. reminiscent of _____ _____   "fluffy cotton balls"
            _____
   b. Reaction to steroids _____.   may completely resolve
   c. CSF is positive for lymphoma cells in   only 10%
       _____%.

8. **True or False. A 70-year-old male with**   44.18
   a homogenously enhancing lesion in
   the central gray matter and corpus
   callosum is suspected of having CNS
   lymphoma. What would make this
   diagnosis more likely and how is it
   properly diagnosed?
   a. hydrocephalus   false
   b. café au lait spots   false
   c. uveitis   true (diagnosed with slit
                                                  lamp)
   d. proximal muscle weakness   false

9. **A 73-year-old male with a history of**   44.1.9
   recently diagnosed CNS lymphoma by
   biopsy presents to the ER with stupor
   and progressively deteriorating
   mental status. CT of the brain reveals
   the mass but no other abnormalities.
   a. True or False.
       i.   emergent surgical excision   false
       ii. radiation therapy   true (CNS lymphomas are
                                                 very sensitive to radiation)
       iii. chemotherapy   false
       iv. steroids   false
   b. followed by _____   chemotherapy

10. **Regarding the prognosis of CNS lymphoma:**   44.1.10
    a. With no treatment, median survival is   1.8 to 3.3 months
        ___ to ___
    b. With radiation therapy, median survival   10 months
        is _____.
    c. With intraventricular methotrexate, the   41 months
        time to recurrence was ____ months.

■ Multiple Myeloma

11. **Complete the following about**   44.2.1
    multiple myeloma (MM):
  a. It is a neoplasm of _____ _____   plasma cells
  b. that produces _____.   M-protein (monoclonal IgG or
                                                IgA)

12. **The characteristic presentation for**   44.2.3
    MM includes:
  a. i_____ s_____ to i_____   increased susceptibility to
                                                infection
  b. a_____   anemia
  c. h_____   hypercalcemia
  d. b____ p____   bone pain
  e. r_____ f_____   renal failure

13. **The evaluation for patients with MM**   44.2.4
    includes:
  a. s_____ r_____ s_____   skeletal radiological survey
                                                (for "punched out" lesions)
  b. C__   CBC
  c. S____   SPEP
  d. A urine test for MM is done to identify
     i. k_____ B_____-J_____ p_____   kappa Bence-Jones protein
     ii. found in _____% of cases.   75%
  e. The most definitive test is b____   bone marrow biopsy
     m_____ b_____.

14. **The treatment of MM includes:**
  a. _____   XRT (MM is very   44.2.5
                                                radiosensitive)
  b. b_____   bisphosphonates
  c. m_____   mobilization
  d. Some lesions may benefit from   kyphoplasty
     k_____.
  e. The median survival for untreated MM is   6 months   44.2.6
     ____ months.

■ Plasmacytoma

15. **Regarding plasmacytoma.**
  a. If a single lesion consistent with MM is   plasmacytoma   44.3.1
     found, it is called p_____.
  b. In 70 to 80% this will progress to
     i. m_____ m_____ in   multiple myeloma
     ii. _____ years.   10

44

45

Pituitary Tumors – General Information and Classification

■ General Tumor Types

1. **Most pituitary tumors are benign tumors that arise from the a_____.** adenohypophysis 45.2.1

2. **Answer the following about pituitary tumors:** 45.2.1
   a. By definition what is the maximal size of a pituitary microadenoma? 1 cm
   b. Larger tumors are called _____. macroadenomas
   c. 50% of pituitary tumors are less than _____ mm. 5 mm

3. **Complete the following about pituitary carcinoma:** 45.2.2
   a. Occurence is _____. rare
   b. They are usually i_____. invasive
   c. They are usually s_____. secretory
   d. The most common hormones are
      i.   A_____ ACTH
      ii. P_____ PRL
   e. True or false. They can metastasize. True
   f. Prognosis of 1-year mortality is _____%. 66%

4. **Neurohypophyseal tumors are tumors of the _____ pituitary** posterior 45.2.3
   a. Occurrence is _____. rare

■ Epidemiology

5. **Epidemiology** 45.3
   a. Pituitary tumors represent approximately _____% of intracranial tumors. 10%
   b. They are most common in the _____ decades of life. 3rd and 4th

c. True or false. The incidence is higher among females.

false

d. Incidence is increased in MEA or MEN, especially type __.

type I

   i. This has an _____ inheritance with _____ penetrance.

autosomal dominant; high

   ii. Also involves p_____ tumors and h_____.

pancreatic islet cell tumors; hyperparathyroidism

   iii. True or False. Pituitary tumors in this syndrome are usually nonsecretory.

true

■ Clinical Presentation of Pituitary Tumors

6. Complete the following about clinical presentation of pituitary tumors:

45.5.2

a. Hormone hypersecretion

   i. _____% of adenomas secrete active hormone.

65%

   ii. prolactin _____%

48%

   iii. growth hormone _____%

10%

   iv. ACTH _____%

6%

   v. thyroid-stimulating hormone (TSH) _____%

1%

b. Prolactin can cause _____-_____ syndrome in females and _____ in males. Etiologies for increased prolactin include:

amenorrhea-galactorrhea; impotence

   i. P_____, which is neoplasia of pituitary _____.

prolactinoma; lactotrophs

   ii. S_____ effect, which may reduce _____ control over PRL secretion.

stalk effect; inhibitory

   iii. With tumors that secrete prolactin, levels are usually > _____.

1000 ng/ml

c. Growth hormone

   i. If elevated it is due to a p_____ a_____

pituitary adenoma

   ii. more than _____% of the time.

95%

   iii. Causes _____ in adults and _____ in prepubertal children.

acromegaly; gigantism

d. Corticotropin

   i. aka _____

ACTH

   ii. excess causes _____ _____

Cushing's disease

   iii. Nelson syndrome can develop only in patients who have had _____.

adrenalectomy

e. Thyrotropin (TSH) causes _____ hyperthyroidism.

secondary (central)

45

7. Complete the following about hormone hyposecretion: 45.5.2

a.   Due to _____ of the normal pituitary.   compression

b.   In order of sensitivity to compression (Hint: *go look for the adenoma*)

    i.   G_____   GH

    ii.   L_____   LH

    iii.   F_____   FSH

    iv.   T_____   TSH

    v.   A_____   ACTH

c.   Most common symptoms include o_____ h_____ and e_____ f_____.   orthostatic hypotension; easy fatigability

d.   Selective loss of one hormone, consider a_____ h_____.   autoimmune hypophysitis

e.   If diabetes insipidus is seen pre-operatively, other etiologies should be sought including

    i.   a_____ h_____   autoimmune hypophysitis

    ii.   h_____ g_____   hypothalamic glioma

    iii.   s_____ g_____ c_____ t_____   suprasellar germ cell tumor

8. Complete the following about mass effect: 45.5.2

a.   The pituitary tumor that gains the greatest size

    i.   is nonsecreting (true or false)   true

    ii.   of the secreting type is the _____   prolactinoma

b.   The tumor that is usually the smallest is the _____ tumor.   ACTH

c.   Structures commonly compressed:

    i.   Optic chiasm classically causing _____ _____.   bitemporal hemianopsia

    ii.   Third ventricle, which can cause _____ _____   obstructive hydrocephalus

    iii.   Cavernous sinus with pressure on the cranial nerves _____ causing: III, IV, V1, V2, VI

        p_____.   ptosis;

        f_____ _____   facial pain;

        d_____   diplopia

9. Patient presents with sudden onset of headache, visual disturbance, ophthalmoplegia, and reduced mental status. Complete the following: 45.5.2

a.   Consider diagnosis of p_____ a_____.   pituitary apoplexy (due to expanding mass in sella turcica resulting from hemorrhage or necrosis)

b.   This may occur in macroadenomas in as many as _____ %   3 to 17%

45

10. **Complete the following about primary brain tumors:**   45.5.2
    a. What are the indications for rapid decompression after pituitary apoplexy?
       i. severe constriction of _____ _____   visual fields
       ii. severe deterioration of _____ _____   visual acuity
       iii. mental status changes due to _____   hydrocephalus
    b. True or False. It is necessary to remove the entire tumor.   true
    c. What else needs to be done?   treat with corticosteroids

■ Specific Types of Pituitary Tumors

11. **Complete the following about the anatomic classification of pituitary adenoma:**   45.6.1
    a. Named the _____ system   Hardy
    b. Suprasellar extension
       i. O: _____   none
       ii. A: expanding into the _____ cistern   suprasellar
       iii. B: anterior recesses of third ventricle _____   obliterated
       iv. C: _____ of third ventricle _____   floor; displaced
    c. Floor of sella
       i. I: intact or _____ _____   focally expanded
       ii. II: sella _____   enlarged
    d. Sphenoid extension
       i. III: localized _____ of sella floor   perforation
       ii. IV: diffuse _____ of sella floor   destruction

12. **Complete the following about functional pituitary tumors:**   45.6.2
    a. What is the most common functional pituitary tumor?   prolactinoma
    b. What are its most common symptoms?
       i. In females: _____-_____   amenorrhea-galactorrhea
       ii. called the _____-_____ syndrome   Forbes-Albright syndrome
       iii. In males: _____   impotence
    c. It arises from anterior pituitary l_____.   lactotrophs
    d. The most common cause of amenorrhea is p_____.   pregnancy

45

13. **Answer the following about Cushing's syndrome:**   45.6.2
a. Which hormone?   ACTH
b. Hypersecretion is called _____ _____.   Cushing's disease
c. Accounts for ___ - ___% of pituitary   10-12%
   adenomas.
d. Other causes of hypercortisolism are   Cushing's syndrome
   known as_____ _____.
e. List the clinical findings in Cushing's
   syndrome:
   Hint: steroids
   i.   s_____   striae
   ii.   t____ _____   thin skin
   iii. e_____   ecchymosis
   iv.   r____ _____   reduced libido
   v.   o_____   obesity
   vi.   i_____, _____ _____   impotence, increased BP
   vii. d_____   diabetes
   viii. s____ _____   skin hyperpigmentation

14. **Complete the following about Nelson Syndrome:**   45.6.2
a. Follows bilateral a_____ in ___ -   adrenalectomy;
   ___% of cases.   10-30%
b. Classic triad includes
   i.   h_____,   hyperpigmentation
   ii.   increase in _____ and   ACTH
   iii. enlargement of the p_____   pituitary
         tumor.
   iv.   Usually occurs __ to ___ years after   1 to 4 years
         adrenalectomy.
c. Hyperpigmentation is due to cross-   melanocyte-stimulating
   reactivity of m_____ s_____   hormone; ACTH
   h_____ and _____.
d. The earliest signs include
   i.   l_____ n_____   linea nigra
   ii.   midline pigmentation from the   umbilicus
         pubis to u_____
   iii. and hyperpigmentation of   scars; gingivae
         s_____, g_____ and areolae.
e. Has an ACTH level greater than   200
   _____ Ng/l. The normal being less   54
   than _____ Ng/l

15. **Answer the following about acromegaly:**   45.6.2
a. > _____% of cases of excess GH result   95%;
   from pituitary _____ adenoma.   somatotroph
b. Ectopic GH secretion may uncommonly
   occur with:
   i.   c_____ t_____   carcinoid tumor
   ii.   l_____   lymphoma
   iii. p_____ i_____-c_____   pancreatic islet-cell tumor
         t_____

45

c. 25% of acromegalics have _____ with normal thyroid studies.   thyromegaly

d. Hypothalamus produces _____ which causes the pituitary to make _____.   GHRH; GH

e. Excess GH induces _____ secretion from the liver, also known as _____.   IGF-1; somatomedin-C

f. What medication can suppress GH release?   somatostatin

g. Mortality rates are _____ to _____ times the expected rate due to: 2 to 3 times
   i.   c_____   cancer
   ii. c_____   cardiomyopathy
   iii. d_____   diabetes
   iv. h_____   hypertension
   v.   i_____   infection
   vi. n_____ _____   neural entrapment

16. **Answer the following regarding TSH-secreting adenomas:**   45.6.2
   a. Comprise of __ to __% of pituitary tumors.   0.5 to 1%
   b. Produces _____ hyperthyroidism   central (secondary)
   c. Elevated _____ and _____ levels with elevated or inappropriately normal _____.   T3 and T4; TSH
   d. True or False. Most of these tumors are invasive and large enough to produce mass effect.   true
   e. Symptoms of hyperthyroidism include
   i.   a_____   anxiety
   ii. p_____   palpitations (due to a-fib)
   iii. h_____ i_____   heat intolerance
   iv. h_____   hyperhidrosis
   v.   w_____ l_____   weight loss

17. **Answer the following regarding pathology of pituitary tumors:**   45.6.2
   a. Chromophobes are most common. May produce _____, _____, or _____.   prolactin, GH, or TSH
   b. Acidophils produce _____, _____, _____.   prolactin, TSH, GH
   c. Basophils produce _____, _____, _____; _____ disease   gonadotropins, β-lipotropin, ACTH; Cushing's disease

18. **Complete the following about tumors of the neurohypophysis and infundibulum:**   45.6.3
   a. The most common tumor in the posterior pituitary is _____.   metastatic
   b. The most common primary tumor is the _____ _____ _____ with a predilection for the _____.   granular cell tumor (GCT) stalk
   c. If this tumor is suspected, operative approach is _____ preferred over _____.   transcranial preferred over transphenoidal

45

46

Pituitary Adenomas – Evaluation and Nonsurgical Management

■ Evaluation

1. **Answer the following regarding visual field deficit patterns:** 46.1.2
   a. The chiasm is located
      i. above the sella in _____% 79%
      ii. posterior to the sella in ____% 4% (postfixed chiasm)
      iii. anterior to the sella in ____ % 5% (prefixed chiasm)
   b. Classic visual field deficit is b_____ bitemporal hemianopsia
      h_____.
   c. Optic nerve compression is more likely postfixed
      with a p_____ chiasm.
      i. Loss of vision in _____ eye. ipsilateral
      ii. There is usually a _____ superior (temporal)
          _____ in the _____ eye quadrantanopsia;
          resulting from compression of the contralateral; anterior knee of
          _____. Wilbrand.
   d. Compression of the optic tract may prefixed;
      occur with _____ chiasm, producing homonymous hemianopsia
      _____ _____.

2. **Answer the following regarding adrenal axis screening:** 46.1.2
   a. Cortisol levels normally peak between __ 7-8 AM
      - __ AM.
   b. ____ AM cortisol better for detecting 8 AM;
      _____. hypocortisolism
   c. Levels < _____ suggestive of adrenal 6 mcg/100 ml
      insufficiency.
   d. Levels between ___ and ____ are 6 and 14 mcg/100 ml
      nondiagnostic.

46

e. _____ is more accurate for _____   24 hr urine free cortisol; hypercortisolism

f. Normally, ____ dose dexamethasone suppresses release of _____ through negative feedback.   low dose; ACTH

    i. 8 AM cortisol < _____ rules out Cushing's syndrome in most patients.   1.8 mcg/dl

    ii. Cushing's syndrome is probably present with cortisol > ____.   10 mcg/dl

    iii. _____ tumors and most cases of ectopic ACTH production will not suppress even with ____ dose dexamethasone.   Adrenal; high dose

3. **Thyroid axis:**   46.1.2

a. Check ____ (total or free) and _____.   T4; TSH

b. Thyrotropin-releasing hormone (TRH) stimulation test is indicated if _____ or borderline.   T4

c. Chronic _____ _____ may produce secondary pituitary hyperplasia indistinguishable from adenoma.   primary hypothyroidism

d. This is due to loss of _____ feedback from _____ _____ causing increase in release of _____ from the _____.   negative; thyroid hormone; TRH; hypothalamus

e. Reduced response to TRH stimulation test indicates _____ _____.   secondary (pituitary) hypothyroidism

f. Etiologies for primary hyperthyroidism include

    i. localized hyperactive _____   thyroid nodule

    ii. circulating ____ that stimulate the thyroid   antibodies

    iii. _____ _____ _____ (AKA ophthalmic hyperthyroidism)   diffuse thyroid hyperplasia

4. **Hormone evaluation in acromegaly:**   46.1.2

a. _____ is the recommended initial test.   IGF-1

b. Checking a single random ____ may not be a reliable indicator and is therefore not recommended.   GH

c. Normal basal fasting GH level is < ____   5 ng/ml

d. Oral glucose suppression test (OGST):

    i. Give ___ oral glucose load and measure _____.   75 gm; GH

    ii. If ____ nadir is not < _____, the patient has acromegaly.   GH; 1 ng/ml

    iii. GH suppression may be absent with _____.   liver disease, uncontrolled DM, and renal failure

46

5. **Inferior petrosal sinus sampling uses a microcatheter to measure _____ levels at baseline then at 2, 5, and 10 minutes after stimulation with IV ____.**   ACTH; CRH   46.1.2

a. Baseline IPS ACTH to peripheral ACTH ratio ____ is consistent with primary Cushing's disease.   1.4:1

b. Post CRH ratio > ____ is also consistent with primary Cushing's disease.   3

c. Complication rate is ____ % including puncture of sinus wall.   1-2%

6. **A potent ACTH analogue _____ can be used to assess cortisol reserve.**   cosyntropin   46.1.2

a. Give _____ and check cortisol levels at 60 mins. Normal response is peak level > ___ AND an increment > ____ or peak >_____ regardless of increment.   cosyntropin; 18 mcg/dl; 7 mcg/dl; 20 mcg/dl

b. Subnormal response indicates _____ _____.   adrenal insufficiency

c. Response may be normal in mild cases of _____ _____ _____ or early after _____ _____ where _____ _____ has not occurred.   reduced pituitary ACTH; pituitary surgery; adrenal atrophy

7. **Complete the following about the insulin tolerance test:**   46.1.2

a. Insulin IV will promptly lower _____.   blood glucose

b. Hypoglycemia is a _____.   stressor

c. In response, the body produces c_____.   cortisol

d. An increment in baseline more than _____ to a peak of _____ mg/dL is normal.   6 mg/dl; 20 mg/dl

e. Peak cortisol = _____: Steroids needed only for stress   16-20 mg/dl

f. Peak cortisol < ___: Glucocorticoid replacement is needed.   16 mg/dl

g. Cushing's syndrome: Increment < ____   6 mg/dl

8. **Characterize the neurohypophysis on MRI.**   46.1.2

a. Normally on T1WI is _____ _____   high signal

b. possibly because it contains p_____.   phospholipids

c. Absence of this sign suggests d_____ i_____.   diabetes insipidus

9. **For pituitary tumors, what is the benefit of coronal CT slices?**   46.1.2

a. sphenoid series _____   midline (can be identified by anatomy of sphenoid sinus septa)

b. sella floor _____   erosion (indicate presence of tumor on one side)

46

■ Management/Treatment Recommendations

10. What is the medical treatment for the following?

a.	growth hormone-secreting tumors	octreotide	46.2.5
b.	ACTH-secreting tumors	ketoconazole	46.2.6
c.	prolactin-secreting tumors	bromocriptine	46.2.4
d.	TSH-secreting tumors	octreotide	46.2.7

11. Complete the following about *nonsecreting* pituitary adenomas: 46.2.3

a. Usual treatment is _____ or _____.   surgery or radiation

b. Bromocriptine may reduce tumor size in only ____% of patients   20%

c. Poor results are due to the paucity of _____ receptors.   dopaminergic

d. Octreotide reduces the tumor size in _____%.   10%

e. Follow-up by MRI at _____, _____, _____, and _____ years.   0.5, 1, 2, and 5 years

12. Complete the following on management of prolactinomas: 46.2.4

a. Prolactin level < ____ in tumors not extensively invasive. Levels may be normalized with surgery.   500 ng/ml

b. Prolactin level > _____: Chances of normalizing with surgery are very low.   500 ng/ml

c. Medical management with _____.   dopamine agonists

d. These drugs work by binding _____ receptors inhibiting synthesis and secretion of _____.   dopamine; prolactin

e. Bromocriptine affects both _____ and _____ receptors.   D1 and D2

f. _____ is a selective _____ agonist.   Cabergoline; D2

g. If response is satisfactory, it is recommended to treat for ___ to ___ years for microadenomas and check _____ yearly.   1 to 4 years; prolactin

h. If prolactin level remains > ___, consider surgery.   50 ng/ml

13. Management of acromegaly: 46.2.5

a. _____ is currently the best initial therapy.   Surgery

b. _____ are used for initial medical therapy.   Somatostatin analogues

c. _____ which is a GH antagonist may be used.   Pegvisomant

46

14. **Management of Cushing's desease:**   46.2.6
    a. _____ _____ is the treatment   Transphenoidal surgery
       choice for most.
    b. Cure rates are ___ for microadenomas   ~85%
       but lower for larger tumors.
    c. For medical therapy, _____ is an   ketoconazole;
       _____ that blocks adrenal steroid   antifungal agent
       synthesis.
    d. What are the indications for total   non-resectable pituitary
       bilateral adrenalectomy? (4)   adenoma; failure of medical
                                        therapy/surgery; life-
                                        threatening Cushing's
                                        disease; Cushing's disease
                                        with no evidence of pituitary
                                        tumor.
    e. Follow-up after bilateral adrenalectomy   Nelson's syndrome
       to rule out _____ syndrome.

15. **Management of TSH-secreting**   46.2.7
    adenomas:
    a. First-line treatment is _____   transphenoidal surgery

       _____.
    b. The tumor may be difficult to remove   fibrous
       and _____.
    c. Medical treatment is with the same   acromegaly;
       agent as for _____ namely,   octreotide

       _____.

■ Radiation Therapy for Pituitary Adenomas

16. **True or False. Radiation therapy**   false   46.3.3
    should be routinely used following
    surgical removal.

46

47

Pituitary Adenomas – Surgical Management, Outcome, and Recurrence Management

■ Surgical Treatment for Pituitary Adenomas

1. **What is the medical preparation for surgery?**   47.1.1
   a. Steroids _____ dose — stress
   b. Hypothyroid patients ideally to be treated before surgery for _____ weeks. — 4 weeks
   c. However, do not replace _____ _____ until the _____ _____ is assessed. Doing so may precipitate _____ _____. — thyroid hormone; adrenal axis; adrenal crisis

2. **Intraoperative disasters during transphenoidal surgery are usually related to _____ of _____.** — loss of landmarks
   a. This may include injury of c_____ _____ typically injured in lateral aspect of opening. — carotid artery   47.1.3
   b. Opening through the c_____ may cause erroneous biopsy of the p_____. — clivus; pons
   c. Opening through floor of _____ _____ may cause injury to _____ _____ with entry into _____ _____ _____. — frontal fossa; olfactory nerves; inferior frontal lobes
   d. The incidence of CSF rhinorrhea (fistula) is ___% — 3.5%   47.1.4

3. **Answer the following regarding post-operative management:**   47.1.6
   a. Avoid _____ _____, which can cause negative pressure on sphenoid sinus and aggravate ____ ____. — incentive spirometry; CSF leak
   b. What are diagnostic criteria for diabetes insipidus? — urine output > 250 for 1-2 hrs and SG < 1.005
   c. Transient DI typically lasts ___ to ___ post-op then normalizes. — ~12 to 36 hours

47

d. Triphasic response involves the following three stages:
   i. _____ due to injury to _____ pituitary   DI (short duration); posterior
   ii. _____ or _____ due to release of _____ from neuron endings from hypothalamus   Normalization or SIADH; ADH
   iii. _____   DI (long-term)
e. Taper and stop hydrocortisone ___ - ___ hrs post-op. Then check _____ AM cortisol.   24-48 hours; 6 AM
f. Cortisol level < _____ suggests _____ deficient.   3 mcg/dl; ACTH
g. Cortisol level > _____ is normal.   9 mcg/dl

■ Outcome Following Transsphenoidal Surgery

4. **Characterize the good outcomes of transphenoidal surgery:**
a. Vision is _____ _____.   significantly improved   47.2.2
b. Cure attained in ___% of prolactinomas.   25%   47.2.3
c. Overall, ____% of all acromegalics had a biochemical cure.   50%
d. Cure rate among Cushing's disease with microadenomas is ____%.   85%
e. Recurrence incidence is ____% with most recurring __ - __ years post-op.   12%; 4 to 8 years

47

48

Cysts and Tumor-Like Lesions

■ Rathke's Cleft Cyst

1. Describe Rathke's cleft cyst (RCC)   48.1
a. Where are the lesions located?   intrasellar-pars intermedia
b. How common are they?   incidental finding in 13-23%
                                           of autopsies
c. Do you find RCC together with pituitary   no
   adenomas?
d. Why?   RCCs have a similar lineage to
                                           pituitary adenomas and are
                                           rarely found together.

e. Appearance on CT
   i.   cystic?   yes
   ii. density?   low density
   iii. enhancement?   may have capsular
                                           enhancement
f. Cell lining is described as s_____ l_____   single layer cuboidal
   c_____ e_____   epithelium
g. Cyst wall is _____.   thin
h. What is the surgical treatment?   partial excision and drainage

■ Colloid Cyst

**2. Complete the following regarding
   Colloid cyst:**
a. Usual age of diagnosis is ___ - ___ years.   20-50 years   48.2.1
b. Most commonly found in _____ _____   third ventricle;   48.2.2
   in the region of _____ of _____. foramen of Monro
c. Pathognomonic hydrocephalus involving   lateral
   only _____ ventricles.
d. On MRI, usually _____ on T1   hyperintense;   48.2.4
   and _____ on T2.   hypointense
e. Symptomatic patients may be more   hyperintense;
   likely to display T2 _____ cysts,   water
   indicating high _____ content, which
   may reflect a propensity for cyst
   expansion.
f. LPs are _____ prior to the   contraindicated;
   placement of shunt due to risks of   herniation
   _____.

3. **Treatment for Colloid cysts:**   48.2.5
    a. The nature of the obstruction requires   bilateral;
        b_____ ventricular shunting.   unilateral;
        Alternatively, one can use u_____   fenestration; septum
        shunt with f_____ of the s_____   pellucidum
        p_____.
    b. Transcallosal approach has higher   venous;
        incidence of v_____ infarction or   forniceal
        f_____ injury.
    c. True or False. Transcallosal approach   false
        depends on dilated ventricles.
    d. Transcortical approach has higher   post-op seizures
        incidence of p_____ s_____.
    e. What are features of colloid cysts that
        correlate with unsuccessful stereotactic
        aspiration?
        i.   high _____ which correlates   viscosity;
             with _____ on CT.   hyperdensity
        ii. d_____ of the cyst from tip   deflection;
             of aspirating needed due to   small size
             _____ ____

■ Epidermoid and Dermoid Tumors

4. **Complete the following regarding**   48.3.1
    epidermoid and dermoid cysts:
    a. Both are d_____, b_____ tumors that   developmental, benign;
        may arise when retained _____ implants   ectodermal;
        are trapped by two fusing _____   ectodermal
        surfaces.
    b. Growth rate is l_____ rather than   linear;
        e_____ as with neoplastic tumors.   exponential
    c. Most common intracranial sites include
        i.   s_____, which commonly   Suprasellar;
             produces b_____ _____ and   bitemporal hemianopsia;
             o_____ a_____.   optic atrophy
        ii. S_____ f_____, which may   Sylvian fissure;
             present with _____.   seizures
        iii. C_____, which can produce   CPA (Cerebellopontine
             _____ _____ especially in   angle); trigeminal neuralgia;
             _____ patients.   young
        iv. b_____-p_____ _____, which   basilar-posterior fossa;
             can produce l_____ c_____   lower cranial nerve;
             n_____ findings or _____   cerebellar dysfunction
             _____.
        v.   Within the _____ system,   ventricular;
             particularly the _____.   4th ventricle
    d. Within the spinal canal, most arise in the
        following locations:
        i.   _____   thoracic spine
        ii. _____   upper lumbar spine

48

e. Epidermoids may occur iatrogenically following _____ _____.

lumbar puncture

f. Dermoids of the spinal canal are usually associated with a d_____ s_____ t_____, which can produce recurrent bouts of spinal _____.

dermal sinus tract; meningitis

5. **Complete the following regarding epidermoid cysts:**

48.3.3

a. Usually arise from e_____ trapped within the _____.

ectoderm; CNS

b. Also known as c_____, which is most often used to describe the lesion in _____ _____ where entrapped epithelium arises from chronic m_____ e_____ i____.

cholesteatoma; middle ear; middle ear infections

c. Epidermoids are lined by _____ _____ epithelium and contain:

stratified squamous

i. _____

keratin

ii. _____

cellular debris

iii. _____

cholesterol

d. Epidermoid cysts are sometimes mistaken for c_____ g_____, which usually occur following c_____ i_____.

cholesterol granulomas; chronic inflammation

e. Rupture of cyst contents may cause recurrent episodes of _____ _____, which may also lead to _____.

aseptic meningitis; hydrocephalus

f. M_____ _____ is a rare variant of _____ which includes the finding of _____ _____ in the CSF.

Mollaret's meningitis; meningitis; large cells

■ Craniopharyngioma

6. **Complete the following regarding craniopharyngiomas:**

48.4.1

a. Usually develop from residual cells of _____ _____ and tend to arise from _____ _____ margin of the p_____.

Rathke's pouch; anterior superior; pituitary

b. Some may arise primarily within the _____ ventricle.

third

c. Fluid in the cysts usually contain c_____ c_____.

cholesterol crystals

d. Peak incidence occurs during age ___ - ____.

5 to 10 years

48

49

Pseudotumor Cerebri and Empty Sella Syndrome

■ Pseudotumor Cerebri

1. Complete the following regarding pseudotumor cerebri: 49.1.1
a. Diagnostic criteria:
  i.   CSF pressure above   20 to 25 cm H_2O
  ii. CSF composition   normal protein, glucose, and cell count
  iii. Symptoms and signs   increased pressure
  iv. Radiologic studies   normal CT and MRI
b. Severe visual defects occur in __ to ___%   4 to 12%
c. Best test to follow vision is _____.   perimetry

2. Describe pseudotumor cerebri treatment. 49.1.9
a. Withdraw patient from _____.   OCPs (oral contraception pills)
b. Medications for treatment include:
  i.   D_____   Diamox
  ii. L_____   Lasix
  iii. D_____   Dexamethasone
c. Procedures to consider include
  i.   serial L_____   LPs
  ii. l_____ _____   lumbo-peritoneal shunt
  iii. o_____ _____ _____ optic sheath fenestration

■ Empty Sella Syndrome

3. Complete the following regarding empty sella syndrome:
a. Herniation of the _____ _____ into   arachnoid membrane; 49.2.2
the _____ _____ can act as a mass, sella turcica;
probably as a result for repeated   CSF pulsation
_____ _____.
b. Female:male ratio is _____.   5:1
c. Associated with _____ and _____.   obesity and hypertension
d. Surgical treatment is usually _____   not indicated;
except in cases of _____.   (CSF) rhinorrhea
e. Secondary causes include: 49.2.3
  i.   t_____   trauma
  ii. r_____ of p_____ t_____ removal of pituitary tumor
  iii. increased i_____ _____ intracranial pressure

50

Tumors and Tumor-Like Lesions of the Skull

■ Skull Tumors

1. **The most common primary bone tumor of the calvaria**   50.1.2
   a. is the o_____.   osteoma
   b. It usually involves only the o_____ t_____.   outer table
   c. Lesions within _____ _____ may present with recurrent _____.   air sinuses; sinusitis
   d. The triad of Gardner's syndrome:
       i. _____   multiple cranial osteomas
       ii. _____   colonic polyposis
       iii. _____   soft-tissue tumors

2. **Complete the following regarding hemangiomas:**   50.1.3
   a. They comprise _____% of skull tumors.   7%
   b. The two types are c_____ (most common) and c_____ (rare)   cavernous; capillary
   c. Accessible lesions may be cured by e___ b____ e_____ or c_____.   en bloc excision; curettage

3. **Complete the following regarding Langerhans cell histiocytosis:**   50.1.5
   a. Most common presenting symptom is _____, _____ _____ _____.   tender, enlarging skull mass
   b. Most common site is the _____ bone.   parietal
   c. True or False. Involves both inner and outer tables.   true
   d. Can differentiate from hemangioma by abscess of _____ appearance.   sunburst

4. **Complete the following on chordomas:**   50.1.6
   a. Chordomas are _____ tumors usually arising from c_____ or s_____.   malignant; clivus or sacrum
   b. Derived from remnants of the p_____ n_____ which normally differentiates into the _____ _____of i_____ d_____.   primitive notochord; nucleus pulposus; intervertebral disks

c. Peak age of cranial chordomas is ____ to ____ years.   50 to 60 years

d. Differential diagnosis of foramen magnum region tumors include:

    i. _____   chondrosarcomas

    ii. _____   chondromas

■ Non-neoplastic Skull Lesions

5. Complete the following regarding hyperostosis frontalis interna: 50.2.2

a. It's a benign irregular nodular thickening of the _____ _____ of the _____ _____ that is almost always _____.   inner table; frontal bone; bilateral

b. Associated with Morgagni's syndrome which includes:

    i. h_____   headache

    ii. o_____   obesity

    iii. v_____   virilism

    iv. n_____   neuropsychiatric disorders

c. Endocrinologic abnormalities include:

    i. a_____   acromegaly

    ii. h_____   hyperprolactinemia

d. Metabolic abnormalities include:

    i. h_____   hyperphosphatemia

    ii. o_____   obesity

6. Complete the following regarding fibrous dysplasia: 50.2.3

a. It is a benign condition in which normal bone is replaced by _____ _____ _____.   fibrous connective tissue

b. Most lesions occur in _____ or craniofacial bones, especially the _____.   ribs; maxilla

c. Can be part of _____-_____ syndrome.   McCune-Albright syndrome

51

Tumors of the Spine and Spinal Cord

■ Compartmental Locations of Spinal Tumors

1. **Compartment locations of spinal tumors and their incidence are**   51.2
    a. extradural in _____%   55%
    b. intradural extramedullary in _____%   40%
    c. intramedullary in _____%   5%
    d. Most metastases are _____.   extradural   51.5.3

■ Differential Diagnosis: Spine and Spinal Cord Tumors

2. **Complete the following regarding extradural spinal cord tumors:**   51.3.2
    a. Arise in _____ _____ or _____ tissue.   vertebral body; epidural
    b. Osteoblastic tumors indicate _____ _____ in men and _____ _____ _____ in women.   prostate metastases; breast cancer metastases

3. **Aneurysmal bone cyst is**   51.3.2
    a. an _____ lesion consisting of a highly vascular honeycomb of blood-filled cavities separated by _____ _____ septa and surrounded by thin _____ _____ which may expand.   osteolytic; connective tissue; cortical bone

4. **Most common intradural extramedullary tumors:**   51.3.4
    a. m_____   meningiomas
    b. n_____   neurofibromas

■ Intradural Extramedullary Spinal Cord Tumors

5. **Characterize spinal meningiomas.**   51.4.1
    a. Peak age is ___ - ___ years.   40-70 years
    b. The female:male ratio is _____.   4:1
    c. Main symptom is _____.   local or radicular pain

51

6. **Characterize spinal schwannomas.**   51.4.2
   a. _____, _____ tumors.   Slow-growing, benign
   b. 75% arise from _____.   dorsal rootlets
   c. Early symptoms are _____.   radicular

■ Intramedullary Spinal Cord Tumors

7. **The most common glioma of the**   ependymoma   51.5.3
   lower cord, conus, and filum is
   _____.
   a. These tumors of the conus and filum are   myxopapillary
      usually of the _____ subtype.

■ Primary Bone Tumors of the Spine

8. **True or False. Regarding osteoid**   51.6.2
   osteomas:
   a. They are benign lesions presenting less   true
      than 1 cm in size.
   b. Osteoid osteomas often degenerate into   false
      osteoblastomas.
   c. Osteoid osteomas occur more   false
      commonly in the pedicle than
      osteoblastomas.
   d. They are expansile destructive lesions.   false (Osteoblastomas are
                                                 expansile destructive lesions.)

9. **The most common primary bone**   osteosarcoma   51.6.3
   cancer is _____.
   a. More common in _____.   children
   b. In the spine, usually occurs in _____   lumbosacral;
      region in males in their _____.   40s
   c. Biopsy needle tract _____ the area.   contaminates
   d. Survival is _____ months.   10

10. **True or False. Vertebral hemangiomas**   51.6.4
    a. are rare tumors.   false (occurs in 9-12%)
    b. May be malignant.   false
    c. are often symptomatic.   false
    d. are radiosensitive.   true (used for the uncommon
                                             painful lesion that can't be
                                             treated by excision or
                                             vertebroplasty)
    e. X-rays show v_____ s_____   vertical striations
    f. or h_____ appearance.   honeycomb

11. **Giant cell tumors of bone**   51.6.5
    a. arise from _____.   osteoclasts
    a. in the same category as _____   aneurysmal bone cysts
       _____ _____.
    b. Almost always b_____ with   benign; pseudomalignant
       p_____ behavior.
    c. Radiation is controversial because of   malignant degeneration
       possibility of m_____ d_____.

52

Cerebral Metastases

■ Metastases to the Brain

1. **Complete the following about cerebral metastases:**   52.2
   a. The most common brain tumor is   cerebral metastases
      _____ _____.
   b. It will be multiple in _____% on MRI.   70%
   c. In patients with no cancer history,   15%
      cerebral metastases are the presenting
      symptom in ____%
   d. The route of metastatic spread to the   hematogenous;
      brain is usually h_____ although   local extension
      l_____ e_____ can occur.
   e. The highest incidence of parenchymal   posterior;   52.4
      metastases is _____ to the Sylvian   MCA
      fissure, likely due to embolic spread to
      terminal _____ branches.

■ Metastases of Primary CNS Tumors. Location of Cerebral Metastases: Clinical Presentation

2. **Complete the following about brain tumors:**
   a. Which primary CNS tumors spread via   52.3.1
      the CSF?
      i.   g_____   glioma
      ii. e_____   ependymoma
      iii. P_____   PNET
      iv. p_____   pineal tumors
   b. The most common primary brain tumor   medulloblastoma   52.3.2
      responsible for extraneural spread is
      m_____.
   c. Solitary brain metastases are the most   posterior fossa   52.4
      common p_____ f_____ tumor in
      adults.

d. Spread to this location may be via
    _____ _____ plexus and
    v_____ v_____.
e. Hemorrhage occurs in
    i.   m_____
    ii.   c_____
    iii. r_____

epidural venous plexus
(Batson's plexus);
vertebral veins

52.6

melanoma
choriocarcinoma
renal cell carcinoma

■ Primary Cancers in Patients with Cerebral Metastases

52

3. **Sources of cerebral mets in children:**   52.5.1
    a. n_____
    b. r_____
    c. W_____

neuroblastoma
rhabdomyosarcoma
Wilm's tumor

4. **Where do brain metastases come**   52.5.1
    from?
    a. l_____
    b. b_____
    c. r_____
    d. i_____ t_____
    e. m_____

lung (44%)
breast (10%)
renal (7%)
intestinal tract (6%)
melanoma (3%)

5. **Complete the following about small**   52.5.2
    cell lung cancer:
    a. aka o_____ c_____ cancer   oat cell
    b. Strongly associated with _____.   smoking (tobacco)
    c. Reaction to radiation is very _____. sensitive
    d. The most common type of non-small cell   adenocarcinoma
        lung cancer is _____.

6. **Complete the following about**   52.5.3
    metastatic melanoma:
    a. Longevity after detected in the brain is   113
        _____ days.
    b. Unless it is a single melanoma   3 years
        metastasis, then patient may live _____
        years.
    c. True or False. Melanoma is responsive to   false
        chemotherapy and radiation.
    d. With chemotherapy for melanoma, the   dacarbazine
        gold standard is d_____.
    e. Immunotherapy that is as effective as   Melacine
        chemotherapy is a vaccine: M_____
    f. Patients with Karnofsky performance   70
        scale (KPS) score < _____ are likely to
        be poor surgical candidates.

■ Management

7. Highly radiosensitive brain metastases include: 52.8.5

a. s_____ _____ ____   small-cell lung Ca
b. g_____ _____   germ-cell tumors
c. l_____   lymphoma
d. l_____   leukemia
e. m_____   multiple myeloma

8. Metastatic tumors highly resistant to radiation therapy include: 52.8.5

a. t_____   thyroid
b. r_____ _____   renal cell
c. m_____   melanoma
d. s_____   sarcoma
e. a_____   adenocarcinoma

9. Complete the following regarding radiation therapy for cerebral metastases: 52.8.5

a. The standard dose is
   i.   _____ Gy in   30
   ii. _____ fractions over   10
   iii. _____ weeks.   2
b. After the usual dose of radiation therapy, what percentage of patients develop dementia at
   i. 1 year: _____%   11%
   ii. 2 years: _____%   50%

■ Carcinomatous Meningitis

10. Complete the following about carcinomatous meningitis:

a. Symptoms include _____ and _____ _____ dysfunction.   headache; cranial nerve   52.10.2
b. CSF is eventually abnormal in _____%.   95%   52.10.3
c. What size sample of CSF is needed?   at least 10 cc of CSF
d. Survival is _____ months without treatment and ___ to ___ months with treatment.   2 months; 5 to 8 months   52.10.4
e. Always include l_____ m_____ in the differential diagnosis.   lymphomatous meningitis   52.10.1

52

53

Spinal Epidural Metastases

■ General Information

1. Complete the following regarding spinal epidural metastasis (SEM):

53.1

a. It occurs in _____% of all cancer patients.

10%

b. It most commonly arises from
- i. l_____ — lung
- ii. b_____ — breast
- iii. p_____ — prostate
- iv. m_____ — myeloma
- v. l_____ — lymphoma

c. One route of metastasis to the spine is by B_____ p_____.

Batson's plexus (spinal epidural veins)

d. The site of metastasis is p_____ to the length of the segment of spine.

proportional

e. First symptom is usually
- i. p_____ which is — pain
- ii. worse in r_____. — recumbency

■ Evaluation and Management of Epidural Spinal Metastases

2. Complete the following regarding conus medullaris SEM and cauda equina lesions:

Table 53.2

a. Conus medullaris lesions
- i. spontaneous pain — rare
- ii. sensory deficit — saddle, bilateral
- iii. motor loss — symmetric
- iv. autonomic symptoms — prominent early
- v. reflexes — only ankle jerk absent
- vi. onset — sudden and bilateral

b. Cauda equina lesions
- i. spontaneous pain — severe, radicular
- ii. sensory deficit — saddle, may be unilateral
- iii. motor loss — asymmetric
- iv. autonomic symptoms — late
- v. reflexes — ankle and knee jerk may be absent
- vi. onset — gradual and unilateral

3. **Complete the following regarding SEM:**

a. Outcome depends on p_____ n_____ s_____.   presenting neurological status   53.4.2

b. Grade   Table 53.3
   i.   mild   patient can walk
   ii. moderate   can move legs, but not antigravity
   iii. severe   slight residual motor and sensory function
   iv. complete   no motor, sensory, or sphincter function below level of lesion

c. Treatment for patient with new symptoms consists of   53.4.4
   i.   d_____   decadron
   ii. s_____   surgery
   iii. r_____   radiation

4. **Complete the following about MRI scans in SEM:**   53.4.3

a. They detect multiple sites of cord compression in ____%.   20%

b. They are _____ on T1WI.   hypointense

c. They are _____on T2WI.   hyperintense

5. **True or False. Regarding diagnostic imaging:**   53.4.3

a. MRI
   i.   is the diagnostic test of choice.   true
   ii. Tumor extension into the spinal canal is common when the patient presents with local back pain.   false

b. Plain x-ray
   i.   Most spinal mets are osteolytic.   true
   ii. Plain x-rays are abnormal as soon as there is bone erosion.   false

c. CT-myelo
   i.   can obtain CSF.   true
   ii. is invasive.   true
   iii. will demonstrate paraspinal lesions.   false
   iv. may require C1-C2 puncture.   true

6. **Regarding the management of SEM:**   53.4.4

a. Group I
   i.   Signs/symptoms?   rapid progression or severe deficit
   ii. When do you evaluate?   immediately

b. Group II
   i.   Signs/symptoms?   mild and stable
   ii. When do you evaluate?   admit and evaluate within 24 hrs

53

53

   c. Group III

      i.   Signs/symptoms?   pain without neurologic involvement

      ii. When do you evaluate?   as an outpatient over several days

7. What is the treatment for SEM?   53.4.5

   a. Chemotherapy is _____.   ineffective

   b. Vertebroplasty/kyphoplasty reduces pain 84%
       by _____%.

   c. radiation treatment

      i.   How soon after diagnosis?   within 24 hours

      ii. After surgery?   within 2 weeks

   d. pre-op embolization

      i.   appropriate for _____   highly vascular
           _____ tumors

      ii. such as r_____ c____   renal cell

      iii. t_____   thyroid

      iv. h_____   hepatocellular

8. Regarding surgery for SEM: 53.4.5

   a. relative contraindications:

      i.   r_____ t_____   radiosensitive tumors

      ii. t_____ p_____ > __ hours total paralysis > 8 hours

      iii. expected survival: < ___ - ___ <3-4 months
          m_____

      iv. m_____ l_____ at   multiple lesions at multiple
          m_____ l_____   levels

   b. indication for surgery:

      i.   greater than _____% block 80%

      ii. r_____ p_____   rapid progression

   c. other indications:

      i.   u_____ p_____   unknown primary

      ii. r_____-r_____ t_____ radio-resistant tumors

9. Characterize surgical treatment: 53.4.5

   a. Laminectomy is a _____ treatment poor

   b. because it _____ the spine.   destabilizes

   c. it is better to do surgery _____ anteriorly

   d. and add _____.   instrumentation

54

General Information, Grading, Initial Management

■ **General Information**

1. In GCS <8, surgical lesions make up ___. With significant head injury, be weary of ___ spine fractures.

   25%;
   C1-C3

   54.1.1

2. With significant head injury, delayed deterioration occurs in ___ %. 75% of these will have an i_____ h_____.

   15%;
   intracranial hematoma

   54.1.2

■ **Grading**

3. Match with mild-moderate-severe

   a. GCS 14 — mild
   b. Focal Neurological defect — moderate
   c. GCS 15 + Impaired Alertness or memory — mild
   d. GCS 5-8 — severe
   e. LOC > 5min — moderate
   f. GCS 15 + Brief LOC — mild

   54.2

■ **Management in E/R**

4. Hypotension (defined as _____) and hypoxia (defined as apnea, cyanosis or PaO$_2$ _____), can _____ the risk of bad outcome.

   SBP <90 mm Hg;
   PaO$_2$ <60 mm Hg;
   triple

   54.4.1

5. Decerebrate or decorticate posturing will usually be _____ to the blown pupil.

   contralateral

   Table 54.2

6. Sedatives and paralytics should be used for i____ h____, i____, t____.

   intracranial hypertension, intubation, transport

   54.4.1

7. Trauma intubation practice guidelines GCS ___.

   GCS<8

   54.4.1

8. True or False.   54.4.1

a. Peri-procedural antibiotics reduce risk of pneumonia and decreases length of stay or mortality.

false (does not alter length of stay or mortality)

b. Hyperventilation should be used prophylactically for severe head trauma patients.

false

9. Ideal PaCO$_2$ should be ____.   30-35mm Hg   54.4.1

10. Hyperventilation can cause _____ (increase or decrease) protein binding of calcium and develop _____ (hyper or hypo) calcemia with tetany.

increase; hypocalcemia   54.4.1

11. Regarding mannitol use.   54.4.1

a. Contraindication to mannitol is h_____ or h_____.

hypotension or hypovolemia

b. In patients with CHF, consider pre-treating with ____ due to transient _____ (increase or decrease) of intravascular volume.

furosemide; increase

12. True or False.   54.4.1

a. AEDs are effective in decreasing early and late post-traumatic seizures.

false (only early)

13. True or False. The following conditions have an increased risk of post-traumatic seizures (PTS):   Table 54.3

a. penetrating brain injuries   true
b. intracranial bleeding   true
c. GCS >13   false (GCS < 10)
d. alcohol abuse   true
e. subgaleal bleed   false

14. Name the condition associated with the following signs: 54.4.2

a. postauricular ecchymosis: b____ s____ f____

basal skull fracture

b. bruit over globe of eye: c____ c_____ f____

carotid cavernous fistula

c. instability of the zygomatic arch: f____ f____

facial fracture (LeFort)

d. bruit over carotid artery: c_____ d_____

carotid dissection

15. CN ___ palsy occurs with increased ICP and clival fractures.   VI (Abducens)   54.4.2

16. Which has higher risk of intracranial injury?   54.4.3

a. frontal or occipital fractures?   occipital
b. upper or lower facial fractures?   upper

■ Radiographic Evaluation

17. **CT findings**   54.5.1
   a. Subdurals are usually _____ in shape, and   crescentic;
      _____ (do or do not) cross suture lines.   do not
   b. Pneumocephalus indicates likely   skull fracture
      underlying s_____ _____.
   c. Traumatic SAH has blood thickest in   Convexity;
      _____ (circle of Willis/Convexity) and   Circle of Willis
      aneurysmal has blood thickest in _____
      (circle of Willis/convexity)

■ Patients with Associated Severe Systemic Injuries

18. **Patients with multi-system injuries**   diagnostic peritoneal lavage   54.7.1
    should receive ____ ____ ____ or ____   or FAST scan
    ____ before receiving a CT scan of the
    head.

19. **Fat embolism clinicial triad:**   54.7.2
    a. a_____ r_____ f_____   acute respiratory failure
    b. g_____ n___ d_____   global neurologic dysfunction
    c. p_____ r____   petechial rash

20. **What are the four segments of the**   54.7.3
    optic nerve and their relative length
    (in mm)?
    a. i_____, ___ mm   intraocular, 1 mm
    b. i_____, ___ - ___ mm   intraorbital, 25-30 mm
    c. i_____, ___ mm   intracanalicular, 10 mm
    d. i_____, ___ mm   intracranial, 10 mm

21. **Which is optic nerve segment is most**   intracanalicular   54.7.3
    commonly damaged?

■ Exploratory Burr Holes

22. **Placement of an emergency burr hole**   ipsilateral   54.8.1
    should be _____ (ipsilateral or
    contralateral) to the blown pupil.

54

55

Concussion, High Altitude Cerebral Edema, Cerebrovascular Injuries

---

■ Concussion

1. By definition, a concussion typically has _____ imaging studies. — normal — 55.1.4

2. True or False. The determination of concussion requires — 55.1.7
a. loss of consciousness from closed head injury. — false
b. brain swelling on computed tomography (CT) of the head. — false
c. altered consciousness as a result of a closed head injury. — true
d. nausea and vomiting after being hit in the head. — false

3. fMRI may be useful in mTBI, by showing dysfunction in f____ l____ compared to control patients. — frontal lobe — 55.1.8

4. Complete the following about concussion: — 55.1.9
a. In concussion, what brain chemical changes in concentration? — glutamate
b. Does it go up or down? — up
c. What mechanism becomes impaired? — cerebral autoregulation
d. It may predispose to m_____ c_____ e_____ — malignant cerebral edema
e. and make the patient susceptible to s_____ i_____ s_____. — second impact syndrome

5. Impaired metabolic state from a concussion can last __ - __ days after injury. — 7-10 days — 55.1.9

6. Post concussive syndrome occurs in ___ - ___% of cases, and often occurs within ___ weeks of injury, and remains ____ after onset of symptoms. — 10-15% / 4 / >1 month — 55.1.10

7. **True or False. When should a player return to the game after a mild concussion?**   55.1.12
   a. the same day   false
   b. only after resolution of symptoms   true
   c. only after CT shows no injury   false
   d. only after being able to walk or run without difficulty   false (A symptomatic patient should not return to competition.)
   e. Steroids should be the primary pharmacologic treatment in PCS.   false

8. **True or False. The second impact syndrome (SIS)**   55.1.13
   a. is rare.   true
   b. requires two head injuries.   true
   c. results from cerebral edema.   true
   d. is responsible for the policy that "no symptomatic player plays."   true
   e. can have severe consequences.   true

9. **Complete the following regarding SIS**   55.1.13
   a. SIS has a mortality of ___ to ____%.   50 to 100% (Second impact syndrome [SIS] mortality occurs in athletes who sustain a second head injury while still symptomatic from an earlier injury. They usually walk off the field, then deteriorate into a coma within minutes.)
   b. What treatment is effective for SIS?   none—condition may be refractory to all treatment

■ Other TBI Definitions

10. **Regarding contusion.**   55.2.1
    a. Low attenuation areas in a TBI in contusions represent e____.   edema
    b. High attenuation areas represent h_____.   hemorrhage

11. **In posttraumatic brain swelling, increased cerebral blood volume occurs from loss of c___ v___ a___, and has a mortality rate near ____%.**   cerebral vascular autoregulation; 100%   55.2.3

12. **Match symptoms mild-moderate-severe for diffuse axonal injury (DAI).**   Table 55.6
    a. Coma 2 hours   none
    b. Coma 30 hours   moderate
    c. flexor and extensor posturing with coma for months   severe
    d. coma with dysautonomia   severe

55

■ High-Altitude Cerebral Edema

13. **In your last trip to Machu Picchu in the high Andes you notice that the passenger sitting beside you in the train starts gasping for air and complains of severe headaches. Within minutes he becomes confused and minutes later becomes paralyzed. You suspect high altitude pulmonary edema (HAPE) with or without cerebral edema (HACE).**   55.3

   a. You pull out your handy ophthalmoscope and find in the fundus:
      i.   p_____   papilledema
      ii. r_____ h_____   retinal hemorrhages
      iii. nerve fiber layer i_____   infarction
      iv. vitreous h_____   hemorrhage
   b. This is compatible with the diagnosis of   HACE—high altitude cerebral
      h_____ a_____ c_____   edema (A milder case of
      e_____.   acute high altitude sickness
                                               [AHAS] that presents without
                                               ocular findings is called
                                               HAPE.)

   c. Prevention
      i. g_____ a_____   gradual ascent
      ii. Avoiding E_____ + h_____   ETOH + hypnotics
   d. Treating cerebral edema
      i.   i_____ d____   immediate descent
      ii. o_____   6-12 L/min O_2
      iii. s_____   steroids may be of use

14. **At the upcoming neurosurgical meeting in the Rockies, one of your colleagues presents with acute onset of inappropriate behavior, hallucinations, ataxia, and reduced mental status. If the breathalyzer is negative, what diagnosis should you consider?**   High altitude cerebral edema   55.3

   a. At 7000 ft you would be correct _____% of the time.   25%
   b. At 15,000 ft you would be correct _____% of the time.   50%

55

■ Traumatic Cervical Artery Dissections

15. **Your family medicine colleague called you after his visit to the chiropractor, and he complains of expanding neck, a whooshing sound in the neck, and some left hemiparesis.**   55.4.1
    a. What are you concerned about? c___ a___ d___   cervical artery dissection
    b. How did this occur? t___ s___ m___   therapeutic spinal manipulation
    c. What test should you order and within what time frame?   CT Angiogram, within 12 hours (if presence of BCVI would alter therapy, and no contraindication to heparin)
    d. Which test is technically the gold standard?   catheter angiogram

16. **Complete the following about blunt cerebrovascular injuries (BCVI):**
    a. The usual injury is _____.   dissection   55.4.1
    b. It occurs in ___ - ___% of BCVI patients.   1-2%   55.4.2
    c. Mortality occurs in _____%.   13%   55.4.1
    d. Which is a better test: MRI or CTA?   CTA   55.4.5
    e. Treatment is with h_____ or occasionally with e_____ techniques.   heparin; endovascular   55.4.6

17. **Traumatic fractures for blunt cerebrovascular injury (BCVI):**   Table 55.7
    a. L__ f____   Leforte fracture II or III
    b. b___ s___ f___   basilar skull fracture
    c. cervical fractures involving ___   C1-C3

18. **Carotid artery dissection occurs in __% of blunt trauma patients, and has a __% mortality rate, and about _____ are untreatable.**   1-2%; 13%; 1/3   55.4.2

19. **Denver grading scale for BCVI. Match description with appropriate grade.**   Table 55.9
    a. pseudoaneurysm   III
    b. transection with free extravasation   V
    c. luminal irregularity with <25% stenosis   I
    d. intraluminal thrombus or raised intimal flap, >25% luminal stenosis   II
    e. occlusion   IV

20. **Match the treatment with the grade.**   55.4.6
    a. endovascular occlusion   IV
    b. ASA or Heparin   I or II
    c. Heparin and repeat MDCTA or catheter angiogram in __ - __ days   III, 7-10 days
    d. urgent surgical repair if accessible   V

55

21. **In grade V BCVI dissections, if lesion is inaccessible, treatment should be**   55.4.6
    a. for complete transections: _____ or _____ e_____   ligate or occlude endovascularly
    b. for incomplete transection s_____   stenting (possible endovascular stenting with concurrent antithrombotics)

22. **Post-injury CTA for grade III was assessed, and the lesion was found to be healed. What is the next step?**   discontinue anticoagulation   55.4.6

23. **If a post-injury CTA shows incomplete lesion, consider ___ (continuing heparin or transitioning to ASA) and do a repeat imaging in ___ months.**   transitioning to ASA; 3 months   55.4.6

24. **PTT goal for heparinization should be ___ - ___ seconds. After trauma, contraindications to anticoagulation are**   40-50 seconds   55.4.6
    a. i____ h____   intracerebral hemorrhage
    b. l___ and s____ injuries   liver and spleen injuries
    c. p____ f_____   pelvic fractures

25. **Carotid artery dissections occur most commonly in _____, and the mechanism involves both h_____ and l____ r____ of the neck.**   MVA (motor vehicle accidents); hyperextension; lateral rotation   55.4.7

26. **True or False. Regarding carotid dissections.**   55.4.7
    a. Most carotid dissections occur at the ICA/ECA origin.   false: often 2cm distal to the ICA origin
    b. Internal bleeding is the most common symptom.   false: ischemic symptoms are the most common
    c. Pseudoaneurysm tends to be more favorable than an incomplete stenosis in patients with ICA dissection.   false: pseudoaneurysm stroke risk is 44% and most will persist despite heparin therapy

27. **What is the odds ratio for vertebral artery dissection caused by spinal manipulation?**   6.62R   55.4.7

28. **Fractures/injuries often associated with blunt vertebral artery injuries are**   55.4.8
    a. f_____ t_____ fractures   foramen transversarium
    b. fractures-dislocation of the _____   facet
    c. v_____ s_____   vertebral subluxation
    d. any type of c____ s____ injury   cervical spine

29. **Complete the following regarding blunt vertebral artery injury:**   55.4.8
   a. Most common etiology is _____.   motor vehicle accident
   b. Treatment to strongly consider is _____   heparin
   c. because strokes were _____ in those patients not treated.   more frequent
   d. Incidence is ____ - ____% but   0.5-0.7%
   e. increases to _____% if cervical fracture or ligament injury.   6%
   f. Is there a warning "TIA"?   no
   g. Can occur from _____ hours to _____ days.   8 hours to 12 days
   h. Is any cervical fracture pattern a predictor of blunt vertebral injury?   no
   i. Overall mortality was _____%   16%
   j. Bilateral VA dissection is highly _____.   fatal

30. **Vertebral artery dissection time from injury to stroke ranges from __ hours to __ days.**   8 hours to 12 days   55.4.8

31. **Treat all blunt vertebral injuries with ___, and restudy chronic occlusion in __ months.**   ASA; 3 months   55.4.8

55

56

Neuromonitoring

■ Intracranial Pressure (ICP)

1. The critical parameter for brain function is adequate c___ b___ f____ to meet C___ demands.

   cerebral blood flow; $CMRO_2$ demands

   56.2.2

2. CPP formula is
   CPP = _____

   CPP = MAP – ICP

   56.2.2

3. Normal CPP is _____ and would have to drop below _____ in a normal brain before CBF is impaired.

   >50mm Hg
   <40mm Hg

   56.2.2

4. If your computer does not give you mean arterial pressure (MAP) how can you calculate it? (Hint: dds/3)

   *MAP = [systolic + (diastolic x 2)] / 3

   56.2.2

5. If CPP is kept in good range, is ICP above 20 mm Hg well tolerated?

   No, it is detrimental

   56.2.2

6. Complete the following:

   56.2.3

   a. The modified _____ hypothesis states that

   Monroe-Kellie

   b. the sum of the intracranial volumes of _____, _____, and _____

   blood, brain, and CSF

   c. and other components is _____.

   constant

   d. An increase in any one must be _____

   offset

   e. by an equal _____ in another

   decrease

   f. or else _____ will rise.

   pressure

   g. Pressure is _____ _____ throughout the intracranial cavity.

   distributed evenly

7. Increased muscle tone and valsalva lead to an

   56.2.5

   a. _____ (increase or decrease) in ICP, by

   increase

   b. _____ (increased or decreased) intrathoracic pressure, leading to

   increased

   c. _____ (increased or decreased) jugular venous pressure, leading to

   increased

   d. _____ (increased or decreased) venous outflow from head.

   decreased

8. **Complete the following regarding intracranial hypertension:**

a. What is Cushing's triad?   Table 56.2

    i.   h_____   hypertension
    ii. b_____   bradycardia
    iii. r_____ i_____   respiratory irregularity

b. Risk factors for IC-HTN with a normal CT: Table 56.3

    i.   age ____   age >40
    ii. SBP ____   SBP <90
    iii. motor exam shows _____.   decerebrate or decorticate
                                          posturing

c. Neurologic Indications for ICP   GCS < 8 and abnormal CTH or   56.2.6
   monitoring: GCS of ___ and _____ or   > risk factors for IC-HTN
   _____.

9. **An important non-traumatic**   acute fulminant liver failure;   56.2.6
   indication for some centers to choose INR > 1.5
   to monitor ICP is a____ f____ l____
   f____ with INR ____ and Grade III of IV
   coma.

10. **These patients frequently require**   factor VII 40 mcg/kg IV over   56.2.6
    _____ prior to administration of   1-2 min;
    subarachnoid bolt. Bolt placement   2 hours
    should occur no more than ____ hours
    after administration.

56

11. **A criterion for discontinuing ICP**   48 to 72 hours   56.2.6
    monitoring is normal ICP for _____
    to _____ hours.

12. **Delayed onset IC-HTN may often start** day 2-3;   56.2.6
    on day ___ with a second peak at days day 9-11 – especially in peds
    ___ - ___.

13. **True or False. In regard to ICP**   56.2.6
    monitoring, it is permissible to

a. use antibiotics   true
b. not use antibiotics   true
c. place monitor in ICU   true
d. place monitor in OR   true
e. Percentage of patients who develop   true
   hemorrhage while ICP is being placed is
   1.4%.

14. **True or False.**   56.2.6

a. EVDs should be changed every 5 days to false – Does not reduce
   reduce rate of infection.   infection rate
b. Subarachnoid bolts are more accurate   false – Surface of brain may
   with higher pressures.   occlude lumen, which often
                                            show lower than actual ICP,
                                            and possible normal
                                            waveform.

15. **Complete the following regarding conversion of mm Hg and cm H_2O:**   56.2.6
    a. Can only work if the AF is concave with the infant upright, and convex when head is flat.   true
    b. Requires the patient to be in supine position.   true
    c. When the anterior fontanelle is flat, the ICP equals atmospheric pressure.   true
    d. The ICP can be estimated in mmHg as the distance from the AF to the point where venous pressure is 0.   false (cm H_2O)

16. **Complete the following regarding conversion of mm Hg and cm H_2O:**   56.2.6
    a. 1 mm Hg equals _____ cm of H_2O 1.36 cm
    b. 1 cm H_2O equals _____ mm of Hg   .735mm
    c. External auditory canal correlates with what intracranial structure?   foramen of Monro

17. **Maximum output from a ventriculostomy would be ___ - ___ml per day, where none of the CSF is absorbed.**   450-700ml   56.2.6

18. **True or False. If an external ventricular catheter no longer functions, the following can be performed safely:**   56.2.6
    a. lower drip nozzle   true
    b. verify clamps are open and air filter is dry   true
    c. flush distal tubing with saline   true
    d. flush IVC with up to 5 mL of saline under gentle pressure   false (up to 1.5ml of preservative-free saline can be used)

19. **True or False. Possible causes of an ICP wave form that is dampened include the following:**   56.2.6
    a. occlusion of the catheter proximal to the transducer   true
    b. catheter pulled out of ventricle   true
    c. collapsed ventricle   true
    d. air in the system   false
    e. intracranial hypertension   false

20. **ICP waveform in a patient with a decompressive craniectomy should appear _____.**   dampened   56.2.6

21. **Regarding normal ICP waveforms.**   56.2.6
   a. Blood Pressure variations
      i. Large (1-2mm Hg) peak corresponds   arterial systolic pressure wave
         to the a____ s___ p___ w___ with
         smaller and less distinct peaks
      ii. followed by a peak corresponding to   central venous "A" wave
         the c____ v___ a____ from the right
         atrium.
   b. Respiratory variations
      i. During expiration, pressure in   increases; decreases
         superior vena cava _____ (increases   (Expiration causes an increase
         or decreases), which _____   in SVC pressure which
         (increases or decreases) venous   decreases venous outflow
         outflow.   leading to increased ICP.)

22. **Lundberg A waves are defined by**   56.2.6
   a. ICP of _____   >50mm Hg
   b. duration of _____   5-20 min
   c. plus _____   increase in MAP

23. **Lundberg B waves are defined by**   56.2.6
   a. ICP of _____   10-20mm Hg
   b. duration of _____   30 secs to 2 minutes
   c. plus _____   periodic respiration

■ Adjuncts to ICP Monitoring

56

24. **An indication for jugular venous**   hyperventilation (pCO_2 = 20-   56.3.1
   oxygen (SjVO$_2$) or brain tissue oxygen   25)
   tension monitoring (pBtO$_2$) is _____.

25. **Jugular venous pressure is**   global;   56.3.1
   representative of g____ oxygen   focal
   content and is insensitive to f____
   pathology.

26. **Normal jugular venous oxygen**   > 60%;   56.3.1
   saturation (SjVO$_2$) is _____ and   < 50%
   desaturations to ____ suggest
   ischemia.

27. **Brain tissue oxygen tension** $pBtO_2$ <15mm Hg;   56.3.2
   monitoring shows death increases $pBtO_2$ <6mm Hg
   with sustained pBtO$_2$ of _____ or brief
   drop to ___ mmHg.

28. **Goal is to maintain pBtO$_2$ above ___.** $pBtO_2$ >25mm Hg   56.3.2

29. **pBtO$_2$ probe placement. Name the**   56.3.2
   correct diagnosis for the following
   techniques:
   a. frontal (2-3cm off midline)   ACA or A-comm aneurysm
      (near the vasospasm risk)
   b. near the site of hemorrhage   ICH
   c. least injured side   TBI
   d. 3cm lateral to midline   ACA-MCA watershed
   e. 4.5-5.5 cm off midline   MCA

30. **Treatment tier based on low pBtO$_2$**   56.3.2
    a. Tier 1
       i.   keep body temp _____ C   temp <37.5 C
       ii. increase CPP to ___ mmHg   increase CPP to >60mm Hg
    b. Tier 2
       i.   increase FIO$_2$ to _____ %   FIO$_2$ to 60%
       ii. increase PaCO$_2$ to _____ mmHg   PaCO$_2$ 45-50mm Hg
       iii. transfuse RBC until Hgb _____ g/dl Hgb >10g/dl
    c. Tier 3
       i.   increase FIO$_2$ to _____ %   FIO$_2$ 100%
       ii. decrease ICP to ___ mmHg   ICP <10 mm Hg
       iii. consider increase in___ if FIO$_2$ @   PEEP
            100%

31. **Bedside monitoring of regional CBF**   fever   56.3.3
    can be limited if patient has a f_____.

■ Treatment Measures for Elevated ICP

32. **Acute ICP crisis - Measures**   Table 56.6
    a. a __ b___ c___   airway breathing circulation
    b. e_____ h_____ of b_____   elevate head of bed
    c. n____ m_____   neck midline
    d. d___ C___ if IVC present   drain CSF
    e. m_____ 1g/kg bolus or _____ 10-   mannitol or 23% saline
       20ml
    f. h_____   hyperventilate
    g. sedation with p_____ or t_____   pentobarbital or thiopental

33. **Patients with hemorrhagic contusion**   surgical excision   56.4.4
    with progressive deterioration may
    benefit from s_____ e_____.

34. **Cushing ulcers are caused by s___**   severe head injury;   56.4.4
    h___ i____ and increased I___.   increased ICP

35. **Fluid volume goal is e_____, even**   euvolemic   56.4.4
    with mannitol.

36. **If ICP remains refractory to mannitol** hypertonic saline   56.4.4
    consider h_____ s_____.

37. **Avoid aggressive hyperventilation,**   PaCO$_2$ goal 30-35;   56.4.4
    with goal PaCO$_2$ at___, and avoid in 24 hours
    the first _____ hours after injury if
    possible.

38. **Before proceeding with "second tier"**   repeat head CT;   56.4.4
    therapy, consider repeating a H_____,   EEG to rule out subclinical
    and possible E_____ to rule out   status epilepticus
    s_____ s_____ e_____.

39. **Decompressive craniectomy should**   12 cm;   56.4.4
    have a flap at least __cm in diameter, duraplasty
    and d_____ is mandatory.

56

40.	PEEP of < ___ does not cause clinically significant increases in ICP. If needed for oxygenation, consider increasing the f_____ of ventilation.	<10 cm H$_2$O; frequency	56.4.4
41.	Prophylactic hypothermia. If used, target temperature is ___ - ____ C, and a non-significant decrease in m_____ if maintained ___ hours.	32-35C; mortality; >48 hours	56.4.4
42.	In the first 24 hours of head injury, C____ is already about h___ of normal.	CBF (cerebral blood flow); half	56.4.4

43. Hyperventilation
56.4.4
a. Avoid use in the first ___ days, and at least in the first __ hours. — 5 days, and at least in the first 24 hours
b. Do not use HPV p_____. — prophylactically
c. If used in IC-HTN, your PaCO$_2$ goal should be ___ - ___. — 30-35
d. If prolonged HPV deemed necessary, consider monitoring of S___, A___, and o/r C___ is recommended. — SjVO$_2$, AVdO$_2$, CBF
e. Do not reduce below ____. — < 25cc

44. Mannitol
56.4.4
a. First reduces IC HTN by r_____, by reducing h____ and b____ v____ then by its o____ e_____. — rheology; hematocrit and blood viscosity; osmotic effect
b. When dosing mannitol, it's important to use the s____ e_____ d_____ as it reduces effectiveness of subsequent doses. — smallest effective dose
c. Mannitol can be enhanced using f_____ as it may reduce c____ e_____ and slow p_____ of C____. — furosemide; cerebral edema; slow production of CSF

45. Hypertonic saline
56.4.4
a. Can be given as a ____ continuous infusion or ___ - ___ bolus through a central line. — 3%; 7.5-23.4%
b. Hold if serum osmolarity is _____. — >320 mOSm/L

46. Steroids
56.4.4
a. Not effective in c_____ edema seen in trauma, but reduces v____ edema seen in brain tumors. — cytotoxic edema; vasogenic edema

47.	Barbiturate therapy is recommended only if IC-HTN is refractory to maximal m___ and s___ ICP lowering therapy.	medical and surgical	56.4.4

a. Main limiting factor is h_____. — hypotension
b. True barbiturate coma requires b____ s_____ on E___. — burst suppression on EEG

56

57

Skull Fractures

■ Depressed Skull Fractures

1. **Indications for surgery in open skull fractures:**   57.3.1
   a. Depressed skull fracture that causes a n_____ d_____.   neurological deficit
   b. c____ s____ f___ l____   cerebral spinal fluid leak
   c. i_____ p_____   intradural pneumocephalus
   d. if depression is greater than __ cm or is greater than the _____   1cm; thickness of the calvarium
   e. Involvement of the f_____ s___.   frontal sinus
   f. c_____ d_____   cosmetic deformity

2. **Indications for surgery in depressed skull fractures:**   57.3.2
   a. Depression greater than ___ cm or greater than the t____ of c____   1 cm; thickness of calvaria
   b. i_____ or g_____ c_____   infection or gross contamination

3. **For contaminated fractures, when excision of depressed bone is necessary, it is recommended to soak fragment in p____ i___.**   povidone iodine   57.3.2

4. **The superior sagittal sinus is often to the ____ of the sagittal suture.**   right   57.3.2

■ Basal Skull Fractures

5. **Temporal bone fracture considerations:**   57.4.2
   a. More common temporal bone fracture is the l_____ fracture, through the p_____-s____ suture and parallel to and through the EAC.   longitudinal fracture; petro-squamosal suture
   b. Peripheral facial nerve palsy may be associated with t_____ p____ fracture due to stretching of the g_____ g_____   transverse petrous fracture; geniculate ganglion

c. Which fracture damages hearing?   transverse fracture
                                                 (horizontal)

6. **Facial EMG's after posttraumatic**   72 hours   57.4.2
    unilateral peripheral facial nerve palsy
    often takes ____ hours to become
    abnormal.

7. **True or False. Glucocorticoids have**   false   57.4.2
    been proven to improve the functional
    outcome of traumatic facial nerve
    palsy.

8. **Clival fracture considerations:**   57.4.2
    a. T_____ a____ can occur with basal skull Traumatic aneurysms
        fractures involving the clivus.
    b. A____ c____ vessels may be affected in   Anterior circulation,
        _____ _____.   transverse fractures
    c. Cranial nerve deficits ___ through ___   CN III through VI; bitemporal
        and b_____ h_____   hemianopsia
    d. Pituitary shear damage associated with   diabetes insipidus
        d_____ i_____
    e. C____ l_____   CSF leak
    f. b_____ i_____   brainstem infarctions

9. **Most sensitive test for detecting skull** CT scan   57.4.3
    base fractures is ____.

10. **Complete the following regarding**
    basal skull fractures:
    a. True or False. Pneumocephalus may be   true   57.4.3
        seen on plain skull x-rays.
    b. Postauricular ecchymosis is called   Battle's sign   57.4.4
        _____.
    c. True or False. Anosmia can be associated false (with frontal bone
        with temporal bone fractures.   fracture)
    d. Sixth nerve palsy can occur with   clival
        _____ fracture.

11. **True or False. The following are**   57.4.4
    clinical signs of basal skull fracture:
    a. CSF otorrhea or rhinorrhea   true
    b. hemotympanum   true
    c. depressed level of consciousness   false
    d. Battle's sign   true
    e. injury to cranial nerve VII   true

57

12. **Management considerations:**   57.4.5
    a. Do NOT place n___ t___, which can be   nasogastric tube;
       fatal in ____% of cases if passed   64%
       intracranially.
    b. Surgery should be considered for
       i.   t_____ a___   traumatic aneurysms
       ii. posttraumatic c____ c____ f_____   posttraumatic cavernous
                                                      carotid fistula
       iii. CSF f_____   CSF fistula
       iv. c_____ d_____   cosmetic deformities
       v.   posttraumatic f___ p___   posttraumatic facial palsy

■ Craniofacial Fractures

13. **Frontal sinus fractures**   57.5.1
    a. Anesthesia of the forehead may be due   supratrochlear and/or
       to s_____ and/or s_____ nerve   supraorbital nerve
       involvement.
    b. Mucocele formation is due to   frontonasal duct
       obstruction of the f_____ d____ or
       chronic inflammation.
    c. Only packing the sinus increases the risk   infection or mucocele
       of i_____ or m_____ formation   formation

14. **Matching. Match the type of LeFort**   57.5.2
    fracture with the structures involved.
    Type of fracture:
    ① LeFort I; ② LeFort II; ③ LeFort III
    Structures involved: (a-g) below
    a. maxilla   ①
    b. inferior orbital rim   ②
    c. orbital floor   ②, ③
    d. nasofrontal suture   ②, ③
    e. zygomatic arches   ③
    f. zygomaticofrontal suture   ③
    g. pterygoid plates   ③

■ Pneumocephalus

15. **Compartments where**   57.6.2
    pneumocephalus can be located in:
    a. e_____   epidural
    b. s____   subdural
    c. s_____   subarachnoid
    d. i_____   intraparenchymal
    e. i____   intraventricular

16. **Craniotomy: risk is higher when**   sitting   57.6.2
    patient is operated with surgery in the
    s_____ position.

57

17. **Congenital skull defects may result in pneumocephalus especially if the defect includes the t_____ t____.**   tegmen tympani   57.6.2

18. **Tension pneumocephalus might occur if**   57.6.5
    a. n_____ o_____ anesthetic is used.   nitrous oxide
    b. c_____ air is trapped.   cool
    c. b_____ v_____ opening occurs.   ball valve
    d. g_____-p_____ organisms are present.   gas-producing

19. **True or False. The presence of intracranial air may produce a characteristic sign known as**   57.6.6
    a. empty delta sign   false
    b. Mt. Hashimoto sign   false
    c. Dawson sign   false
    d. Mt. Fuji sign   true
    e. gas gap   false

20. **Treatment of pneumocephalus.**   57.6.7
    a. ____% O____ for significant or symptomatic post-op pneumocephalus   100% O_2
    b. e_____ of tension pneumocephalus   evacuation

57

58

Traumatic Hemorrhagic Conditions

■ Posttraumatic Parenchymal Injuries

1. **Bifrontal decompressive craniectomy within ____ hours of injury is a treatment option with diffuse, medically refractory posttraumatic cerebral edema and associated IC-HTN.** 48 hours 58.1.1

■ Hemorrhagic Contusion

2. **Surgical evacuation indications:** 58.2.2
   a. m _____ r_____ IC-HTN or mass effect medically refractory
   b. TICH volume _____ ml 50ml
   c. GCS ____, with f____ or t____ contusions with ___ mm MLS and or c_____ b_____ c_____. 6-8; frontal or temporal; > 5; compressed basal cisterns

3. **True or False. Regarding delayed traumatic intracerebral hemorrhage (DTICH).** 58.2.3
   a. The patient typically has GCS ≤ 8. true
   b. Incidence is ≈ 10%. true
   c. Most DTICHs occur within 72 hours of trauma. true
   d. Some patients initially appear well and then deteriorate. true
   e. Coagulopathy contributes to DTICH. true

4. **The following factors contribute to formation of delayed traumatic intracerebral hemorrhage:** 58.2.3
   a. systemic _____ coagulopathy
   b. hemorrhage into an area of n_____ b____ necrotic brain
   c. coalescence of extravasated m_____ microhematomas

■ Epidural Hematoma

5. Complete the following: 58.3.1

a. Incidence of epidural hematoma is   1%
   _____% of all head injuries.

b. Incidence of subdural hematoma is   2%
   _____% of all head injuries.

c. Epidural hematoma male to female ratio   4:1
   is _____.

d. Epidural hematoma arise from arterial   85%
   bleeding in _____%.

e. Epidural hematoma patients develop a   60%
   dilated pupil in _____%.

f. _____% are ipsilateral.   85%

g. _____% had no loss of consciousness.   60%

h. _____% had no lucid internal.   20%

i. Mortality of epidural hematoma is ____ -   20-55%
   ____.

**6. True or False. Regarding epidural   58.3.2
hematomas (EDHs).**

a. The source of bleeding is arterial 99% of   false (85% of the time)
   the time.

b. Women are more commonly affected.   false (Men are more
                                               commonly affected—4:1.)

c. EDHs are rare before age 2.   true (EDHs are rare before
                                               years or greater than 60
                                               years.)

d. The anterior meningeal artery is the   false (middle meningeal
   most common cause of the bleeding.   artery)

e. Patients with epidural hematomas can   true
   present with an ipsilateral hemiparesis.

**7. What is Kernohan notch   58.3.2
phenomenon?**

a. Compression of the _____   contralateral

b. cerebral peduncle on the _____   tentorial notch

c. which can produce _____ _____   ipsilateral hemiparesis
   hemiparesis to the intracranial mass
   lesion.

**8. True or False. Concerning epidural
hematomas.**

a. A dilated pupil is not a good localizing   false (It is a good sign.)   58.3.2
   sign as to the hematoma location.

b. It occurs in more than 15% of head   false 1%   58.3.1
   trauma admissions.

c. No initial loss of consciousness occurs in true   58.3.2
   60%.

d. No lucid interval occurs in 20%.   true

e. In pediatric head trauma, EDH should be   true
   suspected if there is a 10% drop in
   hematocrit after admission.

58

9. **True or False. A 5-year-old girl presents to the emergency room (ER) with a chief complaint of brief posttraumatic loss of consciousness after several hours of playing with her siblings. While she is being worked up in the ER, you get a call from your frantic intern who reports that the patient is now obtunded. You would expect the following signs and symptoms and would include the following statistics in your presumed diagnosis:**   58.3.2

a. early bradycardia   false (Early bradycardia is included in the differential diagnosis of posttraumatic disorder described by Denny-Brown. Late bradycardia may be seen in your presumed diagnosis, epidural hematoma.)

b. Kernohan's notch phenomenon   true (Ipsilateral hemiparesis has been described in EDH.)

c. 85% occurrence of associated ipsilateral pupillary dilation   true (60% of patients with EDH have a dilated pupil and 85% will be ipsilateral to the hematoma.)

d. a crescent-shaped high density lesion on CT   true   58.3.4

10. **What is the mortality rate of EDH?**   20 to 55%   58.3.5

11. **Nonsurgical treatment:**   58.3.6

a. is possible if size is less than _____ and   1 cm

b. patient's symptoms are _____.   mild

c. What may happen between days 5 and16?   increase in size of the hematoma

d. An epidural hematoma thicker than _____ cm should have surgery.   1cm

e. To document resolution repeat CT in ___ to ___ months.   1 to 3

f. A volume of less than _____ cc.   30

12. **Complete the following about delayed epidural traumatic hematoma (DEPTH):**   58.3.7

a. It may occur in as many as ___ - ____% of epidural hematomas.   9-10%

b. It may be related to increasing the patient's _____   BP

c. or reducing the patients _____,   ICP

d. especially following surgical removal of another _____.   epidural

e. _____ is another predisposing factor.   Coagulopathy

58

13. **True or False. Regarding posterior fossa epidural hematoma.**   58.3.7
   a. Nearly 85% will have an occipital skull fracture in adults.   true
   b. Dural sinus tears are common.   true
   c. Abnormal cerebellar signs are common.   false
   d. Overall mortality is over 25%.   true
   e. They represent ~5% of EDH.   true

■ Acute Subdural Hematoma

14. **Regarding acute subdural hematomas (ASDH).**   58.4.1
   a. There is more likely to be an underlying brain injury with an ASDH than with an EDH.   true
   b. On CT, an ASDH typically appears crescentic in shape.   true
   c. One cause of ASDH is the accumulation of blood around a parenchymal laceration.   true
   d. A "lucid interval" may be present.   true

15. **Complete the following about acute subdural hematomas:**   58.4.2
   a. Patient on anticoagulation therapy has a greater chance of ASDH
      i. if the patient is male: ____ fold   7
      ii. if the patient is female: ____ fold   26
      iii. How many days until the subdural membrane begins to form?   4

16. **CT scan in ASDH and time frame**   Table 58.1
   a. acute: ~ ___ - ___ days   1-3 days
   b. subacute: ~___ days to ___ - ___ wks   4 days to 2-3 weeks
   c. chronic: ____ wks to ___ - ___ months   >3 weeks and <3-4 months
   d. lenticular shaped: ___ - ___ months   1-2 months

17. **SDH Treatment**   58.4.3
   a. Surgical indications
      i. ASDH thickness ___ mm or MLS ___   > 10mm or >5
      ii. Do a c_____ not a b___ h___   craniotomy not a burr hole
   b. Surgical indications for smaller ASDH
      i. GCS drops by _____   2 points
      ii. and/or pupils are _____ or fixed and dilated.   asymmetric
      iii. ICP is _____   > 20
   c. Timing of Surgery
      i. Ideally should be operated on within ____ hours.   4 hours

58

18. **True or False. Regarding mortality from ASDH.**   58.4.4
    a. Mortality from an acute subdural hematoma (ASDH) ranges from 50 to 90%.   true
    b. Mortality is from the _____ _____ _____.   underlying brain injury (and not from the extraaxial bleed)
    c. Mortality is higher in young people.   false (Mortality thought to be higher in elderly patients.)
    d. Medication that increases mortality is _____.   anticoagulants

19. **Interhemispheric subdural hematomas**   58.4.5
    a. In children, consider c_____ a____.   child abuse
    b. In adults, usually due to t_____ and can also occur with r_____ a_____.   trauma; ruptured aneurysms
    c. What is falx syndrome?   paresis or focal seizures contralateral to the hematoma
    d. What symptoms can it manifest? (Hint: psadlo)
       i. p_____   paresis
       ii. s_____   seizures
       iii. a_____   ataxia
       iv. d_____   dementia
       v. l_____ difficulties   language
       vi. o_____ palsies   oculomotor

20. **True or False. Regarding infantile acute subdural hematoma.**   58.4.5
    a. Often involves loss of consciousness with initial injury.   false
    b. Skull fractures are often seen.   false
    c. Often presents with g____ s____ after injury.   generalized seizure

21. **Treatment of IASDH**   58.4.5
    a. For minimimally symptomatic cases, you can consider p_____ s____ t____.   percutaneous subdural tap

■ Chronic Subdural Hematoma

22. **What are the risk factors for chronic SDH?**   58.5.1
    (Hint: catss falls)
    a. c_____   coagulopathies
    b. a_____   alcohol abuse
    c. t_____   trauma
    d. s_____   shunts
    e. s_____   seizures
    f. f_____   falls

58

23. **Techniques that promote continued**   58.5.4
    drainage after immediate procedure
    and prevent re-accumulation:
    a. Lay the patient f____.   flat
    b. Place generous burr hole under the   temporalis muscle
        t____ m_____.
    c. Use of a s_____ d_____.   subdural drain
    d. Possible l_____ s_____ i_____ .   lumbar subarachnoid infusion

24. **For twist drill craniotomies for chronic**   58.5.4
    subdurals,
    a. a ventricular catheter is placed into the   subdural
        s_____ space.
    b. ventriculostomy bag is placed ____   20 cm;
        below the _____ _____.   craniotomy site
    c. Catheter is removed when at least _____   ~20%; 1-7 days
        of collection is drained and when patient
        shows signs of improvement which
        occurs within _____ days.

25. **Complete the following regarding**   58.5.4
    chronic subdurals:
    a. Repeat surgery is needed in _____%.   19%
    b. Is the use of a drain recommended?   Yes
    c. With a drain the need to repeat surgery   10%
        is reduced to _____%.

26. **Complete the following about chronic**   58.5.5
    subdural hematoma outcomes:
    a. Persistent fluid at 10 days: _____%   78%
    b. Persistent fluid at 40 days: _____%   15%
    c. How long till full resolution?   May take 6 months
    d. One operation is successful in   80%
        _____% of patients
    e. Two operations are successful in   90%
        _____% of patients.

27. **What are the complications of surgical**   58.5.5
    treatment of chronic SDH?
    (Hint: hherps)
    a. h_____   hemorrhage
    b. h_____   hyperemia
    c. e_____   empyema
    d. r_____   reexpansion failure
    e. p_____   pneumocephalus
    f. s_____   seizures

58

■ Spontaneous Subdural Hematoma

28. **What are the risk factors for spontaneous subdural hematomas?**   58.6.1
    a. h_____   hypertension
    b. v_____ m_____   vascular malformations
    c. n_____   neoplasms
    d. i_____   infection
    e. s_____ a_____   substance abuse
    f. h_____   hypovitaminosis
    g. C_____   coagulopathies
    h. i_____ h_____   intracranial hypotension

29. **In spontaneous SDH, bleeding sites were often a____, often involving c_____ branch of ___.**   arterial;   58.6.3
                                                                                                        cortical branch of MCA

■ Traumatic Subdural Hygroma

30. **Complete the following regarding formation of subdural hygromas:**
    a. Are they associated with trauma?   yes   58.7.1
    b. Do skull fractures occur? _____   yes; 39%
    c. Do they have membranes?   no
    d. Fluid on CT is similar to _____.   CSF   58.7.4
    e. They are created by   58.7.2
        i. a____ t_____ and   arachnoid tear
        ii. b_____ v_____ f_____   ball valve flap
    f. Can be associated post-meningitis often   haemophilus influenzae
       by _____ (species).   meningitis effusion
    g. Recurrent subdural hygromas may   subdural-peritoneal shunt   58.7.5
       benefit from a s____ p____ s_____.

■ Extraaxial Fluid Collections in Children

31. **List the differential diagnosis of extraaxial fluid collections in children.**   58.8.1
    a. a_____ s_____   acute SDH in a child with low Hct
    b. b_____ s_____   benign subdural (extraaxial) collections of infancy
    c. c_____ s_____   chronic symptomatic extraaxial fluid collections
    d. c_____ a_____   cerebral atrophy external hydrocephalus (EH)
    e. c_____ d_____   craniocerebral disproportion
    f. e_____ h_____   external hydrocephalus

32. **What is the mean age of presentation of extraaxial fluid collections of infancy?**   4 months   58.8.2

58

33. **What is the treatment of benign extraaxial fluid collections of infancy?**   58.8.2

   a. o_____   observation (Most cases resolve spontaneously within 8 to 9 months and require no treatment.)

   b. p_____ p_____ e_____   periodic physical examination (Repeat physical exam to identify development of symptoms.)

   c. h_____ c_____   head circumference every 3 to 6 months (Orbital-frontal head circumference [OFC] should be done at 3- to 6-month intervals to monitor head growth that should parallel normal growth and approach normal at 1 to 2 years.)

   d. Most will _____   resolve

   e. by _____.   1-2 years

34. **What are the treatment options for symptomatic chronic extra-axial fluid collections in children?**   58.8.3
   (Hint: otb sp)

   a. o_____   observation with serial orbital frontal head circumferences, ultrasound

   b. t_____   at least one percutaneous tap should be done to rule out infection

   c. b_____   burr-hole drainage ± external drainage

   d. s_____ p_____ s_____   subdural to peritoneal shunt (unilateral with extremely low pressure valve)

58

■ Traumatic Posterior Fossa Mass Lesions

35. **Complete the following about traumatic posterior fossa mass lesions:**   58.9

   a. Head injury that involves the posterior fossa is less than _____%.   3%

   b. The majority are e_____ h_____.   epidural hematoma

   c. Parenchymal hemorrhages can be managed nonsurgically if they are less than _____ cm in diameter.   3

   d. Posterior fossa lesions meeting surgical criteria should be evacuated _____.   asap

59

Gunshot Wounds and Non-Missile Penetrating Brain Injuries

■ Gunshot Wounds to the Head

1. **True or False. Regarding gunshot wounds (GSWs).**   59.1.1

   a. GSWs represent 35% of all deaths from brain injury in the older population (> 45).   false (35% under 45 die)

   b. GSWs are the most lethal type of head injury; one fourth die at the scene.   false (2/3 die)

   c. 90% of victims die.   true

2. **For GSWs to the head, the mechanisms of injury include**   59.1.2
   (Hint: Capone gang shootings land in the East River)

   a. c_____   cavitation, coup-contrecoup

   b. g_____   gas

   c. s_____   shock waves

   d. l_____   low pressure

   e. i_____   impact

   f. e_____   explosive

   g. r_____   ricochet

3. **Cerebral abscess from penetrating wounds can occur from r____ c____ m_____ and p____ c____ with n____ s_____.**   retained contaminated material, persistent communications with nasal sinuses   59.1.4

4. **General initial management in penetrating head injuries**   59.1.6

   a. C____   CPR

   b. evaluation for a_____ i____   additional injuries

   c. s_____ i_____ p_____   spine injury precautions

   d. f____ r_____   fluid resuscitation

5. **Patients with little CNS function in absence of s_____ are unlikely to benefit from craniotomy.**   shock   59.1.6

6. If surgical intervention is necessitated,   59.1.6

a. devitalized tissue around entry and exit wound should be e_____.   excised

b. air sinuses should have mucosa e_____.   exenterated

c. ensure tight d_____ c_____.   dural closure

d. cranioplasty should be delayed ___ - ___ months.   6-12 months

---

■ Non-Missile Penetrating Trauma

7. True or False.   59.2.3

a. It is appropriate to remove the protruding foreign body as soon as possible.   false (stabilize object and only consider removal in the OR)

b. Consider pre-op angiography if object passes near a large named artery or the dural sinuses.   true

c. They have a higher risk of contamination than missile injuries.   true

d. Prophylactic antibiotics are recommended.   true

e. Post-operative arteriograms are recommended.   true (to rule out traumatic aneurysm)

59

60

Pediatric Head Injury

■ General Information

1. Complete the following regarding children hospitalized for trauma: 60.1

a. What percentage have head injury?   75%
b. The overall mortality is ___ - ___%.   10-13%
c. If presenting with decerebrate posturing, mortality is _____%.   71%

■ Home Observation

2. A child with a GCS 14, who is neurologically stable with a negative CT, may be appropriate for h_____ o_____.   home observation   60.2.2

■ Cephalhematoma

3. Indicate if cephalohematoma is more consistent with subgaleal hematoma or subperiosteal hematoma.   60.4.1

a. Bleeding is limited by sutures.   subperiosteal hematoma
b. Do not calcify.   subgaleal hematoma
c. May lead to significant loss of circulating blood volume.   subgaleal hematoma
d. More commonly seen in a newborn, associated with parturition.   subperiosteal hematoma

4. **True or False. A mother brings a 5-day-old baby, born via vaginal delivery, with a large, right-sided, soft scalp swelling that stops at the suture. You should**

60.4.1

a. percutaneously aspirate the lesion.

false (Cephalohematoma is most commonly seen associated with parturition. 80% resorb usually within 2 to 3 weeks. Avoid the temptation of puncturing the lesions because the risk of infection exceeds cosmetic benefits.)

b. tell the mother that 50% of these calcify.

false

c. tell the mother that the baby may develop jaundice as late as age 10 days.

true (Infants may develop hyperbilirubinemia and jaundice as blood is resorbed from this cephalohematoma [subperiosteal hematoma] as late as 10 days after onset.)

d. surgically excise the lesion.

false (Surgery is considered only after 6 weeks if a CT demonstrates calcifications.)

e. consider child abuse.

true (Child abuse needs to be considered always.)

f. treat this differently if the soft area crosses sutures.

false (called subgaleal hematoma)

■ Skull Fractures in Pediatric Patients

5. **Complete the following regarding growing skull fracture:**

60.5.2

a. Leptomeningeal cysts result from a combination of two injuries:

   i.   s_____ f_____   skull fracture
   ii. d_____ t_____   dural tear

b. Why does it grow?

intact arachnoid pulsates and eventually expands

c. If early growth of a fracture line with no subgaleal mass, do _____ in ___ - ___ months to rule out p_____ f_____.

X-ray; 1-2 months; pseudo-growing fracture

d. What is a treatment for true PTLMC?

surgery

6. **What are the surgical indications for pediatric simple depressed skull fracture?**

60.5.3

a. d_____ p____   dural penetration
b. c_____ d_____   cosmetic defect
c. f_____ n_____ d_____   focal neurologic deficit consistent with the site of fracture

60

7. **Fill in the blank regarding ping pong ball fractures**   60.5.3
   a. Usually seen in _____.   newborns
   b. Often no treatment necessary in absence   temporoparietal region
      of underlying brain injury when it occurs
      in the t_____ region

■ Nonaccidental Trauma (NAT)

8. **Answer the following regarding child abuse:**   60.6.1
   a. True or False. There are pathognomonic   false
      findings in child abuse.
   b. Suspicious findings are
      i.   r_____ h_____   retinal hemorrhage
      ii. b_____ c_____ s_____   bilateral chronic subdural
           h_____   hematomas
      iii. s_____ f_____   skull fractures

9. **Retinal hemorrhage differential diagnosis:**   60.6.3
   a. c___ a____   child abuse
   b. b_____ s_____ e_____ in   benign subdural effusion in
      i_____   infants
   c. a_____ h____ a____ s____   acute high altitude sickness
   d. a_____ increase in I_____   acute increase in ICP
   e. P_____ r_____   Purtscher's retinopathy

10. **In skull fractures, the most common**   parietal bone;   60.6.4
    bone affected is the p_____ bone, and overlying hematoma
    can be missed in clinical exam due to
    o_____ h_____.

60

61

Head Injury: Long-Term Management, Complications, Outcome

■ Airway Management

1. Early tracheostomy can reduce the days of m_____ v_____ but does not reduce m_____.

   mechanical ventilation; mortality

   61.1

■ Deep-Vein Thrombosis (DVT) Prophylaxis

2. The risk of developing DVT in untreated severe TBI is ____%.

   20%

   61.2

■ Nutrition in the Head-Injured Patient

3. Nutritional replacement should begin within ____ hours of post-trauma patients with full caloric replacement by _____.

   72 hours; by day 7

   61.3.1

4. IV nutrition has increased risk of h_____ and i_____ compared to enteral nutrition.

   hyperglycemia and infection

   61.3.3

■ Posttraumatic Hydrocephalus

5. What is the incidence of clinically symptomatic hydrocephalus after traumatic SAH?

   12%

   61.4.1

6. Hydrocephalus ex vacuo is v_____ e_____ due to atrophy secondary to ____ _____ _____ in TBI patients.

   ventricular enlargement; diffuse axonal injury

   61.4.2

61

7. **When should a shunt be considered in posttraumatic hydrocephalus?**   61.4.3
   a. e_____ p_____ on 1 or more LPs   elevated pressure
   b. p_____   papilledema
   c. t_____ a_____   transependymal absorption

■ Outcome from Head Trauma

8. **The basal cisterns is evaluated on axial CT scan at the level of the m_____, and 3 limbs, which are _____.**   midbrain; quadrigeminal cistern, 2 lateral limbs (posterior portion of the ambient cisterns)   61.5.2

9. **Compression of the basal cisterns is associated with a ____ fold risk of _____ _____.**   3 fold risk; increased ICP   61.5.2

10. **Midline shift measurements are done at the level of the f_____ of M_____.**   foramen of Monro   61.5.2

11. **Complete the following:**   61.5.2
    a. What is the genotype associated with head injury?   apolipoprotein E4 allele
    b. It is also a risk factor for A_____ d_____.   Alzheimer's disease

■ Late Complications from Traumatic Brain Injury

12. **The three most common symptoms associated with postconcussive syndrome are:**   61.6.2
    a. h_____   headache
    b. d_____   dizziness
    c. m_____ d____   memory difficulty

13. **Treatment for postconcussive syndrome is generally s_____.**   supportive   61.6.2

14. **Neuropathology in chronic traumatic encephalopathy shows**   61.6.3
    a. n_____ t_____ and   neurofibrillary tangles
    b. a_____ a_____.   amyloid angiopathy
    c. These changes are similar to A_____ disease, however the n_____ t_____ are more s_____ in CTE.   Alzheimer's disease; neurofibrillary tangles; superficial

61

15. **True or False. Chronic traumatic encephalopathy is more likely in boxers who**

    a. have more than 20 fights.   true

    b. fight for more than 10 years.   true

    c. have the apolipoprotein E4 allele   true

    d. have cerebral atrophy.   true

    e. have cavum septum pellucidum.   true (13%, may be acquired condition)

    f. It is also known as d_____ p_____.   dementia pugilistica

61.6.3

61

62

General Information, Neurologic Assessment, Whiplash and Sports-Related Injuries, Pediatric Spine Injuries

■ Introduction

1. **Complete the following:**   62.1
   a. What must you look for in a patient with a major spinal injury?   a second spinal injury
   b. It occurs in _____%.   20%

■ Terminology

2. **Complete the following:**   62.2.3
   a. In spinal cord injury, any residual motor or sensory function more than three segments below the level of injury represents an _____ lesion.   incomplete
   b. Signs of this being the case include
      i. s_____   sensation (include position sense)
      ii. v_____ m_____   voluntary movement in the lower extremities;
          s_____ s_____   sacral sparing (Preserved sacral reflexes alone do not qualify as incomplete injury. Also requires preserved sensation around the anus or voluntary rectal sphincter contraction, or voluntary toe flexion.)
   c. Types of this lesion include these syndromes:
      i.   c_____ c_____   central cord syndrome
      ii. B_____-S_____   Brown-Séquard syndrome
      iii. a_____ c_____   anterior cord syndrome
      iv. p_____ c_____   posterior cord syndrome

3. A complete spinal cord lesion   62.2.3
a. is defined as no
  i.   m_____ or   motor
  ii.   s_____ function   sensory
  iii. t_____ levels below lesion.   three
b. What percentage of patients with no   3%
    function on initial exam will develop
    some recovery within 24 hours?
c. A complete spinal cord injury that   No distal recovery will occur.
    persists for 72 hours indicates what?

4. Complete the following regarding   62.2.3
spinal shock:
a. hypotension:
  i.   interruption of s_____   sympathetic activity
        a_____
  ii.   loss of v_____ t_____   vascular tone
  iii. implies injury above which level?   T1
b. bradycardia: unopposed p_____   parasympathetic
    activity
c. relative hypovolemia:
  i.   loss of _____   muscle skeletal tone below
                                              injury
  ii.   resulting in _____ _____   venous pooling
d. true hypovolemia: loss of _____   blood
e. neurogenic spinal shock is:
  i.   transient loss of _____   neurological function
  ii.   resulting in _____   flaccid paralysis, loss of
                                              reflexes
  iii. loss of _____ reflex   bulbocavernosus

■ Whiplash-Associated Disorders

5. What is the most common nonfatal   whiplash   62.3.1
automobile injury?

6. Describe the five grades of whiplash-   Table 62.1,
associated disorders and clinical   Table 62.2,
evaluation of each.   Table 62.3.
a. Grade 0
  i.   clinical   no complaint
  ii.   radiological studies   none required
  iii. treatment   none
b. Grade 1
  i.   clinical   neck pain
  ii.   radiological studies   no x-rays
  iii. treatment   optional collar/rest (not more
                                            than 72 hours)
c. Grade 2
  i.   clinical   reduced ROM/point
                                            tenderness
  ii.   radiological studies   flexion-extension x-rays
  iii. treatment   optional collar/rest (not more
                                            than 96 hours)

62

d. Grade 3
    i.   clinical   neurological deficits
    ii. radiological studies   CT/MR
    iii. treatment   treatment as SCI
e. Grade 4
    i.   clinical   fracture/dislocation
    ii. radiological studies   CT/MR
    iii. treatment   treatment as SCI
f. What percentage of whiplash injuries   76%   Table 62.4
    recover within 1 year?

■ Pediatric Spine Injuries

**7. Complete the following about
    pediatric spine injuries:**
a. Due to ligamentous laxity together with   ligamentous   62.4.1
    immaturity of paraspinal muscles and
    underdeveloped uncinate processes,
    pediatric spinal injury tends to involve
    _____ injuries.
b. In the age group ≤ 9 years, the_____   cervical   62.4.3
    spine is the most vulnerable segment.
c. Of all cervical spine injuries in the   upper 3
    pediatric population, 67% occur in the
    _____ segments of the cervical spine.

**8. Complete the following about   62.4.3
    pediatric spine injuries:**
a. "Pseudospread of the atlas" is a   Jefferson fracture
    phenomenon occurring in children – but
    it could be confused with what kind of
    fracture?
b. Normal total offset of the total overlap of
    2 C1 lateral masses on C2 on AP open
    mouth view is
    i.   ____mm at 1 year of age   2
    ii. ____mm at 2 years of age   4
    iii. ____mm at 3 years of age   6
    iv. and should never be more than   8
         ____mm

**9. Answer the following about Jefferson   62.4.3
    fractures:**
a. True or False. Jefferson fractures are   false
    common in pediatric cervical spine
    injury.
b. They are more common during the   teenage
    _____ years.

■ Sports-Related Cervical Spine Injuries

10. Complete the following about football-related cervical spine injuries: 62.7.2

a. stinger
  i.   involves _____   one extremity
  ii. represents _____   compression of root
b. burning hands
  i.   involves _____   bilateral upper extremities
  ii. represents _____   mild central cord syndrome
c. neuropraxia
  i.   involves _____   all four extremities
  ii. represents _____   cervical cord injury
  iii. must rule out _____   cervical stensosis
  iv. by performing an _____   MRI

11. Complete the following: 62.7.2

a. A football player who uses his helmet as   spear tackler
   a battering ram is called a _____.
b. What evidence may be present on his
   spine x-rays?
  i.   loss of _____   lordosis
  ii. evidence of _____   prior trauma
  iii. presence of _____   cervical spinal stenosis
c. When may the athlete resume play?   when lordosis returns

12. True or False. Contact sports are permitted in   Table 62.7

a. Klippel-Feil with symptoms   false
b. Klippel-Feil without symptoms   true
c. spina bifida   true
d. status post-anterior cervical discectomy true
   and fusion (ACDF) 1 level
e. status post-ACDF 2 levels   false
f. status post-ACDF 3 levels   false

■ Neurological Assessment

13. Complete the following: 62.8.1

a. Cervical nerves exit _____ their like-   above
   numbered vertebra.
b. Thoracic and lumbar nerves exit   below
   _____ their like-numbered vertebra.
c. For a segment of cord that lies under a   two cord levels
   given vertebra, T2 to T10 add _____
   _____ _____.
d. Under T11, T12, L1 lie the _____ ___   lowest 11 spinal segments
   _____ _____.
e. The conus lies at _____.   L1-2

62

14. **Give the location of the key sensory landmarks.**   Table 62.11

a.	occipital protuberance	C2
b.	supraclavicular fossa	C3
c.	shoulders	C4
d.	lateral side of antecubital fossa	C5
e.	thumb	C6
f.	middle finger	C7
g.	little finger	C8
h.	medial side of antecubital fossa	T1
i.	nipples	T4
j.	xyphoid	T6
k.	umbilicus	T10
l.	inguinal ligament	T12
m.	medial femoral condyle	L3
n.	medial maleolus	L4
o.	great toe	L5
p.	lateral maleolus	S1
q.	popliteal fossa in midline	S2
r.	ischial tuberosity	S3
s.	perianal area	S4-5

15. **Write out the American Spinal Injury Association (ASIA) motor scoring system—upper extremity—for the indicated root, muscle, and action to test.**   Table 62.10

a. root C5
   i.   muscle: d_____ or b_____   deltoid or biceps
   ii. action: s_____ a_____ or   shoulder abduction; elbow
        e_____ f_____   flexion
b. root C6
   i.   muscle: w_____ e_____   wrist extension
   ii. action: e_____ w_____   extend wrist
c. root C7
   i.   muscle: t_____   triceps
   ii. action: e_____ e_____   extend elbow
d. root C8
   i.   muscle: f_____ d_____   flexor digitorum profundus
        p_____
   ii. action: s_____ h_____   squeeze hand
e. root T1
   i.   muscle: h_____ i_____   hand intrinsics
   ii. action: a_____ l_____   abduct little finger
        f_____

62

16. **Write out the American Spinal Injury Association (ASIA) motor scoring system—lower extremity—for the indicated root, muscle, and action to test.**   Table 62.10
    a. root L2
        i.   muscle: i_____   iliopsoas
        ii. action: f_____ h_____   flex hip
    b. root L3
        i.   muscle: q_____   quadriceps
        ii. action: s_____ k_____   straight knee
    c. root L4
        i.   muscle: t_____ a_____   tibialis anterior
        ii. action: d_____ f_____   dorsiflexion
    d. root L5
        i.   muscle: e_____ h_____   extensor hallucis longus
             l_____
        ii. action: d_____ g_____   dorsiflex great toe
             t_____
    e. root S1
        i.   muscle: g_____   gastrocnemius
        ii. action: p_____ f_____   plantar flex foot
             f_____

17. **Name the main nerve root responsible for the following motor action:**   Table 62.10
    a. great toe extension   L5
    b. ankle dorsiflexion   L4
    c. knee extension   L3
    d. ankle plantar flexion   S1

18. **Complete the following regarding Beevor's sign:**   Table 62.10
    a. It tests the level of spinal cord injury at   T9
       about T_____.
    b. It is performed by
        i.   flexing the _____.   neck – patient activates
                                                     rectus abdominus
        ii. Note that the _____ moves   umbilicus
             cephalad.

19. **Complete the following regarding the abdominal cutaneous reflex:**   Table 62.10
    a. What is it?   Stroking quadrants of
                                        abdomen causes abdominal
                                        muscle contraction, umbilicus
                                        deviation towards quadrant
                                        of stimulus
    b. The upper quadrant is served by   T8-9
       _____.
    c. The lower quadrant is served by   T10-12
       _____.
    d. Its presence indicates (at least some)   spinal cord
       function of the _____ _____.

62

e. There is _____ _____ spinal cord injury   no complete

f. because the reflex _____ to the _____ and then _____ to the abdominal muscles.   ascends to the cortex and descends

20. **There is a sensory region that is not represented on the trunk.**   62.8.3

a. It jumps from C_____ to T_____.   C4 to T2

b. These levels are distributed exclusively on the u_____ e_____.   upper extremity

21. **Give the motor and sensory descriptions for each class in the ASIA impairment scale as modified from the Frankel neurologic performance scale.**   Table 62.13

a. class A   Complete cord injury: no motor or sensory function preserved

b. class B   Incomplete cord injury: sensory but no motor function preserved below the neurological level (includes sacral segments S4-5)

c. class C   Incomplete cord injury: motor function preserved below the neurologic level (more than half of key muscles below the neurologic level have a muscle strength grade <3)

d. class D   Incomplete cord injury: motor function preserved below the neurologic level (more than half of key muscles below the neurologic level have a muscle strength grade ≥ 3)

e. class E   Normal: sensory and motor function normal

■ Spinal Cord Injuries

22. **True or False. Regarding central cord injuries.**   62.9.3

a. They usually result from a hyperflexion injury.   false (hyperextension)

b. Motor deficit is greater in the arms than legs.   true

c. Hyperpathia is uncommonly seen.   false (hyperpathia is common)

d. It's the most common type of incomplete spinal injury.   true

e. The cord's centermost region is a watershed zone.   true

62

f.	Somatotopic organization places fibers to lower extremities more medial.	false (more lateral)
g.	BP must be maintained at an MAP of 85 to 90 for at least 1 week.	true
h.	Prompt surgery for decompression is advised.	false

23. **A 45-year-old alcoholic male trips and falls, briefly losing consciousness. He was unable to move for 15 minutes, but currently complains only of weakness of both hands. He has an abrasion of his forehead. Computed tomographic (CT) scan of his head was negative. X-ray of C-spine reveals only spondylosis. True or False. Regarding this lesion.**   62.9.3

a.	It has the best prognosis of all incomplete spinal cord injuries.	false (Brown-Séquard is the best)
b.	There may be sparing of sensation around the anus with an intact voluntary anal sphincter.	true
c.	Immediate surgery is recommended even for patients without spinal instability.	false
d.	Urinary catheterization is recommended for patients in spinal shock.	true

24. **Complete the following about surgical intervention in patients who have had a central spinal cord injury:**   62.9.3

a. Indications for surgical intervention are

i.	spine _____	instability
ii.	continued spinal cord compression in a patient who fails to _____ or _____	improve; progressively worsens

b.	What surgery should be done?	decompressive laminectomy + fusion

25. **What is the prognosis in patients with central cord injury?**   62.9.3

a.	_____% will recover enough to ambulate.	50%
b.	Bowel and bladder function _____.	recover
c.	Upper extremities (do/don't) _____ recover well.	don't
d.	Elderly patients (do/don't) _____ recover well.	don't

62

26. **Answer the following about anterior cord syndrome:**   62.9.3
    a. True or False. Motor findings are those of hemiplegia below the lesion.   false (paraplegia)
    b. True or False. There is loss of pain sensation, with preservation of deep pressure sensation.   true
    c. It may result from _____.   occlusion of anterior spinal artery
    d. Sensory pattern is termed "dissociated" because there is loss of
        i. _____ _____ _____ and preservation of   spinal thalamic tract
        ii. _____ _____.   dorsal columns

27. **Answer the following about a Brown-Séquard syndrome:**   62.9.3
    a. True or False. There is contralateral pain loss beginning 1 to 2 levels above the lesion.   false (1-2 levels below lesion)
    b. True or False. Contralateral position sense is preserved.   true
    c. Prognosis compared with all other incomplete cord lesions is _____.   best of all incomplete cord injuries
    d. What % will eventually walk?   90%

63

Management of Spinal Cord Injury

■ General Information

1. Complete the following: 63.1
a. The major causes of death in spinal cord
   injury are
   i. _____ and _____.   aspiration and shock
b. Associated findings suggestive of spinal
   cord injury include
   i. _____ breathing and   abdominal
   ii. _____.   priapism (autonomic
                                                  dysfunction)

■ Management in the Field

2. True or False. In caring for an injured   false   63.2
   athlete, prompt removal of the helmet
   is recommended.

3. Complete the following: 63.2
a. In spinal cord injury with hypotension in   dopamine
   the field, the agent of choice is

   _____.

b. Avoid _____.   phenylephrine –
                                                 noninotropic, possible reflex
                                                 bradycardia

4. In evaluating spinal cord injury in the   63.2
   field, hypopnea may be related to
   three conditions:
a. paralyzed i_____ m_____   intercostal muscles
b. paralyzed d_____   diaphragm
c. depressed _____   LOC

■ Management in the Hospital

5. Complete the following: 63.3.1
a. True or False. Spinal cord injury can   true
   cause loss of temperature regulation.
b. This is called p_____   poikilothermy
c. and is caused by v_____ p_____.   vasomotor paralysis

63

6. **Complete the following about initial management of spinal cord injuries:**   63.3.1

a. True or False. Spinal cord injury can cause electrolyte disturbances   true

b. due to what changes to blood pressure and volume?   hypotension & hypovolemia

c. which cause an increase in what plasma hormone?   aldosterone

d. which leads to what electrolyte changes?   hypokalemia

7. **Should methylprednisolone be given for the treatment of acute SCI?**   no   63.3.3

8. **Should GM-1 ganglioside (sygen) be given for the treatment of acute SCI?**   no   63.3.3

9. **True or False. Methylprednisolone protocol has been shown to be useful for patients with**   63.3.3

a. cauda equina syndrome   false

b. gunshot wounds to the spine   false

c. children   false

d. pregnant women   false

10. **True or False. Regarding deep vein thrombosis (DVT) in spinal cord injury (SCI):**   63.3.5

a. Heparin 5000 U subcutaneous (SQ) twice a day is more effective than SQ heparin to titrate partial thromboplastin time (PTT) to 1.5 times normal.   false — better to titrate to 1.5x PTT

b. Pneumatic boots should be used initially.   true

11. **Complete the following about spinal cord injury and deep vein thrombosis:**   63.3.5

a. incidence: _____%   100%

b. mortality: _____%   9%

c. What medication can cause thrombocytopenia and osteoporosis?   heparin

---

■ Radiographic Evaluation and Initial C-Spine Immobilization

12. **Matching. In assessing C-spine in these categories of trauma patient, perform the following tests:**   63.4.3
① none needed; ② CT from occiput to T1; ③ plain C-spine x-rays; ④ flexion-extension; ⑤ MRI
Category of trauma patient: (a-e) below

a. alert, denies neck pain   ①

b. alert, complains of neck pain   ②

c. obtunded or inebriated   ②

d. abnormal CT   ⑤

e. neurological deficit   ② and ⑤

63

13. **When do we do plain 3-view C-spine x-ray?**   63.4.3
   a.   If _____ is not available.   CT
   b.   Flexion extension views
      i.   in an _____ patient   awake
      ii.   who complains of _____   neck pain
         _____
      iii.   and in whom _____ is normal   CT
      iv.   and _____ is not available.   MRI

14. **Factors associated with increased risk of failing to recognize spinal injuries during radiographic evaluation include**   63.4.3
   a.   decreased _____ of _____   level of consciousness
   b.   multiple _____   injuries

15. **Radiographic signs of C-spine trauma include**   Table 63.2
   a.   retropharyngeal space > _____ mm   7mm
   b.   retrotracheal space > _____ mm in adult   14 mm
   c.   or > _____ mm in pediatrics   22 mm
   d.   atlantodental interval (ADI) > _____ mm in adult   3mm
   e.   > _____ mm in pediatrics   4mm
   f.   In the neurologically intact patient, subluxation up to _____ mm may be normal.   3.5 mm
   g.   To prove it is normal do _____.   flexion-extension views

16. **When should we order anteroposterior (AP) and lateral views of the thoracic and lumbosacral spine?**   63.4.3
   a.   clinical symptoms?   back pain
   b.   mechanism of injury?   high grade: MVA, fall > 6 feet, LOC

17. **Complete the following:**   63.4.3
   a.   How can we tell an old injury from an acute one?   bone scan
   b.   We should test between _____ and _____ days.   2 and 21
   c.   Test will remain abnormal for _____.   1 year

18. **During evaluation of occult cervical spine trauma, what are the contraindications for flexion-extension cervical spine x-rays?**   63.4.3
   a.   patient who is not _____   cooperative/awake
   b.   patient who has _____ impairment   cognitive
   c.   subluxation of _____mm or more   3.5
   d.   neurologic deficit of _____   any degree

63

19. **True or False. A normal flexion-extension of the cervical spine x-ray may demonstrate slight anterior subluxation distributed over all cervical levels with preservation of the normal contour lines.**

true

63.4.3

20. **Complete the following:**

63.4.3

a. Lumbar puncture (for myleogram) is dangerous in complete spinal block and may cause deterioration in _____%.

14%

b. Avoid this with a _____ _____ _____ or _____.

lateral cervical puncture or MRI

21. **Indications for emergent myelogram or magnetic resonance imaging (MRI) in spinal cord injury includes neurologic deficit**

63.4.3

a. that is not _____.

explained

b. after closed _____.

reduction

c. after _____ surgery.

spinal

22. **Complete the following about MRI in spine:**

63.4.3

a. It is appropriate when
   i. CT of spine is _____,

inconclusive

   ii. patient has neurological _____.

deficits

b. It should be done within _____ - _____ hours.

48-72

c. Most useful sequences are
   i. _____ and

T2

   ii. _____.

STIR

■ Traction/Reduction of Cervical Spine Injuries

23. **Contraindications to traction/reduction of cervical spine injuries include**

63.5.1

a. atlanto-occipital _____.

disassociation

b. types of axis fractures called _____ or _____.

type IIA or III hangman's fractures

c. a defect in the _____

skull at pin site

d. the patient is less than _____ years of age.

3

24. **Complete the following:**

63.5.2

a. After placing the patient in tongs we must obtain a _____

lateral c-spine x-ray

b. and measure the distance between the _____ and the _____,

basion; odontoid

Table 64.1

   i. which should be less than _____ mm in adults

12mm

   ii. and less than _____ mm in children.

10mm (unreliable <13 yrs because of variable ossification/fusion of odontoid tip)

63

25. **What is considered proper pin care?** 63.5.2

a. Clean with _____. half strength hydrogen peroxide

b. Apply _____. povidone-iodine

c. This may reduce the incidence of osteomyelitis

_____.

26. **Complete the following:** 63.5.2

a. Closed reduction of cervical dislocations retropulsed cervical disc

may be associated with neurologic

deterioration, and this may be due to a

r_____ c_____ d_____.

b. If neurologic deterioration occurs after MRI

closed reduction what tests must you do

immediately?

■ Indications for Emergency Decompressive Surgery

27. **Complete the following:** 63.6.1

a. True or False. Patient with recent onset false (May worsen injury.)

of loss of function due to spinal cord

injury should have a decompressive

laminectomy.

b. If surgery is done, it is usually combined stabilization procedure

with _____ _____.

28. **Contraindications to emergent** 63.6.1

operation for acute spinal cord injury

include:

a. complete _____ _____ _____ spinal cord injury;

for more than 24 hours without evidence spinal shock

of _____ _____

b. unstable _____ medically

c. central _____ _____ cord syndrome

(controversial)

63

64

Occipitoatlantoaxial Injuries (Occiput to C2)

■ Atlanto-Occipital Dislocation

1. Complete the following: 64.1.1

a. Incidence in spinal injury is approximately ____%.   1%

b. Are they more common in pediatrics or in adults?   pediatrics

c. Mortality results from _____ _____.   respiratory arrest (bulbar cervical disassociation)

d. They may demonstrate what type of paralysis?   cruciate

2. Complete the following about the three types of atlanto-occipital dislocation: 64.1.1

a. Type I: occiput in relation to atlas is dislocated ____   anteriorly

b. Type II: occiput in relation to atlas is dislocated ____   superiorly

c. Type III: occiput in relation to atlas is dislocated ____   posteriorly

3. Name the ligaments at the following sites: 1.8

a. atlas to occiput

   i. a_____ a_____-o_____ m_____   anterior atlanto-occipital membrane (ALL)

   ii. p_____ a_____-o_____ m_____   posterior atlanto-occipital membrane

   iii. a_____ b_____ (of c_____ l_____)   ascending band (cruciate ligament)

b. axis to occiput (via dens)

   i. t_____ m_____   tectorial membrane

   ii. a_____ l_____   alar ligaments

   iii. a_____ l_____   apical ligament

c. atlas to axis

   i. t_____ l_____   transverse ligament (part of cruciate)

   ii. a_____ l_____   alar ligament

   iii. d_____ b_____ (of c_____ l_____) descending band (cruciate ligament)

4. Complete the following: 1.8

a. What structure is the cephalad extension of the

   i.   anterior longitudinal ligament?   anterior atlanto-occipital membrane

   ii. posterior longitudinal ligament?   tectorial membrane

b. Which structures are most important in maintaining atlanto-occipital stability?

   i.   t_____ m_____   tectorial membrane

   ii. a_____ l_____   alar ligaments

5. Complete the following: 1.8

a. Name the horizontal component of the cruciate ligament.   transverse ligament

b. What does it hold together?   odontoid and atlas

c. What is the strongest ligament in the spine?   transverse ligament

6. Complete the following:

a. What is the best method by which to measure AOD?   BAI-BDI   64.1.3

b. It is considered normal if each is less than _____ mm.   12

c. Another method is called the _____ _____.   Powers' ratio   64.1.4

d. Traction may be used but _____% of patients deteriorate.   10%   64.1.5

7. Complete the following:

a. A measurement used in evaluating atlanto-occipital dislocation (AOD) is called _____ _____.   Power's ratio   64.1.4

   i.   divide distance from basion to _____   posterior arch of the atlas

   ii. by distance from opisthion to _____   anterior arch of the atlas

b. It is considered normal if below _____.   0.9   Table 64.2

c. It is definitely abnormal if above _____.   1

8. Power's ratio greater than _____ is diagnostic of atlanto-occipital dislocation.   1   Table 64.2

9. AOD is suspected if

a. the atlanto-occipital interval is greater than _____ mm and/or   2 mm   Table 64.1

b. there is blood in the _____ _____.   basilar cistern   64.1.3

64

■ Occipital Condyle Fractures

10. **Complete the following:**
    a. Can they involve the hypoglossal nerve?   yes   64.2.1
    b. List the types.   Table 64.4
        i. I is a _____ fracture.   comminuted (axial loading)
        ii. II has a _____fracture.   linear (extension of basilar
            skull fracture)
        iii. III has an _____ fracture.   avulsion (traction)
    c. Treatment is with _____.   collar   64.2.1
    d. What are the indications for halo or   craniocervical misalignment,
       fusion?   occiput-C1 interval > 2mm
    e. Incidence in trauma patients is   0.4%
       _____%.

■ Atlantoaxial Subluxation/Dislocation

11. **Answer the following about atlanto-axial dislocation:**
    a. True or False. It has less morbidity and   true   64.3.1
       mortality than atlanto-occipital
       dislocation.
    b. Name and describe the three types.   rotatory, anterior, posterior   Table 64.5
        i. rotatory atlanto-axial dislocation
           type I
           transverse ligament _____   intact
           facet capsule _____ _____   bilateral injured
           treatment _____ _____   soft collar
           type II
           transverse ligament _____   injured
           facet capsule _____ _____   unilateral injury
           treatment _____, _____   fusion, halo
           type III
           transverse ligament _____   injured
           facet capsule _____ _____   bilateral injury
           treatment _____, _____   fusion, halo
        ii. anterior atlanto-axial dislocation
            o_____ f_____   odontoid fracture
            c_____ h_____   congenital hypoplasia
            d_____ of t_____ l_____   disruption of transverse
            ligament

12. **Complete the following regarding   64.3.2
    atlanto-axial rotatory subluxation:**
    a. Name four causes. Hint: stur
        i. s_____   spontaneous
        ii. t_____   trauma
        iii. u_____   upper respiratory tract
            infection (Grisel syndrome)
        iv. r_____   rheumatoid arthritis
    b. Competence of the _____ _____   transverse ligament
       must be assessed.

64

c. What is the characteristic head position?   "cock robin" (20 degrees lateral tilt, 20 degrees rotation opposite, slight flexion)

d. Patients are usually _____.   young

e. It can occlude the _____ arteries.   vertebral

13. **Complete the following regarding the rule of Spence:**   64.3.3

a. It is designed to determine if the transverse ligament _____ _____   is disrupted

b. If disrupted what effect does it have on treatment?   requires immobilization (surgical, halo, or collar, based on type of disruption)

c. It is performed by studying what view?   open-mouthed AP

d. To assess what structures?   lateral masses of C1-C2 overhang

e. The critical reference number is ___mm sum of both sides.   7mm

■ Atlas (C1) Fractures

14. **Complete the following:**   64.4.1

a. isolated fracture: _____%   56%

b. combined with C2 fracture: _____%   44%

c. additional spine fracture: _____%   9%

d. combined with head injury: _____%   21%

15. **True or False. Regarding a Jefferson fracture:**   64.4.3

a. It involves a single fracture through the ring of C1.   false (at least 2 fracture sites)

b. It is generally a stable fracture.   false (But without neurologic deficit.)

c. "Rule of Spence" assesses displacement.   false

d. Treatment is generally surgical (fusion).   false (usually collar/halo)

■ Axis (C2) Fractures

16. **Complete the following about acute fractures of the axis:**   64.5.1

a. Represent _____% of cervical fractures.   20%

b. Neurologic deficit occurs in _____%.   10%

64

17. **Complete the following:**   64.5.3
    a. True or False. Regarding hangman's   false – hyperflexion, axial
       fracture: loading
       i.   In contrast to judicial hanging,
            modern-day hangman's fractures
            result from hyperextension and
            distraction.
       ii. This is usually a stable fracture.   true
    b. There is a common occurrence of   false (usually heal with collar)
       nonunion, hence the need for surgery.
    c. Hangman's fracture results in a fracture   pars of C2;
       through the _____. It is also known   traumatic spondylolisthesis of
       as _____.   the axis

18. **Complete the following regarding**   64.5.3
    hangman's fracture:
    a. Subluxation of C2 on C3 by more than   3; disc
       _____ mm indicates _____
       disruption.
    b. This is a marker for _____ and usually instability; surgery
       requires _____.

19. **Classify hangman's fractures**   Table 64.7
    a. Type I: vertical pars fractures
       i.   subluxation: _____   <3mm
       ii. angulation: _____   0
       iii. treatment   collar
    b. Type IA: nonparallel fractures
       i.   subluxation: _____   2-3 mm
       ii. angulation: _____   0
       iii. treatment   collar
    c. Type II: vertical fracture through pars
                                                     with disruption of C2/3 disc
                                                     and PLL
       i.   subluxation: _____   >3mm
       ii. angulation: _____   significant
       iii. treatment   traction/halo vs surgery
    d. Type IIA: type II with oblique fractures
       i.   subluxation: _____   >3mm
       ii. angulation: _____   >15 deg
       iii. treatment   NO TRACTION. Halo.
    e. Type III: type II + bilat C2-3 facets
                                                     disrupted
       i.   subluxation: _____   yes
       ii. angulation: _____   facets locked
       iii. treatment   NO TRACTION. Surgery
    f. A special caution for Type IIA and III   traction
       fractures is to avoid the use of _____.
    g. What is the name of the classification   Effendi
       system?

20. **Most hangman's fracture patients**   64.5.3
    a. present neurologically _____ and   intact
    b. need MRI to assess _____ disc.   C2-3

64

c. It can be treated with _____ for   immobilization; 12
    _____ weeks.

d. Average time to heal is _____ weeks   11.5

21. **Describe the radiologic criteria of**   64.5.3
    good fusion.

a. Across the fracture site we should see   trabeculations
    _____.

b. Flexion-extension radiographs should   movement
    show no _____.

22. **Complete the following about**   64.5.4
    odontoid fractures:

a. Odontoid fractures represent   10-15%
    approximately ____ - ____% of all
    cervical spine fractures.

b. Mechanism of injury is usually _____.   flexion

c. They are fatal in about ____ - ____%.   25-40%

d. Major deficits in type II is _____%.   10%

e. In Type III it is _____ to have   rare
    neurologic deficit.

f. A displacement

    i. of _____ mm   6mm

    ii. results in a nonunion rate of   70%
    _____%.

    iii. Therefore, the treatment advised is   surgical
    _____.

23. **True or False. Regarding odontoid**   64.5.4
    fractures:

a. They are a hyperflexion injury in most   true
    instances.

b. Most patients have presenting   false
    neurological deficit.

c. Neck pain is infrequent.   false

24. **Complete the following:**

a. Regarding odontoid fractures: Table 64.9

    i. Type I is fracture through the _____   apical dens
    _____.

    ii. Type II is fracture through the _____   base of dens
    of _____.

    iii. Type III is fracture through the   body of C2
    _____ of _____.

b. True or False. The spinal cord occupies   false (1/3)   64.5.4
    50% of the canal at C1.

c. True or False. The ossiculum terminale   false – from nonunion
    results from posttraumatic fracture of
    the apical dens.

64

25. **Complete the following:**   64.5.4
   a. List indications for surgical treatment of
      Type II odontoid fractures.
      i.   displacement of dens more than   5mm
           _____ mm
      ii. despite halo there is _____   instability
      iii. despite immobilization there is   nonunion
           _____
      iv. patient is older than _____   50
      v.   disruption of the _____   transverse ligament
           _____
   b. True or False. Most odontoid type III   false – 90% heal
      fractures should be treated surgically
      due to low union rate by rigid external
      immobilization (halo).

26. **The appearance of os odontoideum is**   64.5.4
   a. a _____ bone   separate
   b. with _____ borders   smooth
   c. near a _____ odontoid peg.   short
   d. It may fuse with the _____.   clivus
   e. It may mimic a _____ fracture.   type II odontoid

27. **Complete the following about os**   64.5.4
   odontoideum:
   a. Postulated etiologies
      i. c_____   congenital
      ii. a_____   avulsion of alar ligament
   b. Does treatment depend on the etiology?   no
   c. Myelopathy correlates with an AP canal   13 mm
      diameter of less than _____mm.
   d. Will immobilization result in fusion?   no
   e. Treatment
      i. p_____ w_____   posterior wiring
      ii. t_____ s_____   transarticular screw
   f. Do we need a halo with each of these   Not with transarticular screws
      procedures?

■ Combination C1–2 Injuries

28. **Complete the following about**
   combined C1 and C2 fractures:
   a. Treatment is decided based on type of   C2   64.6.2
      _____ fracture.
   b. An odontoid fracture type II that is   5mm;   Table 64.13
      displaced more than _____ mm is   unstable
      considered _____.
   c. Treatment is _____ _____.   posterior fusion

65

Subaxial (C3 through C7) Injuries / Fractures

■ Classification Systems

1. **Matching. For the following conditions, choose the most appropriate mechanism producing the cervical fracture.**
   Mechanism: ① hyperextension; ② vertical compression; ③ hyperflexion; ④ flexion plus rotation

   Table 65.3

   a. burst fracture   ②
   b. unilateral locked facet   ④
   c. bilateral locked facet   ③
   d. laminar fracture   ①

2. **Guidelines for determining clinical instability include:**

   65.1.4

   a. Compromise of the anterior elements produces more instability in _____.   extension
   b. Compromise of the posterior elements produces more instability in _____.   flexion

3. **Give radiographic criteria for clinical instability.**

   Table 65.4

   a. a sagittal plane displacement of _____ mm and   >3.5mm
   b. relative sagittal plane angulation of _____ degrees(on neutral position lateral C-spine films)   >11

■ Clay Shoveler's Fracture

4. **Clay shoveler's fracture usually involves the spinous process of _____.**   C7

   65.2

65 ■ Flexion Injuries of the Subaxial Cervical Spine

5. **True or False. The following is true of teardrop fractures:**   65.4.3
   a. They usually result from
      i.   hyperflexion injuries   true
      ii. compression flexion injury   true
      iii. hyperextension injury   false
   b. They are stable fractures.   false
   c. The fractured vertebra is usually   true
      displaced posteriorly into the spinal
      canal.
   d. They are often associated with a fracture true
      through the sagittal plane of the
      vertebral body.
   e. The patient is often quadriplegic.   true
   f. A "teardrop" chip of bone is at the   false – anterior-inferior
      anterior-superior edge of the vertebral
      body.

6. **Complete the following:**   65.4.3
   a. A teardrop fracture must be   avulsion fracture
      distinguished from an _____

      _____.
      i.   _____ _____ is unstable and   Teardrop fracture;
           requires _____,   surgery
      ii. _____ _____ is stable.   avulsion fracture
   b. How can we distinguish them? A
      teardrop will have:
      i.   size of fracture   small chip
      ii. alignment   displaced
      iii. neurological _____   deficits
      iv. soft tissue   swelling
      v.   fracture   through vertebra
      vi. height of disc   reduced
      vii. height of vertebral body   reduced/wedged
   c. If in doubt, perform _____ views.   flexion-extension
   d. If negative, repeat _____ in ___ -   flexion-extension;
      ___ days.   4-7 days
   e. The fractured vertebra is displaced   posteriorly
      _____.
   f. True teardrop fractures should be   combined anterior and
      treated with c_____ a_____ and   posterior fusions.
      p_____ f_____.

7. **Quadrangular fractures have four   65.4.5
   features.**
   a. Feature 1: an _____ fracture   oblique
      i.   from _____-_____   anterior-superior
      ii. to _____ _____   inferior endplate
   b. Feature 2: subluxation of superior   posteriorly
      vertebral body (VB) on the inferior VB
      _____
   c. Feature 3: with angular _____   kyphosis

d. Feature 4: disruption of
    i. _____   disc
    ii. _____   ALL
    iii. _____   PLL
e. Treat with _____ _____ _____   combined anterior and
    _____ _____.   posterior fusions.

■ Distraction Flexion Injuries

8. Describe distraction flexion injuries.

a. Flexion injuries include _____, _____, _____ _____.   strain, subluxation, locked facets   65.5.1

b. Which ligament is injured early?   posterior ligamentous complex

c. X-rays demonstrate this by showing _____.   widening of interspinous distance

d. We may need to test by performing _____.   flexion-extension views or MRI   65.5.2

e. If symptoms persist 1 to 2 weeks we should _____.   repeat flexion-extension views

f. Ligamentous instability is confirmed if there is a   65.5.3
    i. subluxation of _____ mm or angulation of   3.5
    ii. _____ degrees.   11

9. Describe locked (aka jumped) facets.   65.5.4

a. Normally the inferior facet of the level above is _____ to the superior facet of the level below.   posterior

b. In locked facets there is _____ of the facet _____.   disruption; capsule

c. Flexion and rotation produces _____ _____.   unilateral locked facets

d. Hyperflexion produces _____ _____.   bilateral locked facets

e. Neurological injury is _____ for cord and/or root injury.   frequent

f. In patients with locked facets the inferior facet of the level above is _____ to the superior facet of the level below.   anterior

10. Describe evidence of locked facets on x-ray.   65.5.4

a. In unilateral locked facets the spinous process is rotated to the side of the _____ _____.   locked facet

b. Facets look like a _____.   bow tie

c. Interspinous space is _____.   widened

d. Neural foramen is _____.   blocked

e. Articular surfaces of the facets are _____.   on the wrong side

65

11. **Complete the following regarding locked facets:**   65.5.4

a. When the articulating surfaces of the facets are on the wrong side, this is called the "_____ _____ sign."   naked facet

b. In bilateral locked facets traumatic disc herniation is found in _____%.   80%

c. Attempt at closed reduction of locked facets by traction must not exceed _____ lb per vertebral level.   10

d. Disc space height must not exceed _____mm.   10

e. If neurologic worsening occurs, you should suspect _____ _____ and plan for _____.   disc hernation; surgery

f. Closed reduction is _____ until MRI assesses for _____ _____.   contraindicated; disc hernation

12. **Answer the following about locked facets:**   65.5.4

a. True or False. Stabilization is more likely to be successful in halo if there are
   i. multiple fractures of the facets.   true
   ii. no fractures of the facets.   false

b. Halo alone is successful for good anatomical result in _____%.   23%

c. Failure of good anatomical result occurs in ___%.   77%

d. True or False. Surgical fusion is therefore clearly indicated in cases without facet fracture fragments.   true

■ Extension Injuries of the Subaxial Cervical Spine

13. **Complete the following about subaxial (C3 - C7) injuries/fractures:**   65.6.1

a. Extension injuries can produce
   i. _____ _____ _____ in adults and   central cord syndrome
   ii. _____ in children.   SCIWORA

b. The ligament that is most often injured in extension injuries is the _____.   ALL

c. Is disc injury possible?   yes

d. What vascular injury can occur?   carotid artery dissection

■ Treatment of Subaxial Cervical Spine Fractures

14. Complete the following: 65.7.3
a. When combined anterior and posterior   anterior
    cervical fusion is needed which should be
    done first?
b. When the mechanism of injury is flexion   posterior fusion
    what is the procedure of choice?
c. When the mechanism of injury is
    extension what is the procedure of
    choice for
    i.   teardrop fracture   combined anterior/posterior
                                               fusion
    ii. burst fracture   combined anterior/posterior
                                               fusion

15. Complete the following about cervical   65.7.3
    corpectomy:
a. Decompression of the cord usually   16mm
    requires corpectomy that is at least
    _____ mm wide.
b. It is advised to note position of _____. vertebral arteries

■ Spinal Cord Injury Without Radiographic Abnormality (SCIWORA)

16. True or False. Answer the following   65.8.1
    about SCIWORA (spinal cord injury
    without radiographic abnormality):
a. There is a higher incidence in age ≤ 9   true
    years.
b. There is a risk of SCIWORA among young   true
    children with asymptomatic Chiari I.
c. Dynamic flexion/extension films are   true
    normal.
d. 54% of children have a delay between   true
    injury and the onset of objective
    sensorimotor dysfunction.

66

Thoracic, Lumbar and Sacral Spine Fractures

■ Assessment and Management of Thoracolumbar Fractures

1. Matching. Match the following structures with the appropriate Denis column:

66.1.2

① anterior; ② middle; ③ posterior

a.	anterior half of disc	①
b.	posterior half of disc	②
c.	posterior arch	③
d.	anterior half of vertebral body	①
e.	posterior half of vertebral body	②
f.	facet joints and capsule	③
g.	anterior anulus fibrosus	①
h.	posterior anulus fibrosus	②
i.	interspinous ligament	③
j.	supraspinous ligament	③
k.	anterior longitudinal ligament	①
l.	posterior longitudinal ligament	②
m.	ligamentum flavum	③

2. True or False. The following are considered minor fractures of the lumbar spine:

66.1.2

a.	fracture of transverse process	true
b.	fracture of spinous process	true
c.	fracture of superior articular process	true
d.	fracture of inferior articular process	true
e.	fracture of superior end plate of vertebral body	false

3. True or False. Major injuries of the spine include:

66.1.2

a.	compression fracture	true
b.	burst fracture	true
c.	seat belt fracture	true
d.	fracture of articular process	false
e.	fracture dislocation	true

66

4. True or False. Subtypes of burst fracture include the following: 66.1.2

a. fracture of both end plates   true
b. fracture of superior end plate   true
c. fracture of inferior end plate   true
d. fracture of pars interarticularis   false
e. burst rotation   true

5. True or False. Regarding burst fracture.   66.1.2

a. It occurs mainly at thoracolumbar junction.   true
b. Mechanism—axial load   true
c. Mechanism—flexion and compression   false – usually pure axial load
d. It is a consequence of fracture of the anterior and middle column.   true
e. The most common subtype is fracture of the superior end plate.   true

6. True or False. Radiographic evaluation of burst fracture might show the following: 66.1.2

a. lateral x-ray—cortical fracture of posterior vertebral wall   true
b. AP x-ray—increase in interpedicular distance   true
c. lateral x-ray—loss of posterior vertebral height   true
d. CT—fracture posterior wall with retropulsed bone   true
e. myelogram—large central defect   true

7. True or False. Seat belt fracture has all of the following subtypes: 66.1.2

a. chance fracture, one-level through bone   true
b. one-level through ligaments   true
c. two-level, bone in middle column, ligaments in anterior and posterior columns   true
d. pedicle fracture   false
e. two-level through ligaments in all three columns   true

8. State which of the following are stable or unstable fractures of the spine: 66.1.2

a. three or more consecutive compression fractures   unstable
b. a single compression fracture with loss of > 50% of height with angulation   unstable
c. kyphotic angulation > 40 degrees at one level or > 25%   unstable
d. progressive kyphosis   unstable

66

9. State whether the following are stable or unstable fractures of the spine: 66.1.2
    a. middle column fracture above T8 below T1 if ribs and sternum intact   stable
    b. middle column fracture below L4 if posterior column is intact   stable
    c. posterior column fracture   stable acutely, as long as middle column intact
    d. compression fracture in three consecutive segments   unstable

10. True or False. Regarding burst fractures.   66.1.2
    a. Surgical treatment is recommended if angular deformity > 20 degrees.   true
    b. Surgical treatment is recommended for patients with neurologic deficit.   true
    c. Surgical treatment is recommended for anterior body height reduction ≥ 50% compared with the posterior body height.   true
    d. Surgery is recommended for canal reduction ≥ 50%.   true
    e. The anterior approach is recommended if a dural tear is present.   false – posterior recommended

11. Burst fractures are unstable if   66.1.2
    a. K—Kyphosis is more than _____.   20%
    b. I—Interpendicular distance is _____.   increased
    c. P—Progressive _____ occurs.   kyphosis
    d. H—Height of anterior body is less than_____% posteriorly.   50%
    e. D—Deficit in n_____ status.   neurological

12. True or False. Regarding L5 burst fractures.
    a. They are very common.   false   66.1.2
    b. It is difficult for instrumentation to maintain alignment at this level.   true
    c. Patients will lose ~15 degrees of lordosis between L4 and S1 even with instrumentation.   true
    d. If treatment is nonsurgical, a thoracolumbar-sacral orthosis (TLSO) brace is recommended for 4 to 6 months.   true
    e. If treatment is surgical a posterior approach with fusion and fixation L5-S1 is recommended.   true
    f. If "ligamentotaxis" is expected, distraction should be done within _____ hours.   48   66.2.1

■ Surgical Treatment

13. Complete the following about post-spinal fusion wound infections: 66.2.5

a. They are usually due to _____.   staph aureus

b. They may respond to _____ alone.   antibiotics

c. Rarely _____ may be necessary.   debridement

d. Only occasionally must instrumentation   removed
be _____.

■ Osteoporotic Spine Fractures

14. Complete the following regarding demographics of osteoporotic spine fractures:

a. True or False. There are ~700,000   true   66.3.1
osteoporotic fractures per year in the
United States.

b. True or False. Risk factors include weight.   true – weight < 58kg   66.3.2

c. There is a risk with the use of which   phenytoin
anticonvulsant?

d. There is a risk with the use of which   warfarin
anticoagulant?

e. There is a risk with consumption of   alcohol
which beverage?

f. There is a risk with the use of c_____.   cigarettes

g. There is a risk with the use of which anti-   steroids
inflammatory drug?

15. Complete the following regarding osteoporotic spine fractures:

a. The most likely population is _____.   elderly white and Asian   66.3.1
females

b. Can these fractures occur in   yes
premenopausal women?

c. The lifetime risk for women is _____%.   16

d. The lifetime risk for men is _____%.   5

e. The best predictor of fractures is _____   bone mineral density;   66.3.3
_____ _____ test measured at   femur
the _____.

16. True or False. Regarding bone mineral density (BMD).   66.3.3

a. It is not the correct predictor of bone   false
fragility.

b. It is measured by DEXA Scan at the   true
proximal femur.

c. The AP view of the lumbosacral spine   false- overestimates
underestimates BMD.

d. The T-score of BMD compares to normal   true
subjects.

e. The Z-score defines osteoporosis   true
compared with subjects of the same age
and sex.

66

17. **True or False. Regarding sodium fluoride.**   66.3.4
   a. 75 mg/d increases bone mass.   true
   b. 75 mg/d decreases fracture rate.   false
   c. 25 mg PO BID (slow fluoride) increases   true
      the fragility of the bone.
   d. Fluoride increases the demand for Ca.   true
   e. If you use fluoride also use Ca and   true
      vitamin D.

18. **True or False. The following drugs reduce bone resorption:**   66.3.4
   a. estrogen   true
   b. calcium   true
   c. vitamin D   true
   d. calcitonin   true

19. **Calcitonin is derived from _____.**   salmon   66.3.4

20. **How do the bisphosphonates work?**   66.3.4
   a. They inhibit _____   bone resorption
   b. by destroying _____.   osteoclasts

21. **True or False. The following are bisphosphonates that inhibit bone resorption:**   66.3.4
   a. etidronate (Didronel)   true
   b. alendronate (Fosamax)   true
   c. risedronate (Actonel)   true

22. **True or False. Recommended treatment for osteoporotic vertebral body fracture:**   66.3.4
   a. sufficient pain medications   true
   b. bed rest for 3 to 4 weeks   false (7 to 10 days only)
   c. DVT prophylaxis is contraindicated.   false
   d. Start physical therapy in 7 to 10 days.   true
   e. lumbar brace for pain control and   true
      comfort

23. **True or False. Regarding PVP.**   66.3.4
   a. PVP stands for percutaneous   true
      vertebroplasty.
   b. It involves injection of   true
      polymethylmethacrylate (PMMA) into
      compressed bone.
   c. Goals include prevention of progression   true
      of kyphosis.
   d. Goals include correction of kyphosis.   false
   e. Goals include shortened duration of   true
      pain.
   f. PMMA injection is FDA approved for   false – not for trauma, PMMA
      treatment of compression fractures due   may inhibit healing
      to tumor, osteoporosis and trauma.

24. True or False. Indications for PVP include the following: 66.3.4

a. severe pain that interferes with activity — true

b. painful osteoporotic compression fracture with < 10% of height reduction — false

c. failure to control pain with pain medications — true

d. progressive vertebral hemangioma — true

e. pedicle screw salvage — true

66

25. True or False. Vertebroplasty contraindications include   66.3.4

a. coagulopathy — true

b. chronic injury — true

c. active infection — true

d. burst fracture — true – concern for PMMA leakage

26. Matching. Match the complications of PVP with the order in which they are more likely to occur.   66.3.4
① highest; ② second highest; ③ least
Complications: (a-c) below

a. vertebral hemangiomas — ②

b. pathologic fractures — ①

c. osteoporotic compression fractures — ③

27. True or False. Complications of PVP include   66.3.4

a. PMMA leak — true

b. pedicle fracture — true

c. transverse process fracture — true

d. spinous process fracture — false

e. rib fracture — true

28. True or False. Post-PVP recommendations include the following: 66.3.4

a. discharge home the same day — false – usually admitted overnight

b. watch for chest pain — true

c. watch for fever — true

d. watch for neurologic deficit — true

e. gradual mobilization after 2 hours — true

■ Sacral Fractures

29. **Complete the following:**

a.	Look for in patients who have _____ pelvic fractures	pelvic	66.4.1
	i. because _____% will also have sacral fractures	17%	
b.	accompanied in _____% by neurologic deficits.	20-60	
c.	Sacral fractures are divided into _____ zones.	3	Table 66.6
	i. I involves _____ _____	ala only	
	ii. II involves _____ _____	sacral foramina	
	iii. III involves _____ _____	neural canal	
d.	The fractures that involve neurologic deficits are those involving zones ____ and ____	II and III	66.4.3
e.	Which fracture can cause bowel and bladder incontinence?	III	
f.	Which fracture can cause L5 root injury?	I	

67

Penetrating Spine Injuries and Long Term Management / Complications

■ Gunshot Wounds to the Spine

1. **True or False. Indications for surgery in gunshot wounds to the spine include the following:**   67.1.2
   a. injury to cauda equina if root compression is demonstrated — true
   b. to remove copper-jacketed bullets from the spine — true – cause local reaction
   c. CSF leak — true
   d. compression of nerve root — true
   e. vascular injury — true
   f. to improve spinal cord function — false
   g. spinal instability — true

■ Penetrating Trauma to the Neck

2. **True or False. Regarding vascular injuries of the neck:**   67.2.2
   a. Venous injuries occur in ≈ 30% of penetrating neck trauma. — false – 18%
   b. Arterial injuries occur in ≈ 12% of penetrating neck trauma. — true
   c. 72% of vertebral artery injuries had no neurological deficits on exam. — true
   d. Common carotid artery injury is the most common vascular injury. — true

3. **Matching. Penetrating wounds of the neck are divided into three zones by anatomical boundaries.**   67.2.3
   Zone:
   ① zone I; ② zone II; ③ zone III
   Anatomical boundaries: (a-e) below
   a. clavicle — ②
   b. angle of mandible — ②-③
   c. head of clavicle — ①
   d. thoracic outlet — ①
   e. base of skull — ③

67

4. **True or False. Treatment of penetrating trauma to the neck includes the following:**   67.2.5
   a. immediate prophylactic intubation to protect airway | false
   b. cricothyroidotomy if apparent mechanical instability of the neck | true
   c. Surgical exploration is recommended for all wounds piercing the platysma and entering the anterior triangle of the neck. | true
   d. Patients in coma are poor candidates for surgical vascular reconstruction. | true – high mortality

5. **Complete the following regarding vertebral artery (VA) trauma:**   67.2.5
   a. It is more common to treat by _____ than by direct repair. | ligation
      i. What must you know about other vessels before you decide on treatment of VA injury? | patency
      ii. Which vessels? | contralateral VA, PICA
   b. What minimally invasive treatment is available? | covered stent placement
   c. Is arterial bypass ever indicated? | no

■ Delayed Cervical Instability

6. **Delayed cervical instability is defined as instability identified after ___ days.** | 20   67.3.1

■ Chronic Management Issues with Spinal Cord Injuries

7. **True or False. Syndromes associated with spinal cord injuries include all of the following:**   67.5.1
   a. autonomic hyporeflexia | false – hyperreflexia
   b. DVT | true
   c. syringomyelia | true
   d. spasticity | true
   e. osteoporosis | true
   f. shoulder-hand syndrome | true

8. **True or False. In autonomic hyperreflexia the following is found:**   67.5.3
   a. exaggerated autonomic response to stimuli | true
   b. only in patients with lesion above T6 | true
   c. complaints of headache, flushing, and diaphoresis | true
   d. extreme hypertension | true
   e. epinephrine is released causing this syndrome | false – norepinephrine

9. **True or False. Regarding autonomic hyperreflexia in SCI.**   67.5.3

a. It occurs only in patients with SCI below T6. false – above T6

b. Patients complain of pounding headache. true

c. It can be life threatening. true

d. It occurs in ≈ 30% of quadriplegic patients. true

e. There is a lag time of 3 to 4 months. true

67

10. **True or False. Regarding autonomic dysreflexia in SCI.**   67.5.3

a. It often occurs in the first 3 to 4 months after SCI. false – occurs after first 3-4 mos.

b. Bladder distension may cause onset. true

c. Colorectal distension may cause onset. true

d. DVT may cause onset. true

11. **True or False. Presentation of autonomic hyperreflexia in SCI includes**   67.5.3

a. paroxysmal hypertension true

b. anxiety true

c. miosis false – mydriasis

d. penile erection true

e. Horner's syndrome true

12. **Complete the following about autonomic hyperreflexia:**   67.5.3

a. What is the triad of presenting symptoms?

  i. h_____ headache

  ii. s_____ sweating

  iii. facial f_____ facial flushing

b. It could be confused with _____. pheochromocytoma

68

Low Back Pain and Radiculopathy

■ General Information

1. Complete the following about low back pain and radiculopathy:

a. True or False. Bed rest beyond 4 days is more helpful than harmful for patients with low back pain.

false (Bed rest beyond 4 days may be more harmful than helpful.)

68.1

b. True or False. 60% of patients with low back pain will improve clinically within 1 month even without treatment.

false (89-90% will improve within 1 month without treatment, including patients with sciatica from disc herniation.)

c. Pure radicular symptoms will include upper motor neuron (UMN) signs or lower motor neuron (LMN) signs?

LMN signs (Radiculopathy will/may show associated decreased reflexes, weakness, and atrophy.)

2. True or False. The percentage of low-risk back pain patients who will improve without treatment in 1 month's time is

68.1

a. 10%   false

b. 20%   false

c. 90%   true (Most low back patients will resolve and no specific diagnosis can be made in 85% despite aggressive workup.)

d. 0%   false

■ Intervertebral Disc

3. The nucleus pulposus is a remnant of the embryonic _____.

notocord

68.2.2

■ Nomenclature for Disc Pathology

4. **True or False. The following may be considered a non-pathological condition:** — 68.3

a. degenerated disc — false
b. annular fissure — false
c. bulging disc generalized > 50% — true (Bulging disc is a circumferential symmetrical extension of the disc beyond the endplates. Incidence increases with age.)
d. focal herniation — false
e. protruding disc — false

5. **True or False. Gas in the disc usually is a sign of** — Table 68.1

a. disc infection — false
b. disc degeneration — true
c. AKA v_____ d_____ — vacuum disc

6. **An extruded disc where the free fragment is contained by the posterior longitudinal ligament is called a _____ disc.** — sequestered — Table 68.1

7. **Give the definition of a sequestered disc.** — Table 68.1

a. _____ disc — extruded
b. loss of _____ with its disc of _____ — continuity; origin
c. also known as a _____ _____ — free fragment

■ Vertebral Body Marrow Changes

8. **Provide the Modic's classification of vertebral body marrow changes:** — Table 68.2

a. Type 1: T1WI ___, T2WI ___ — ↓ ↑ (bone marrow edema associated with acute or subacute inflammation)
b. Type 2: T1WI _____, T2WI _____ — ↑ ↑ (chronic change- bone marrow replaced by fat)
c. Type 3: T1WI _____, T2WI _____ — ↓ ↑ (chronic- reactive osteosclerosis)

■ Disability, Pain and Outcome Determinations

9. **Oswestry disability index** — Table 68.3

a. Is a scale used for ____ ____. — back pain
b. A score of _____% is essentially totally disabled. — 45%
c. A functional score is below _____%. — 20%

■ Initial Assessment of the Patient with Back Pain

68

10. True or False. Cauda equina syndrome may include the following: 68.8.2

a. bladder dysfunction (incontinence or retention)   true

b. Faber sign or Patrick-Faber sign (flexion abduction external rotation)   false (Positive in hip joint disease and does not exacerbate true nerve root compression.)

c. saddle anesthesia   true
d. unilateral/bilateral leg weakness or pain   true
e. fecal incontinence   true

11. Name the associated nerve root for each of the following: 68.8.3

a. great toe strength   L5 and some L4
b. dorsal foot sensation   L5
c. lateral foot sensation   S1
d. medial foot sensation   L4
e. plantar foot sensation   S1
f. achilles reflex   S1

12. For patients with low back pain, red flags for a serious underlying pathology would include signs consistent with what conditions?
(Hint: CISC)   68.8.4

a. C_____   cauda equina syndrome
b. I_____   infection
c. S_____   spinal fracture
d. C_____   cancer

13. Signs of cauda equina syndrome include   Table 68.5

a. _____   saddle anesthesia
b. _____   bladder overflow incontinence or retention
c. _____   fecal incontinence or loss of anal sphincter tone
d. _____   leg pain (unilateral/bilateral)
e. _____   leg weakness (unilateral/bilateral)

14. Electromyography (EMG) is not helpful to evaluate for myelopathy, myopathy, or nerve root dysfunction unless the symptoms have been present for at least ___ - ___ weeks.   3 to 4 (results are variable before this time)   68.8.5

■ Radiographic Evaluation

15. **True or False. Regarding plain lumbosacral spine x-rays.**   68.9.2

a. Are recommended for routine evaluation of back pain.   false

b. When indicated, AP and Lateral views are usually adequate.   true

c. Unexpected findings occur frequently.   false

d. Gonadal radiation is insignificant.   false

e. Appropriate in patients who have "red flags."   true

16. **True or False. Red flags include**   68.9.2

a. patients under age 20   true

b. patients over age 50   false (>70)

c. drug users   true

d. diabetics   true

e. post-op urinary tract patients   true

f. persistent pain for more than 1 week   false (>4 weeks)

17. **Complete the following about low back pain and radiculopathy:**   68.9.3

a. Signs on MRI that indicate disc degeneration include

   i. increase or decrease of signal intensity on T2-weighted imaging (T2WI)?   decrease

   ii. increase or decrease of disc height?   decrease

b. Signs on computed tomography (CT) that indicate disc herniation include

   i. increase or decrease of the normal epidural fat   decrease

   ii. _____ of the thecal sac   indentation

c. CT will show loss of _____ (concavity/convexity) of the thecal sac?   convexity   68.9.4

18. **Other useful tests include the following:**   68.9.5

a. Myelogram-CT: Identifies contribution to cause of pressure by _____.   bone

b. In terms of discography

   i. reliability?   controversial

   ii. interpretation?   equivocal

   iii. false positives?   high

   iv. May help in cases of multiple discs when?   one produces pain

68

■ Psychosocial Factors

19. **List five signs of psychosocial distress in back pain, remembering that inappropriate response to any three suggests psychological distress is present.**
(Hint: PIAMP)

   68.13

   a. P*   physical exam over reaction
   b. I*   inconsistent performance (straight leg test changes from sitting to standing, etc.)
   c. A*   axial loading produces pain
   d. M   motor/sensory exam inconsistent with anatomy
   e. P   pain on superficial palpation

■ Treatment

20. **Clear indications for urgent lumbar surgery include**

   68.14.1

   a. c_____ e_____   cauda equina syndrome
   b. p_____ n_____ d_____   progressive neurological deficit
   c. p_____ w_____   profound weakness (motor)

21. **True or False. The following conservative therapy treatments have proven beneficial for patients with back pain:**

   68.14.2

   a. epidural steroids   false
   b. transcutaneous electrical nerve stimulation (TENS)   false
   c. traction   false
   d. oral steroids   false
   e. spinal manipulation   false
   f. muscle relaxants   false

22. **Is there a risk to the use of Parafon Forte? If so, what is the risk?**   yes; fatal hepatotoxicity   68.14.2

23. **Is lumbar fusion for LBP without stenosis or spondylolisthesis ever recommended?**   yes, for patients with LBP due to 1 or 2 level DDD for ≥ 2 years who failed medical therapy, with disease at L4-L5 and/or L5-S1   68.14.3

24. **When is lumbar spinal fusion indicated according to current practice guidelines?**   68.14.3

   a. fracture/dislocation   yes
   b. instability due to tumor or infection   yes
   c. following disc excision for HLD or 1st time recurrence   no

d.	as potential adjunct to discectomy in HLD with preoperative deformity or instability	yes
e.	Pain associated with Modic type 1 changes? Modic type 2 or 3?	yes; no

25. True or False. Standard discectomy and microdiscectomy are of similar efficacy.   true   Table 68.6

■ Chronic Low Back Pain

26. The patient's chances of returning to work if off for   Table 68.7

a.	6 months is _____%	50%
b.	1 year is _____%	20%
c.	2 years is _____%	< 5%

■ Coccydynia

27. True or False. Coccydynia is related to the following:

a.	Is worse when standing.	false (worse when sitting or rising from sitting)	68.16.1
b.	Is most common in females.	true	
c.	Differential involves local trauma, neoplasms, and prostatitis.	true	68.16.2
d.	Needs nuclear bone scan for workup.	false (CT for bony pathology, and MRI for detecting soft tissue masses)	68.16.3

■ Failed Back Surgery Syndrome

28. Failure rate for lumbar discectomy to provide long-term pain relief is ___ - ___%   8-25%   68.17.1

29. Common etiologies of failed back surgery syndrome include but are not limited to: 68.17.2

a.	incorrect initial diagnosis	true (clinical findings not correlating with imaging abnormality, imaging consistent but actually symptomatic from other diagnosis (e.g. trochanteric bursitis, diabetic amyotrophy, etc.))
b.	continued nerve root compression	true (residual compression, recurrent pathology, adjacent pathology, peridural scar, epidural hematoma, etc.)

68

c. temporary nerve root injury | false (associated with permanent injury from original compression)

30. Discitis usually produces back pain ___ - ___ weeks post-op. 2-4   68.17.2

31. Arachnoiditis: 68.17.3
a. Also known as _____ arachnoiditis. adhesive
b. Inflammatory fibrosis of which meningeal layers? pia, arachnoid, dura
c. Increased risk associated with which of the following:
   i. spinal anesthesia true
   ii. spinal meningitis true
   iii. autoimmune diseases false
   iv. trauma true

32. MRI findings in arachnoiditis typically are in 3 patterns: 68.17.3
a. c_____ a_____ separating nerve roots into 1 or 2 chords Central adhesion
b. e_____ t_____ s_____: only CSF signal visible intrathecally Empty thecal sac- roots adhere to meninges around periphery
c. thecal sac filled with i_____ t_____ inflammatory tissue; no CSF signal, candle-dripping appearance

33. At 6-month follow up, ___% of patients will have extensive peridural scar, but ___% of the time, these are asymptomatic. 43%; 84%   68.17.4

34. Peridural scar is best evaluated by what imaging modality? MRI with and without IV gadolinium   68.17.4
a. True or False. Unenhanced MRI shows scar that becomes more enhanced from T1WI to T2WI. false (Becomes less intense whereas HLD becomes more intense with this transition.)
b. True or False. Enhanced MRI shows enhancement of scar. true (Enhances inhomogeneously, whereas disc does not enhance at all.)

69

Lumbar and Thoracic Intervertebral Disk Herniation / Radiculopathy

■ Lumbar Disc Herniation and Lumbar Radiculopathy

1. **Radiculopathy typically presents with _____.**	pain and/or subjective sensory changes (numbness, tingling) in nerve root dermatome	69.1.1
2. **True or False. Radiculopathy causes hyperreflexia.**	false (sometimes accompanied by weakness and decreased reflex changes)	69.1.1
3. **Typical disc herniation compresses the nerve exiting the neural foramen at the level _____.**	below	69.1.1
4. **True or False. Surgical indications include**		69.1.1
a. cauda equine syndrome	true	
b. numbness of foot	false	
c. progressive symptoms	true	
d. abnormal MRI	false	
e. neurologic deficits	true	
f. abnormal discogram	false	
g. failed conservative treatment	true	
h. pain when coughing	false	
i. severe radicular pain for 2 weeks	false (6 weeks)	
j. severe back pain	false	
5. **Why do disc herniations tend to occur slightly off midline posteriorly to one side within the central canal?**	Posterior longitudinal ligament is strongest in midline, and posterolateral annulus bears disproportionate load from above.	69.1.3

6. **Complete the following regarding lumbar disc herniation:**   69.1.5

a. Occurrence of voiding dysfunction in lumbar disc herniation varies from ___ to ___%.   1 to 18%

b. Concerning bladder symptoms, what is the sequence of events from the earliest findings?

    i.   d_____ b_____ s_____   decreased bladder sensation
    ii. u_____ u_____   urinary urgency
    iii. i_____ f_____   increased frequency (due to increased postvoid residual)
    iv. e_____ and i_____   enuresis (bed wetting) and incontinence are rare

c. Urinary retention with overflow incontinence is suggestive of what diagnosis?   cauda equina compression

7. **What is the most sensitive sign of herniated lumbar disc?**   Lasègue's sign   69.1.6

8. **Regarding the significance of a positive crossed straight-leg raising sign.**

a. Specificity for nerve root compression of ___%.   90%   Table 69.1

b. It suggests a more _____ HNP.   central   69.1.6
c. It may correlate with a disc fragment within the _____ of the contralateral root.   axilla

d. Lasègue specificity for root compression is ___%   83%

e. For crossed Lasègue, the percentage increases to ___%   90%

9. **Describe a positive Lasègue's sign:**   69.1.6
a. patient positioned _____   supine
b. raise leg by the ankle until _____   pain elicited, specifically in leg (paresthesias or pain). Back pain alone is negative SLR.

c. pain occurs below ___ degrees   60
d. positive in ___% herniated nucleus pulposus (HNP)   83% (most likely to be positive in patients under 30)

10. **Describe the following techniques to elicit indications of nerve root tension:**   69.1.6

a. Lasègue's sign   straight leg raising by ankle
b. Cram test   extend knee with leg already raised

c. Fajersztajn's sign   crossed SLR (central disc). 97% HNP had this be positive
d. Femoral stretch test   prone, knee maximally flexed = L2, L3, L4 root lesions

e. Bowstring sign   flex knee after SLR: Hip pain persists but sciatic pain ceases

f. Sitting knee extension   sitting SLR

11. Describe the FABER test   69.1.6

a. also known as _____ _____   Patrick's test

b. performed by _____   flexion abduction, external rotation; lateral malleolus on contralateral knee, with downward pressure on flexed knee

c. positive sign indicative of ____ _____   hip pathology

12. Complete the following regarding the Trendelenburg sign: 69.1.6

a. The affected hip _____ when the patient is walking,   dips

b. which indicates the contralateral thigh adductors are _____.   weak

c. This causes the contralateral pelvis to _____,   tilt

d. which is caused by a lesion of the _____ root.   L5 (Affected hip dips when walking to indicate weakness of contralateral thigh adductors, or while standing on leg with weak adductors causes pelvis to tilt contralateral to weakness.)

13. Complete the following about crossed adductors sign: 69.1.6

a. Crossed adductors sign is positive when knee jerk is elicited and the contralateral thigh _____ _____.   adductors contract

b. If knee jerk is

     i. hyperactive, it suggests ____ _____   UMN lesion

     ii. hypoactive, it suggests _____ _____   pathological spread due to nerve root irritation

14. Complete the following about Hoover's sign: 69.1.6

a. It is a test to learn if patient's leg weakness is _____.   functional (vs. organic)

b. Examiner places hand under patient's normal _____.   heel

c. When asked to lift the weak leg, lack of effort to move the _____ leg _____ is indication that weakness is functional.   normal; down

15. For the listed lumbar disc level, what is the frequency of herniated disc syndrome?   Table 69.3

a. L5-S1: ___ - ___%   45-50%

b. L4-5: ___ - ___%   40-45%

c. L3-4: ___ - ___%   3-10%

69

16. **Name physical findings associated with a L5-S1 disc herniation and where pain radiates.**   Table 69.3

a. Reflex: absent a_____ r_____   achilles reflex
b. Motor: _____ weakness   gastrocnemius (plantar flexion)
c. Sensory: decreased at l_____ m_____ and l_____ f_____   lateral malleolus and lateral foot
d. Pain: posterior aspect of ____ and _____   calf and ankle

17. **Name three indicators for emergency lumbar surgery.**   69.1.9
(hint: ces, pmd, ip)

a. ces   cauda equina syndrome (urinary retention and/or overflow incontinence, saddle anesthesia)
b. pmd   progressive motor deficit (i.e. foot drop)
c. ip   intolerable pain (urgent)

18. **List potential findings for cauda equina syndrome.**   69.1.9
(Hint: cauda-s)

a. C   Can't function sexually (sexual dysfunction)
b. A   Ankle jerk absent
c. U   Urinary retention/incontinence (most consistent finding)
d. D   Diminished sphincter tone
e. A   Anesthesia of saddle area (most common sensory deficit)
f. S   Strength decreased

19. **True or False. The following is classically recognized as a cause of the cauda equina syndrome:**   69.1.9

a. tumor   true
b. epidural spinal hematoma   true
c. free fat graft following discectomy   true
d. trauma/fracture   true
e. lumbar stenosis   false (more chronic process/ would not classically give an acute/subacute presentation of CES)

20. **True or False. In cauda equina syndrome, surgery should be performed**   69.1.9

a. stat   false
b. within 24 hours   false
c. within 48 hours   true
d. within 72 hours   false
e. within a week   false

69

21. **True or False. Comparing microdiscectomy to standard discectomy for lumbar disc herniation, which of the following are true?**   69.1.9
    a. shorter incision   true
    b. shorter hospital stay   true
    c. less blood loss   true
    d. better efficacy   false (Efficacy has been shown to be equivalent between the two techniques.)
    e. may be more difficult to retrieve large fragments   true

22. **Success rate at 1 year for surgical discectomy is ___%.**   85%   69.1.9

23. **True or False. Intradiscal procedures such as chemonucleolysis are used more than discectomy.**   false   69.1.9

24. **Complete the following about intradiscal procedures:**   69.1.9
    a. What percentage of lumbar disc patients considered for surgery could be candidates for intradiscal procedures?   10-15%
    b. What is the success rate of intradiscal procedures (pain free and return to work)?   37-75%

25. **True or False. Following discectomy:**   69.1.9
    a. Epidural steroids prior to closure have no benefit.   true
    b. Systemic steroids and bupivacaine may reduce hospital stay and postop narcotic requirements.   true

26. **True or False. Regarding epidural free fat graft.**   69.1.9
    a. It can cause nerve root compression.   true
    b. It is believed to reduce epidural scar formation.   mixed (opinions vary)
    c. Some believe it may increase epidural scar.   true
    d. It increases the incidence of postoperative infection.   false
    e. It may cause cauda equina syndrome.   true but rare

27. **Characterize complications of lumbar disc surgery.**   69.1.9
    a. Mortality: ___%   0.06% (1/1800 patients)
    b. Superficial infection: __ - __% with _____ organism   0.9-1%, S. aureus
    c. Deep infection: ___%   <1% (discitis, spinal epidural abscess)
    d. Discitis: ___%   0.5%
    e. Motor deficit: __ - __%   1-8% (some transient)

69

f.	Durotomy: __ - __%	0.3-13%
g.	Durotomy after redo: ___%	18%
h.	Surgical repair: ___	1/1000 patients
i.	Pseudomeningocele: __ - __%	0.7-2%
j.	Recurrent disc: ___%	4% (with 10 year follow-up)

28. Complete the following about durotomy: 69.1.9

a. What is the incidence of incidental durotomy in lumbar laminectomy? — 0.3-13% (increases to 18% on redos)

b. Give four possible complications related to incidental durotomies.

    i.   C_____ — CSF fistula-requiring repair in 10/10,000 patients

    ii. p_____ — pseudomeningocele 0.7-2%

    iii. h_____ — herniation of nerve roots

    iv. i_____ — increased epidural bleeding

29. What is the incidence of recurrent herniated lumbar disc?   69.1.9

a.	same level either side in first 10 years ___%	~4%
b.	any level over 10 years	3-19%
c.	first year same level either side ___%	1.5%
d.	any different incidence depending on level	2x more common at L4-5
e.	same level recurrence ___%	74%
f.	different level recurrence ___%	26%

30. Complete the following regarding the anterior longitudinal ligament: 69.1.9

a.	Asymptomatic perforations occur in ___% of discectomies.	12%
b.	Depth of disc space is ___.	3.3 cm
c.	Vascular injury produces bleeding into operative field only ___% of the time.	50%
d.	Great vessel injury mortality is ___%.	37-67%

31. Enumerate five complications related to positioning for lumbar discectomies.   69.1.9

Hint: tecup

a.	t_____	tibialis anterior compartment syndrome
b.	e_____	eyes pressure
c.	c_____	cervical spine injury
d.	u_____	ulnar nerve compression
e.	p_____	peroneal nerve compression

32. True or False. Regarding unintended durotomy.   69.1.9

a. Normal ambulation is not considered a cause for failure of dural repair.   true

b. Risk of a cerebrospinal fluid (CSF) leak is increased in

    i. revision surgery   true

    ii. removal of ossification of the posterior longitudinal ligament (OPLL)   true

    iii. high-speed drills   true

c. It is not considered an act of malpractice.   true

d. The use of fibrin glue to close is advantageous.   true

e. It can be due to thinned dura by longstanding stenosis.   true

69

33. Enumerate four signs of postoperative cauda equina syndrome (i.e., from epidural hematoma).   69.1.9

Hint: pain

a. p_____   pain out of the ordinary

b. a_____   anesthesia of saddle area

c. i_____   inability to void

d. n_____   numerous muscle groups weak

34. True or False. Regarding the outcome of surgical treatment of lumbar herniated disc.   69.1.9

a. 5% will be classified as having failed back syndrome.   true

b. At 1 year the surgical group had a better outcome than with conservative treatment.   true

c. The benefit persisted at 10 years.   false (Surgery group had better outcome at 1 year but benefit was no longer statistically significant at 4-year follow-up. At 10 years neither surgical nor conservative treatment group complained of sciatica or back pain.)

d. 63% had complete relief of back pain at 1 year post-op.   true

e. At 5- to 10-year follow-up 86% felt improved.   true

35. **True or False. The percentage of patients with L3-4 disc herniation having a past history of L4-5 or L5-S1 disc herniation is**   69.1.10
   a. < 10%   false
   b. approximately 25%   true
   c. approximately 50%   false
   d. 60 to 80%   false
   e. almost 90%   false

36. **Characterize a herniated upper lumbar disc.**   69.1.10
   a. What is the incidence?
      i.   L1-2: _____%   0.28%
      ii. L2-3: _____%   1.3%
      iii. L3-4: _____%   3.6%
   b. Most common muscle involved?   quadriceps femoris
   c. Femoral stretch test _____.   may be positive
   d. Knee jerk _____.   reduced in 50%

37. **Characterize extreme lateral lumbar disc herniations.**   69.1.11
   a. What is the incidence?   3 to 10%
   b. What level is most commonly involved?
      i.   L4-5: _____%   60%
      ii. L3-4: _____%   24%
      iii. L5-S1: _____%   7%
   c. Enumerate four differences compared with other common disc herniations.
      i.   Straight leg raising (SLR) is negative in ___ - ___%.   85 to 90%
      ii. Pain is increased by lateral bending in _____%.   75%
      iii. Pain is more _____.   severe
      iv. Extruded fragments are _____ _____.   more frequent

38. **Distinguishing features concerning far lateral disc herniation include the following:**   69.1.11
   a. The root involved is the root _____ _____ _____ _____.   exiting at that level
   b. SLR is _____.   negative
   c. Lateral bending is _____.   likely to produce pain
   d. Severity of pain is _____ because _____ _____ _____ is compressed.   greater; dorsal root ganglion
   e. Most common levels are _____ and _____.   L4-5 and L3-4
   f. Best surgical approach is _____ _____.   standard hemilaminectomy (and follow nerve laterally; perform medial facetectomy)

39. **Zones in which disc herniation can occur are:**   69.1.11
   a. c_____   central
   b. s_____   subarticular
   c. f_____   foraminal
   d. e_____   extraforaminal

40. **True or False. One third of extreme lateral lumbar disc herniations are missed on initial radiologic exams.**   true   69.1.11

41. **To test for far lateral disc, what is the value of post-discography CT scan?**   may be the most sensitive test—94%   69.1.11

42. **Give the incidence of surgery for herniated discs in pediatric patients.**   69.1.12
   a. under 20 years of age: _____%   less than 1%
   b. under 17 years of age: _____%   less than 1/2 of 1%

43. **Characterize intradural disc herniation.**   69.1.13
   a. What is the incidence?   0.04 to 1.1%
   b. Can it be diagnosed preoperatively?   rarely
   c. It is suspected at surgery because of a n_____ e_____.   negative exploration
   d. Does it require a surgical dural opening?   rarely

44. **Regarding intravertebral disc herniations, answer the following:**   69.1.14
   a. It is also known as _____ _____.   Schmorl's nodes
   b. Herniation occurs through what structure?   through the cartilaginous end plate into cancellous bone of the vertebral body
   c. True or False. Presentation is similar to typical herniated disk with radiculopathy.   false - Presents with low back pain aggravated by axial weight load bearing.
   d. Radiographically on MRI
      i. Symptomatic (acute) lesions present as _____ on T1WI and _____ on T2WI.   low; high
      ii. Asymptomatic (chronic) lesions present as _____ on T1WI and _____ on T2WI.   high; low
   e. Treatment?   conservative therapy with NSAIDs. Symptoms generally improve within 3-4 months.

45. **Characterize recurrent herniated disc.**   69.1.15
   a. second herniation: ___ - ____%   3 to 19%
   b. 10 years same level: _____%   4%
   c. 1 year same level: _____%   1.5%

69

46. **Does it take a larger or smaller disc herniation to cause symptoms in recurrent disc? Why? Because s_____ t_____ prevents the nerve from moving away.**   smaller; scar tissue   69.1.15

■ Thoracic Disc Herniation

47. **Characterize thoracic disc herniation.**   69.2.1
    a. It usually occurs below the level of_____.   T8
    b. Because many are calcified it is wise to get a _____ _____.   CT scan
    c. The incidence is ____ to ____% of all disc herniations.   0.25 to 0.75%
    d. _____% occur between ages 30 and 50.   80%
    e. History of trauma is _____%.   25%

48. **Characterize access to the thoracic spine.**
    a. upper: _____   sternal splitting   96.1.1
    b. mid: _____   right thoracotomy (heart not in way)   96.2.2
    c. lower: _____   left–easier to mobilize aorta than vena cava   96.2.3
    d. thoracolumbar: _____   right to avoid liver unless pathology is far on left side   96.4.1
    e. lumbar: _____   transabdominal   96.5.1

49. **Complete the following concerning the thoracic spine and spinal cord anterior access to:**
    a. lower thoracic spine   96.2.3
        i.   use _____ side thoracotomy   left
        ii. avoid _____ _____   vena cava
        iii. easier to mobilize _____   aorta
    b. thoracolumbar spine   96.4.1
        i. use _____ side retroperitoneal approach   right
        ii. thereby avoiding _____   liver

70

Cervical Disc Herniation

■ General Information

1. **Where does the cervical root exit in relation to the pedicle?** — in close relation to the undersurface of the pedicle — 70.1

■ Cervical Nerve Root Syndromes (Cervical Radiculopathy)

2. **Complete the following table concerning cervical disc syndromes:** — Table 70.1

Table 70.1 Cervical disc syndromes

Syndrome	Cervical disc syndromes			
	C4–5	C5–6	C6–7	C7-T1
% of cervical discs				
compressed root				
reflex diminished				
motor weakness				
paresthesia & hypesthesia				

Table 70.1 (incomplete)

Table 70.1 Cervical disc syndromes

Syndrome	Cervical disc syndromes			
	C4–5	C5–6	C6–7	C7-T1
% of cervical discs	2%	19%	69%	10%
compressed root	C5	C6	C7	C8
reflex diminished	deltoid & pectoralis	biceps & bra-chioradialis	triceps	finger-jerk
motor weakness	deltoid	forearm flexion	forearm ext (wrist drop)	hand intrinsics
paresthesia & hypesthesia	shoulder	upper arm, thumb, radial forearm	fingers 2 & 3, all fingertips	fingers 4 & 5

Table 70.1 (complete)
(Reprinted with permission from Greenberg MS, Handbook of Neurosurgery. 8th ed. New York: Thieme; 2016.)

3. **Complete the following about intervertebral disc herniation:**
   a. C6-7 disc causes a C_____ radiculopathy. — C7 — 70.2.1
   b. C5-6 disc causes a C_____ radiculopathy. — C6 — 70.2.2
   c. It may simulate a _____. — myocardial infarction

4. **A left C6 radiculopathy can simulate an _____ _____ _____.** — acute myocardial infarction — 70.2.2

5. **C8 or T1 nerve root involvement (i.e., a C7-T1 or T1-T2 disc) may produce a partial _____ syndrome.** — a partial Horner syndrome — 70.2.2

6. **The most common scenario for patients with herniated cervical discs is that the symptoms were first noticed upon _____.** — awakening in the morning (without identifiable trauma and stress) — 70.2.2

7. **Complete the following about intervertebral disc herniation:**   Table 70.1
   a. C4-5 disc compresses C _____ root_____.   C5 root
   b. C7-T1 disc compresses C _____ root   C8 root

■ Physical Exam for Cervical Disc Herniation

8. **Narrowing the cervical foramen mechanically is called _____ _____.**   Spurling's sign   70.5.2

9. **Complete the following about the Spurling's sign:**   70.5.2
   a. Performed by
      i.   examiner exerting pressure on the_____   vertex
      ii. while patient tilts head toward the_____ _____   symptomatic side
      iii. with neck _____.   extended
   b. Reproduces _____ _____.   radicular pain
   c. analogous to _____   SLR for lumbar disc—a mechanical sign

■ Radiologic Evaluation

10. **Give the accuracy of radiological workups.**
    a. MRI is ____ to ____%.   85 to 90%   70.6.1
    b. CT myelogram is _____%.   98%   70.6.2

■ Cervical Myelopathy and SCI due to Cervical Disc Herniation

11. **True or False. Regarding fusion.**   70.7.3
    a. a plate reduces pseudoarthrosis.   true
    b. a plate reduces graft problems.   true
    c. a plate maintains lordosis.   true
    d. improves clinical outcome.   false
    e. improves arm pain.   true
    f. provides more rapid relief of arm pain.   true
    g. maintains foraminal height.   false
    h. maintains disc space height.   false
    i. reduces post-op kyphosis.   true
    j. improves fusion rate.   true

12. **What is the incidence of vocal cord paresis due to injury of the recurrent laryngeal nerve (RLN)?**   70.7.3
    a. Temporary: _____ %   11%
    b. Permanent: _____ %   4%

70

13. **True or False. A good way to treat vertebral artery injury is by**   70.7.3
    a. packing   false
    b. direct suture   true
    c. endovascular trapping   true

14. **The rare complication of sleep-induced apnea can occur with anterior cervical discectomy and fusion (ACDF) at the level of _____.**   C3-4   70.7.3

15. **Characterize dysphagia following ACDF.**   70.7.3
    a. Incidence early is _____%,   60%
    b. at 6 months only _____%.   5%
    c. Most serious cause is _____.   hematoma
    d. Permanent recurrent laryngeal nerve injury occurs in _____%.   1.3%

16. **Characterize pseudoarthrosis following ACDF. On flexion extension cervical spine x-rays:**   70.7.3
    a. movement of more than _____ mm   2
    b. between the _____ _____   spinous processes
    c. lack of _____ across the fusion   trabeculation
    d. l_____ around the screws   lucency
    e. t_____ of the screws on flexion extension films   toggling
    f. n_____ uniformly associated with symptoms   not

17. **For patients in certain professions we prefer to do posterior cervical surgery instead of anterior.**   70.7.3
    a. Which two professions?   speaker and singer
    b. The reason is that there is a _____% incidence of _____ _____ after anterior cervical surgery.   4%; voice change

18. **Indications for posterior keyhole laminotomy are**   70.7.3
    a. s_____ l_____ d_____   soft lateral disc
    b. occupation of s_____ or s_____   singer or speaker
    c. l_____- or u_____-l_____ d_____   lower- or upper-level disc

70

19. **Matching. Match the recommended sequence of bone removal with the recommended sequence for posterior keyhole laminotomy.**
    Sequence of bone removal recommended:
    ① superior facet of the vertebra below;
    ② inferior facet of the vertebra above;
    ③ lateral aspect of lamina above
    Recommended sequence: (a-c) below

    a. 1st area of bone removal   ③
    b. 2nd area of bone removal   ②
    c. 3rd area of bone removal   ①

    70.7.3

20. **The success rate of posterior keyhole laminectomy is in the range of _____ to _____ %.**   90 to 96%   70.7.3

70

71

Degenerative Cervical Disc Disease and Cervical Myelopathy

■ General Information

1. Cervical degenerative disc disease is generally discussed in terms of "_____ _____," a term which is sometimes used synonymously with "cervical spinal stenosis."

cervical spondylosis

71.1

■ Clinical

2. Cervical spondylosis is the most common cause of myelopathy in patients >___ yrs of age.

55

71.3.1

3. Characterize the frequency of symptoms for the following reflexes
   a. hyperreflexia: ___%
   b. Babinski: ___%
   c. Hoffman: ___%

87%
54%
12%

Table 71.1

4. Complete the following about degenerative disc/spine disease:
   a. What reflex test is said to be pathognomonic of cervical spinal myelopathy?

   b. Elicited by performing the _____ _____

   c. and obtaining a response of f_____ of the f_____.

inverted radial reflex

brachioradialis reflex

flexion of the fingers

71.3.4

5. Complete the following regarding hyperactive jaw jerk:
   a. Significant is that it indicates an u_____ m_____ n_____ l_____

   b. located a_____ t_____ m_____.

upper motor neuron lesion

above the midpons (It distinguishes this from UMN lesions due to lower-level causes, i.e., cervical myelopathy.)

71.3.4

■ Differential Diagnosis

6. **Complete the following table to differentiate amyotrophic lateral sclerosis (ALS) from cervical myelopathy:**

71.4.2

	ALS	CM
Sensory loss		
Sphincter loss		
Jaw jerk		
Dysarthria		
Tongue fasciculations		

Table 71.1 (incomplete)

	ALS	CM
Sensory loss	No	Yes
Sphincter loss	No	Yes
Jaw jerk	Yes	No
Dysarthria	Yes	No
Tongue fasciculations	Yes	No

Table 71.1 (complete)

7. **True or False. Concerning ALS:**
   a. Jaw jerk is present.
   b. Tongue fasciculations are present.

71.4.2

true (may be first clue)
true (as seen on EMG or visible fasciculations)

■ Evaluation

71

8. **Complete the following about degenerative disc/spine disease:**
   a. cervical spine myelopathy, spinal canal diameter
      i. myelopathic at _____ mm or less
      ii. symptomatic at _____ mm
      iii. increased risk at _____ mm
   b. not symptomatic at _____ mm or more

71.5.1

10 mm or less
11.8 mm
14.0 mm
14 mm

9. **True or False. Regarding MRI abnormalities that correlate with poor prognosis in cervical spondylitic myelopathy.**
   a. T2W1 hyperintensity within the cord
   b. A "banana" shaped cord on axial images has no correlation with the presence of CSM.
   c. "snake eyes" on axial T2W1

71.5.2

true
false

true

10. **True or False. Preop SSEP testing can aid in decision making.**

true

71.5.5

■ Treatment

11. Contraindications to posterior decompression are
71.6.2

a. kyphotic angulation, also known as _____ _____.   swan neck

b. subluxation of greater than _____ mm   3.5 mm

c. or rotation in the sagittal plane of more than _____ degrees.   20 degrees

12. Characterize cervical spondylitic myelopathy.
71.6.2

a. Post-op palsy after anterior or posterior decompression occurs in ____ to ____%.   3 to 5%

b. It involves the d_____ or b_____ muscles   deltoid, biceps

c. and C5 region, which provides sensation to the _____ area.   shoulder

d. It usually occurs within _____ _____ of surgery.   1 week

e. Prognosis for recovery is _____.   good

71

72

Thoracic and Lumbar Degenerative Disc Disease

■ General Information about Degenerative Disc Disease (DDD)

1. Since structures outside of the disc are usually also involved, the term degenerative spine disease (DSD) may be preferable to _____ _____ _____.

degenerative disc disease   72.1

■ Anatomic Substrate

2. Enumerate the changes that occur in the intervertebral disc with increasing age.
   (Hint: ddddisc)   72.2.1
   a. d_____   decrease disc height
   b. d_____   decrease in proteoglycan content
   c. d_____   desiccation (loss of hydration)
   d. d_____   degeneration of mucoid
   e. i_____   ingrowth of fibrous tissue
   f. s_____   susceptibility to injury
   g. c_____   circumferential tears of the annulus

3. What level is most commonly the site of lumbar stenosis?   L4-5 and then L3-4   72.2.2

4. Characterize lateral recess stenosis.   72.2.4
   a. Is the pain unilateral or bilateral?   can be either
   b. It is due to _____ of the   hypertrophy
   c. _____ _____ facet.   superior articular
   d. The most common level is at _____.   L4-5

5. **Complete the following about**   72.2.5
    degenerative disc/spine disease:
    a. Spondylolisthesis or anterior subluxation   subluxation
        of one vertebral body on another is
        graded according to the percent of
        _____.

    b. List the % for the following grades.
        i.   I _____%   < 25%
        ii. II ____ to ____%   25 to 50%
        iii. III ____ to ____%   50 to 75%
        iv. IV _____%   75% to complete

6. **What posture may elicit pain in**   hyperextension   72.2.5
    lumbar stenosis in adolescents and
    teens?

7. **Complete the following about**   72.2.5
    degenerative disc/spine disease:
    a. True or False. It is common for listhesis   false
        to cause root compression.
    b. If it does do so it compresses the nerve   exits
        root that _____ at that level
    c. below the _____ above   pedicle
    d. compressed by the _____ _____   superior articular facet
        _____
    e. being displaced _____.   upward

8. **What is a pseudo disc?**   72.2.5
    a. It is the appearance on _____   MRI
    b. in a patient with _____.   listhesis
    c. It is more common to see a herniated   above
        disc at the level _____ the listhesis

72

■ Associated Conditions

9. **What two congenital conditions are**   achondroplasia and   72.4
    associated with spinal stenosis?   congenitally narrowed canal

10. **Paget's disease and ankylosing**   acquired   72.4
    spondylitis are examples of _____
    conditions that are associated with
    spinal stenosis?

■ Clinical Presentation. Differential Diagnosis

11. **Matching. Match the condition with the appropriate clinical feature(s).**
    Clinical feature:
    ① pain is dermatomal; ② sensory loss stocking; ③ sensory loss is dermatomal; ④ pain with exercise; ⑤ pain with standing; ⑥ rest relieves pain promptly; ⑦ rest relieves pain slowly; ⑧ relief with standing; ⑨ relief only with stooping or sitting; ⑩ achiness over thigh; ⑪ pain on pressure over hip; ⑫ Faber sign positive
    Condition: (a-c) below

    a. neurogenic claudication   ①, ③, ④, ⑤, ⑦, ⑨   72.5.2
    b. vascular claudication   ②, ④, ⑥, ⑧
    c. trochanteric bursitis   ⑩, ⑪, ⑫   72.6.1

■ Diagnostic Evaluation

12. **Give the normal lumbar spine CT measurements for each of the following:**   72.7.1

    a. anteroposterior (AP) diameter   > 11.5 mm
    _____mm
    b. ligamentum flavum thickness   < 4 to 5 mm
    _____mm
    c. height of lateral recess _____mm   > 3 mm

13. **State the AP diameter of the normal lumbar spine canal on plain films.**   72.7.1
    a. lower limits of normal: _____mm   15 mm
    b. severe lumbar stenosis: _____mm   less than 11 mm
    c. average: _____mm   22–25mm

14. **Give the dimensions of lateral recess on CT.**   72.7.1
    a. lateral recess height: _____ mm   3 to 4 mm
    b. suggestive of lateral recess syndrome: < 3 mm
    _____ mm
    c. diagnostic of lateral recess syndrome: < 2mm
    _____ mm

■ Treatment

15. **Is treatment for asymptomatic moderate stenosis at adjacent levels appropriate?**   yes (They have a likelihood of progressing to become symptomatic.)   72.8.4

16. **True or False. Patients who undergo decompressive laminectomies are likely to develop lumbar instability?**   false - Less than 1%   72.8.4

72

17. **Complete the following:**   72.8.4
    a. Stability is thought to be maintained if   >50-60%
       ____ - ____% of the facets are preserved
       during surgery
    b. and the _____ space is not violated.   disc
    c. Younger or more active patients are at   higher
       _____ risk of subluxing.

18. **Matching. Following decompression in**   72.8.4
    a patient, which procedures are
    appropriate?
    ① no fusion; ② posterolateral fusion;
    ③ adding pedicle screw instrumentation
    a. no instability preop   ①
    b. instability preop   ②
    c. spondylolisthesis preop   ②, ③

■ Outcome

19. **Give the lumbar spinal stenosis**
    outcomes.
    a. mortality: _____%   .32%   72.9.1
    b. superficial infection: _____%   2.3%
    c. deep infection: _____%   5.9%
    d. deep vein thrombosis (DVT): _____%   2.8%
    e. postural pain relief: _____%   96%   72.9.3
    f. recurrence after 5 years: _____%   27%
    g. long-term success at 1 year and 5 years: 70%
       _____%

20. **Non-union risk factors include**   72.9.2
    a. s_____   smoking
    b. number of _____ fused   levels
    c. use of _____ type medications   NSAIDs

72

73

Adult Spinal Deformity and Degenerative Scoliosis

■ General Information

1. **Adult degenerative scoliosis:**   73.1
   a. Spinal deformity with a Cobb angle > ___   10 degrees
      degrees.
   b. Causes include asymmetric d_____   asymmetric disc
      d_____, h_____ p_____, o_____   degeneration, hip pathology,
                                                   osteoporosis

■ Epidemiology

2. **Adult degenerative scoliosis is more**   60 years; 68%   73.2
   prevalent in patients over ___ years
   old, and incidence of asymptomatic
   burden is over ___ % in the same age
   group.

■ Clinical Evaluation. Diagnostic Testing

3. **Evaluation of ADS includes:**
   a. Unlike lumbar spinal stenosis in the   not improved   73.3
      absence of scoliosis, spinal stenosis
      secondary to adult deformity is usually
      _____ by flexion,
   b. True or False. Diagnostic testing includes   73.4
      all of the following.
      i.   CT   true
      ii. MRI   true
      iii. myelogram   false
      iv. DEXA scan   true
      v.   standing x-rays   true

■ Pertinent Spine Measurements

4. Scoliosis nomenclature   73.5.2

a. What are end vertebrae?   Defined as top and bottom of scoliotic curve on AP x-ray.

b. What does the Cobb angle measure?   Angle made between a horizontal line through the superior endplate of the superior end vertebrae, and another line through inferior end plate of inferior vertebra.

c. Which side of curve determines naming properties?   Convex side (convex to right=dextroscoliosis, convex to left=levoscoliosis)

d. What is the difference between a structural and non-structural curve?   Non-structural curve can correct on side bending.

e. Major vs. fractional curve?   Major is the largest structural curve. Fractional is curve below major curve.

5. Spino-pelvic parameters are important to understand ADS correction. Regarding the following measurements: 73.5.3

a. Sagittal vertical alignment (SVA)

    i.   Define it.   horizontal distance from posterior edge of S1 endplate to plumb line (from mid C7 vertebrae)

    ii. What is normal?   <5cm

    iii. Is this susceptible to error?   yes, depending on patient pain level and accommodation

b. Pelvic Tilt (PT)

    i.   Define it.   angle between vertical reference line (midpoint of femoral head) to midpoint of S1 endplate

    ii. What is normal?   10-25 degrees (goal is <20 degrees)

c. Pelvic incidence (PI)

    i.   Define it.   angle between line perpendicular to S1 endplate, and line from midpoint of femoral head to middle of S1 endplate

    ii. What is normal?   approximately 50 degrees

    iii. Does this change?   no, not once skeletal maturity is reached

d. Sacral Slope (SS)

    i.   Define it.   angle between the horizontal reference line and S1 endplate

    ii. What is normal?   36-42 degrees

    iii. SS = ___ - ___   PI - PT

73

e. Lumbar lordosis (LL)
    i.   Define it. — angle between top of S1 and top of L1
    ii. What is normal? — 20-40 degrees
    iii. What is the goal? — LL = PI ± 9 degrees
f. Thoracic kyphosis (TK)
    i.   Define it. — angle between top of T4 and bottom of T12
    ii. What is normal? — 41 degrees, ± 12 degrees

■ SRS-Schwab Classification of Adult Spinal Deformity

6. **What is the SRS-Schwab classification?** — Scoliosis classification based on regional radiographic features as well as spino-pelvic parameters as it relates to quality of life. — 73.6

■ Treatment/Management

7. **Indications for surgery?** — axial back pain ± neuropathic symptoms deleterious to ADLs — 73.7.2

8. **Summary of spino-pelvic objectives:** — 73.7.2
a. LL: _____ degrees — LL= PI ± 9 degrees
b. PT: _____ degrees — <20 degrees
c. SVA: _____cm — <5cm

9. **What is generally considered an appropriate goal for sagittal correction of lumbar lordosis, given retroverting the pelvis for compensation?** — Increase in LL needed is approximately equal to (PI – LL – 9 degrees) + (PT – 20 degrees) — 73.7.2

73

74

Special Conditions Affecting the Spine

■ Paget's Disease of the Spine

1. **Characterize Paget's disease.**   74.1.1
   a. Also known as o_____ d_____.   osteitis deformans
   b. Disorder of o_____.   osteoclasts
   c. Results in r_____ of bone.   resorption
   d. Reactive osteoblasts o_____produce   over
      bone.
   e. This results in sclerotic, radiodense,   ivory bone
      brittle bone called i_____ b_____.

2. **Which spinal nerve is most commonly**   CN VIII   74.1.5
   compressed as it exits through its
   bony foramina?

3. **Most common symptom of Paget's**   bone pain   74.1.6
   disease is?

4. **Typical presentation to a**   74.1.6
   neurosurgeon includes:
   a. Neural compression due to
      i. expansion of w_____ b_____,   woven bone
      ii. o_____ t_____,   osteoid tissue
      iii. pagetic extension into l_____   ligamentum flavum;
          f_____ and e_____ f_____.   epidural fat
   b. Typically present for longer than _____.   12 months
   c. If symptoms progress over a timeframe
      < 6 months, then what is differential?
      i. m_____   malignancy (sarcomatous)
      ii. p_____ f_____   pathological fracture
      iii. compromise of n_____ s_____   neurovascular supply
                                    (compression or pagetic
                                    vascular steal)

5. **Recommended laboratory tests**   74.1.7
   include:
   a. a_____ ph_____   alkaline phosphatase
   b. ur_____ hy_____   urinary hydroxyproline
   c. bone scan _____ _____ areas of   lights up (localized
      abnormality   enlargement of bone, cortical
                      thickening, sclerotic changes,
                      and osteolytic areas)

74

d. Spinal Paget's disease involves s_____   several contiguous levels
    c_____ l_____   (pedicles/lamina thickened,
    vertebral bodies dense, discs
    replaced by bone)

e. Treatment with c_____ and b_____   calcitonin;   74.1.8
    may reverse neurologic deficit in 50% of   bisphosphonates
    cases.

6. **What are the neurosurgical**   74.1.8
    indications in Paget's disease of the
    spine?
    a. spinal _____   instability
    b. uncertain _____   diagnosis
    c. failure of _____ _____   medical management

■ Ankylosing Spondylitis

7. **Characterize ankylosing spondylitis.**   74.2.1
    a. It is also known as M_____-   Marie-Strümpell disease
        S_____ d_____.
    b. Locus of involvement at the e_____   entheses
    c. Replacement of _____ with   ligaments with bone
        _____.
    d. Bone is very o_____.   osteoporotic
    e. On x-ray it is called b_____   bamboo spine
        s_____.
    f. To differentiate from rheumatoid   negative for rheumatoid
        arthritis (RA), serum is n_____ for   factor
        r_____ f_____.
    g. Fracture may occur with _____   minimal trauma
        _____.
    h. Screws for fusion may _____   not hold
        _____.
    i. Enthesis
        i. is the _____ _____   attachment point
        ii. of ligaments, tendons or capsules on   bones
            _____.

8. **True or False. Ankylosing spondylitis**   74.2.3
    usually presents as:
    a. radiating low back pain   false (non-radiating low back
        pain)
    b. evening back stiffness exacerbated by   false (Morning back stiffness.
        inactivity and improved by exercise   Everything else is accurate)
    c. Patrick's test is performed by   true (Positive test will elicit
        compressing the pelvis with patient in   pain.)
        lateral decubitus position.

9. **What are radiologic considerations in**   74.2.5
    ankylosing spondylosis?
    a. Rotary s_____ may occur in high   subluxation
        cervical area.
    b. Last area to stay mobile is the   occipito-atlanto
        o_____-a_____

74

c. and a_____ joints.   atlantoaxial

d. Minor trauma may result in spine   fracture
    _____.

e. Vertebral fractures occur through the   ossified disc
    _____ _____.

f. An early site of involvement is the   SI joint (This is the sine qua
    _____ joint.   non for definite diagnosis.)

g. If suspicious, x-ray the _____   entire spine
    _____.

■ Ossification of the Posterior Longitudinal Ligament (OPLL)

10. **Insert a term starting with the   74.3.2
    indicated letter to characterize the
    pathologic process of ossification of
    the posterior longitudinal ligament
    (OPLL).**

a. c_____   calcification

b. d_____   dura

c. e_____   evolves from C3-4

d. f_____   fibrosis

e. g_____   grows 0.6 mm/year in the AP
                                                    direction and 4.1 mm/year in
                                                    the longitudinal direction

f. h_____   hypervascular

g. p_____   periosteal

h. o_____   ossification

11. **True or False. OPLL progresses in the   74.3.2
    following order:**
    ① ossification;
    ② fibrosis;
    ③ calcification

a. ①, ③, ②   false

b. ②, ①, ③   false

c. ③, ①, ②   false

d. ②, ③, ①   true

74

12. **OPLL grows at a rate of   74.3.2**

a. _____ mm in the anterior posterior   0.6 mm
    (AP) direction and

b. _____ mm longitudinally per year.   4.1 mm

13. **Provide the pathologic classification.   74.3.2**

a. Confined to space behind vertebral body   segmental
    is called_____.

b. Extends from body to body spanning   continuous
    disc is called _____.

c. Combines both of the above and has skip   mixed
    areas is called _____.

14. Describe the evaluation of OPLL.   74.3.6
a. Plain x-rays _____ _____ to   often fail
   demonstrate OPLL.
b. MRI:
   i. OPLL is difficult to appreciate until it   5mm
       is _____ mm thick.
   ii. T2W1 may be very _____.   helpful
c. CT, especially with 3D reconstruction, is   best
   the _____ method.

15. List the clinical grading of OPLL.   74.3.7
a. Class I   x-ray only—radiographically
              evident; no symptoms or
              signs
b. Class II   minimal—myelopathy A/O
               radiculopathy minimal or
               stable deficit
c. Class IIIA   myelopathy—moderate to
                 severe myelopathy
d. Class IIIB   quadriplegia—moderate to
                 severe quadriplegia

16. Complete the following regarding   74.3.7
    Nurick grades of cervical spondylosis:
a. Assess the extent of _____.   disability
b. Surgery showed no benefit for Nurick   1 and 2
   grades _____ and _____.
c. Surgery was valuable for Nurick grades   3 and 4
   _____ and _____.
d. Surgery was ineffective for Nurick grade   5
   _____.

74

■ Diffuse Idiopathic Skeletal Hyperostosis (DISH)

17. Characterize diffuse idiopathic skeletal   74.5
    hyperostosis (DISH).
a. The following areas of the spine are
   affected in what percentage of cases?
   i.   thoracic: _____%   97%
   ii. lumbar: _____%   90%
   iii. cervical: _____%   78%
   iv. all three segments: _____%   70%
b. Area spared?   sacroiliac joints
c. Is the area spared in ankylosing   no
   spondylitis?

■ Scheuermann's Kyphosis

18. **Complete the following regarding Scheuermann's kyphosis:**   74.6.1
   a. It is defined as
      i. _____ wedging   anterior
      ii. of at least _____ degrees   5
      iii. of _____ or more _____   3; adjacent
      iv. _____ vertebral bodies.   thoracic
   b. Which age group does it affect?   adolescents   74.6.2

■ Spinal Epidural Hematoma

19. **What is the most common cause of**   74.7.1
   spinal epidural hematoma?
   a. _____ plus   trauma - almost exclusively in
                                                  patients with
   b. h_____ b_____ t_____   higher bleeding tendency
                                                  (anticoagulated, bleeding
                                                  diathesis, etc.)

20. **Complete the following about spinal**   74.7.1
   epidural hematoma:
   a. The most common area of occurrence is   thoracic
      _____.
   b. Is it anterior or posterior?   often posterior (which
                                                  facilitates removal)
   c. The most common category of patient is   anticoagulated
      _____.

21. **What is the usual presentation of**   severe back pain (with   74.7.3
   spinal epidural hematoma?   radicular component)

74

■ Spinal Subdural Hematoma

22. **Complete the following regarding**   74.8
   spinal subdural hematoma:
   a. They occur _____.   rarely
   b. They are often related to _____.   trauma
   c. Patients are usually on _____   anticoagulant
      medication.
   d. It may sometimes be managed   conservatively
      _____.

75

Other Non-Spine Conditions with Spine Implications

■ Rheumatoid Arthritis

1. **Name four upper cervical spine abnormalities associated with rheumatoid arthritis.**
   a. b_____ i_____
   b. a_____ s_____
   c. s_____ s_____

   d. v_____ a_____ i_____

   basilar impression
   atlantoaxial subluxation
   subaxial subluxation (less common)
   vertebral artery insufficiency—due to changes at the craniocervical junction (less common)

   75.1.2

2. **What are the three stages in pathophysiology that lead to atlantoaxial subluxation in rheumatoid arthritis?**
   (Hint: iel)
   a. infl_____ at a_____ s_____
      j_____
   b. ero_____ c_____ in o_____
   c. loo_____ of the t_____
      l_____

   inflammation at atlantoaxial synovial joints
   erosive changes in odontoid
   loosening of the transverse ligament

   75.1.3

3. **What percentage of rheumatoid arthritis patients develop subluxation?**

   Atlantoaxial subluxation occurs in 25% of patients with rheumatoid arthritis.

   75.1.3

4. **Complete the following regarding atlantoaxial subluxation in rheumatoid arthritis:**
   a. The odontoid C1 interval is normal when less than _____ mm.

   4 mm

   75.1.3

   b. The asymptomatic patient needs surgery if distance is greater than _____ mm.

   8 mm

   c. To do transoral odontoidectomy, the mouth needs to open at least _____ mm.

   25 mm

   d. Mortality of C1-C2 wiring is ___ to ____%.

   5 to 15%

   75.1.4

5. **Characterize posterior atlantodental interval (PADI).**   75.1.3
   a. Correlates with the presence of _____.   paralysis
   b. Predicts neurologic recovery following _____.   surgery

   c. No recovery occurs if the PADI is less than _____ mm.   10
   d. An indication for surgery is a PADI less than _____ mm.   14

6. **What degree of atlantodental interval is a generally accepted surgical indication in asymptomatic patients?**   8 mm (6 to 10 mm is the range)   75.1.3

7. **What is the percentage of nonfusion for C1-C2 fusions in rheumatoid arthritis?**   18 - 50%   75.1.4

8. **Characterize basilar impression in rheumatoid arthritis.**   75.1.6
   a. Changes in lateral masses are called e_____.   erosive
   b. Permitting relationship of C1-C2 to change is called t_____.   telescoping
   c. Position of dens moves u_____   upward
      i. causes compression of p_____ and m_____   pons and medulla
      ii. contributes to b_____ compression   brainstem

9. **Matching. List the most common symptoms and signs of basilar impression of patients with rheumatoid arthritis and match with their order of frequency.**   Table 75.3
   ① 100%; ② 80%; ③ 71%; ④ 30%; ⑤ 22%
   a. limb paresthesias   ③ 71%
   b. Babinski, hyperreflexia   ② 80%
   c. bladder incontinence/retention   ④ 30%
   d. cranial nerve dysfunction   ⑤ 22%
   e. headache   ① 100%
   f. ambulatory problems   ② 80%

10. **Characterize basilar impression in rheumatoid arthritis.**   75.1.6
    a. Pain may be a result of c_____ of C1 and C2 nerves.   compression
    b. Cranial nerve dysfunction results from compression of the m_____.   medulla

75

11. **What is the treatment for basilar impression?**   75.1.6
    a. if reducible with t_____   traction
        i.   C1 d_____ l_____ followed   decompressive laminectomy
             by
        ii. o_____-c_____ f_____   occipital-cervical fusion
    b. in nonreducible patients
        i.   t_____ o_____ r_____   transoral odontoid resection
             followed by
        ii. o_____-c_____ f_____   occipital-cervical fusion

■ Down Syndrome

12. **Down syndrome is associated with l_____ l_____ of the spine.**   ligamentous laxity   75.2.1

13. **Incidence of AAS in Down syndrome is _____%**   20%   75.2.2

76

Special Conditions Affecting the Spinal Cord

■ Spinal Vascular Malformations

1. **Characterize spinal AVM classification.**   76.1.2
   a. Type I
      i.   known as d_____ A_____   dural AVM
      ii. IA: has a s_____ arterial feeder   single
      iii. IB: has _____ or _____   2 or more
           arterial feeders
      iv. formed at the d_____ r_____   dural root
           sleeve
   b. Intradural AVMs
      i.   flow is _____   high
      ii. _____% with acute symptoms   75%
   c. Type II
      i.   aka spinal g_____ AVM   glomus
      ii. located i_____   intramedullary
      iii. true A_____ of the cord   AVM
      iv. has a c_____ n_____   compact nidus
      v.   prognosis is _____ than dural   worse
           AVM
   d. Type III
      i.   aka _____ spinal AVM   juvenile
      ii. essentially on enlarged _____   glomus
      iii. occupies the e_____ cross   entire
           section
   e. Type IV
      i.   aka _____ spinal AVM   perimedullary
      ii. aka _____ fistula   arteriovenous
      iii. presents with _____ hemorrhage   catastrophic

2. **What is the most common type of   76.1.2
   spinal AVM?**
   a. type _____   type 1
   b. dural _____   AVM
   c. fed by a r_____ a_____   radicular artery
   d. and draining into a s_____   spinal vein
      v_____
   e. on the _____ aspect of the cord   posterior
   f. _____ % are males   90%

76

3. **What is the most common presentation of a spinal AVM?**   76.1.3
    a. onset of _____ pain   back pain
    b. progressive lower extremity _____ and _____ _____   weakness and sensory loss—
                                                                    acute onset of back pain
                                                                    associated with progressive
                                                                    LE weakness and sensory loss
                                                                    (may be over months to
                                                                    years)

4. **Spinal AVM with pain may have this syndrome.**   76.1.3
    a. Onset of subarachnoid hemorrhage (SAH), and sudden excruciating back pain is also called c_____ d_____ p_____ of Michon.   Coup de Poignard of Michon
    b. This is considered clinical evidence of _____ _____.   spinal AVM

5. **What is Foix-Alajouanine syndrome?**   76.1.3
    a. Acute or subacute _____ _____   neurologic deterioration
    b. in a patient with _____ _____   spinal AVM
    c. without evidence of _____   hemorrhage
    d. caused by _____ _____   venous hypertension
    e. with secondary _____   ischemia

■ Spinal Meningeal Cysts

6. **What is a Tarlov's cyst?**   spinal meningeal cyst   76.2.1

7. **What are the different types of spinal meningeal cyst, and which compartment are they located in?**   76.2.1
    a. Type I   superficial compartment
                                                              extradural without root fibers
    b. Type II   middle compartment
                                                              extradural with spinal root
                                                              fibers—diverticulum
    c. Type III   central compartment
                                                              intradural arachnoid cyst

8. **Complete the following statements about spinal meningeal cyst:**   76.2.1
    a. Type II spinal meningeal cyst is also known as _____ _____.   Tarlov's cyst
    b. It occurs on the _____ roots.   dorsal

9. **What are the treatment options for spinal meningeal cyst?**   76.2.4
    a. e_____   excise the cyst
    b. o_____   obliterate the ostium
                                                              between cyst and
                                                              subarachnoid space
    c. m_____   marsupialize if excision is not
                                                              possible

76

■ Syringomyelia

10. Complete the following about syringomyelia: 76.4.1

a. _____ cavitation of the spinal cord   cystic

b. associated with Chiari I in _____%   70%

c. Affects upper or lower extremities first?   upper

d. More rapid neurologic progression is   5 mm; edema
predicted by a cavity more than
_____mm in diameter and with
associated cord _____.

11. **Rostral extension into brainstem is**   syringobulbia   76.4.1
called _____.

12. **Communicating syringomyelia is**   76.4.2
commonly associated with what
congenital conditions?
(Hint: bCDe)

a. b_____   basilar impression

b. C_____   Chiari malformation

c. D_____   Dandy-Walker syndrome

d. e_____   ectopia of cerebellum

13. **What are the main presenting**   76.4.6
symptoms and signs of a syrinx?
(Hint: accC)

a. a_____ w_____   arm/hand weakness

b. c_____ s_____ l_____   sensory loss with suspended
"cape" dissociated sensory
loss (loss of pain and
temperature with preserved
joint position sense)

c. c_____/o_____ p_____   cervical/occipital pain

d. C_____ j_____ (p_____   Charcot's joints—painless
a_____)   arthropathies

14. **Distinguish from similar entities.**   76.4.8

a. Tumor cyst

i. Most e_____.   enhance

ii. Fluid is p_____.   proteinaceous

iii. Syrinx fluid has MRI characteristics of   CSF
C_____.

b. Residual spinal canal

i. Central canal usually _____.   involutes

ii. Is not more than _____ to   2 to 4
_____ mm wide.

iii. Is perfectly _____ on cross   round
section.

iv. Is perfectly in the _____ on axial   center
MRI.

15. **Dilatation of central canal with**   hydromyelia   76.4.8
ependymal cell lining is called
_____.

76

■ Posttraumatic Syringomyelia

16. **True or False. The level of spinal injury that has the highest incidence of posttraumatic syringomyelia is**   76.5.2
    a. cervical   false
    b. thoracic   true
    c. lumbar   false

17. **Characterize posttraumatic syringomyelia.**   Table 76.6
    a. Most common symptom is _____.   pain - not relieved by analgesics
    b. Most common sign is _____ _____ _____.   ascending sensory level

18. **What may be the only feature of descending syringomyelia in patients with complete cord lesions?**   hyperhidrosis   76.5.3

19. **Complete the following statements about traumatic syringomyelia:**
    a. Incidence is _____.   3.2%   76.5.2
    b. Latency is _____.   average 9 years after injury
    c. What should raise the index of suspicion for a syrinx in a patient who is paraplegic from trauma?   76.5.3
        i. The _____ development   late
        ii. in a _____   paraplegic patient
        iii. of _____ _____ weakness.   upper extremity

■ Spinal Epidural Lipomatosis (SEL)

20. **Characterize spinal epidural lipomatosis (SEL).**
    a. due to h_____ of epidural fat   hypertrophy   76.7.1
    b. due to
        i. o_____ and/or   obesity
        ii. exogenous s_____   steroids
    c. Symptoms
        i. first is _____ _____   back pain
        ii. progressive _____ _____ _____   lower extremity weakness
        iii. and _____ changes.   sensory
    d. Most occur in the _____ spine.   thoracic
    e. Diagnose by using _____ or _____. CT or MRI   76.7.2
    f. Should be at least _____ mm thick to be SEL.   7
    g. Treatment   76.7.3
        i. Reduce the use of _____ or   steroids
        ii. lose _____.   weight
        iii. Remove _____.   surgically
    h. Complication rate is _____.   high   76.7.4

76

77

Introduction and General Information, Grading, Medical Management, Special Conditions

■ Definition

1. **Complete the following about aneurysmal SAH:**   77.1.3
   a. What percentage of patients die before reaching the hospital?   10-15%
   b. What is the risk of rebleeding within 2 weeks?   15-20%
   c. What is the risk of death from vasospasm?   7%
   d. What is the risk of severe deficit from vasospasm?   7%
   e. What is the 30-day mortality rate?   about 50%
   f. What is the strongest prognostic indicator?   severity of clinical presentation

■ Etiologies of SAH

2. **True or False. Etiologies of subarachnoid hemorrhage (SAH) include the following:**   77.2
   a. arteriovenous malformation (AVM) rupture   true
   b. vasculitis   true
   c. encephalitis   false
   d. drug use   true
   e. coagulopathy   true
   f. dural sinus thrombosis   true

■ Incidence

3. **What is the incidence of aneurysmal SAH?**   9.7-14.5 per 100,000   77.3

77

■ Risk Factors for SAH

4. **True or False. Risk factors for SAH include the following:**   77.4

a. hypertension   true
b. genetic syndromes   true
c. cigarette smoking   true
d. pregnancy   false

■ Clinical Features

5. **True or False. SAH may present as any of the following:**   77.5.1

a. meningismus   true
b. photophobia   true
c. hearing loss   false
d. low back pain   true
e. ptosis   true

6. **True or False. Formal angiography is indicated in**   77.5.2

a. sentinel hemorrhage   true
b. crash migraine (thunderclap headache)   false
c. benign orgasmic cephalgia   false

7. **The incidence of sentinel hemorrhage is ____ - ____%.**   30-60%   77.5.2

8. **True or False. Regarding benign thunderclap headache.**   77.5.2

a. Can be distinguished from SAH.   false
b. Reaches maximal intensity in one minute.   true
c. Is accompanied by vomiting.   true
d. Never recurs.   false
e. Is related to vascular cause.   true
f. CT and LP show no blood.   true
g. Require angiography.   false

9. **Complete the following about reversible cerebral vasoconstrictive syndrome:**   77.5.2

a. Has a s_____ onset.   sudden
b. Associated with n_____ deficit.   neurological
c. Angiography shows _____ appearance,   string of beads
d. which clears within _____ months.   1-3 months
e. Associated with v_____ drugs.   vasoconstrictive
f. May occur p_____.   post-partum

10. **Complete the following about benign orgasmic headache:**   77.5.2

a. Occurs just before or at time of o_____.   orgasm
b. Workup is the same as for t_____ headache.   thunderclap

77

11. **Complete the following about meningismus:**   77.5.3
   a. aka n_____ r_____   nuchal rigidity
   b. Signs
      i.   Bend neck and hip flexes called   Brudzinski's sign
           _____ sign
      ii. Knee bent then straightened causes   hamstring; Kernig's sign
           _____ pain and is called _____ sign

12. **True or False. Coma in SAH may be due to the following:**   77.5.3
   a. seizure   true
   b. increased intracranial pressure (ICP)   true
   c. intraparenchymal hemorrhage   true
   d. hydrocephalus   true
   e. low blood flow   true

13. **What percentage of patients with subarachnoid hemorrhage have funduscopic abnormalities?**   20-40%   77.5.3

14. **Matching. Match the type of ocular hemorrhage with the associated characteristic(s).**   77.5.3
   Ocular hemorrhage: ① subhyaloid; ② retinal; ③ vitreous
   Characteristic: (a-e) below
   a. bright red blood near optic disc   ①
   b. vitreous opacity   ③
   c. blood obscures the retinal vessels   ①
   d. surrounds the fovea   ②
   e. may result in retinal detachment   ③

15. **True or False. The following are characteristics of SAH:**   77.5.3
   a. Subhyaloid hemorrhage from SAH occurs near the optic disc.   true
   b. Retinal hemorrhage occurs near the fovea.   true
   c. The prognosis for vision recovery in Terson syndrome is poor.   false
   d. Vitreous hemorrhage may occur with nonaneurysmal causes for increased ICP.   true
   e. Ocular hemorrhage from SAH may be associated with retinal detachment.   true

77

■ Work-Up of Suspected SAH

16. **Complete the following:**   77.6.2
   a. A good-quality computed tomographic (CT) scan will detect SAH in what percentage of patients?   ≥95%
   b. If scanned within how many hours?   48 hours
   c. Ventriculomegaly (hydrocephalus) occurs acutely in _____%.   21%

17. **True or False. Regarding head CT for SAH.**   77.6.2
   a. Ventricular size needs to be assessed because hydrocephalus can occur acutely.   true
   b. There may be intracranial hemorrhage requiring urgent craniotomy.   true
   c. The amount of SAH correlates with vasospasm risk.   true
   d. If there are multiple aneurysms, the distribution of SAH may reveal which aneurysm ruptured.   true
   e. Head CT is a poor predictor of aneurysm location.   false

18. **Regarding prediction of aneurysm location.**   77.6.2
   a. Blood in the ventricles suggests _____ _____ aneurysm.   posterior fossa
   b. Anterior interhemispheric fissure suggests an _____ aneurysm.   A-Comm
   c. Sylvian fissure is compatible with a
      i. _____ or a   P-Comm
      ii. _____ aneurysm   MCA

19. **Complete the following:**   77.6.2
   a. The most sensitive test for SAH is _____ _____.   lumbar puncture
   b. Lowering the cerebrospinal fluid (CSF) pressure might precipitate rebleeding because it causes an _____ _____ _____ _____.   increase in transmural pressure
   c. Therefore, as a precaution
      i. use only a _____-_____ _____ and   small-gauge needle
      ii. remove only a _____ _____ of _____.   small amount of fluid

20. **True or False. The following CSF findings are expected with SAH:**   77.6.2
   a. elevated opening pressure   true
   b. nonclotting bloody fluid   true
   c. xanthrochromia   true
   d. red blood cells (RBCs) > 100,000   true
   e. elevated glucose   false

21. **Complete the following about xanthochromia:**   77.6.2
   a. Used to differentiate SAH from _____.   traumatic tap
   b. Does not show up until _____ hours after bleeding.   2-4
   c. Is present in 100% of patients by _____ hours.   12
   d. Lingers for up to _____ weeks.   4

77

22. Complete the following about MRI: 77.6.2
  a. Most sensitive sequence for detecting   FLAIR
     blood in the subarachnoid space is the
     _____ sequence.
  b. It is most reliable for detecting SAH after   4-7 days
     ___ - ___ days.

23. Complete the following about MRA: 77.6.2
  a. Can detect aneurysm larger than   3;
     _____ mm with approximately   90
     _____% accuracy.

24. CTA has an accuracy of _____% and   97;   77.6.2
  shows a _____-dimensional image.   three

25. Complete the following: 77.6.2
  a. Angiography demonstrates the source of   80-85
     SAH in ___ - ___%.
  b. To call an angiogram negative for
     aneurysm you must see what two areas?
     i.   Take off both _____ and   PICAs
     ii.   _____   A-Comm
  c. What percentage of aneurysms occur at   1-2%
     the posterior inferior cerebellar artery
     (PICA) origin?

26. Complete the following about the   77.6.2
  infundibulum:
  a. The three criteria are
     i.   _____ shape   triangular
     ii.   size of mouth less than _____   3
           mm
     iii. _____ at apex   vessel
  b. The most common site is at the   P-Comm
     _____.

27. Infundibula are found in   10   77.6.2
  approximately what percentage of
  normal angiograms?

28. If infundibulum is located near SAH,   exploration   77.6.2
  _____ is advisable.

■ Grading SAH   77

29. Matching. Match the hemorrhage   77.7.2
  grade with when to operate.
  ① manage till patient improves;
  ② immediately; ③ promptly within 24
  hours
  a. Hunt and Hess grade 1   ③
  b. Hunt and Hess grade 2   ③
  c. Hunt and Hess grade 3, 4, or 5   ①
  d. Patient with large hematoma   ②
  e. Patient with multiple bleeds   ②

30. **What is the Hunt and Hess grade in a patient who has a headache and SAH seen on CT scan**   Table 77.2
    a. and a third nerve palsy?   Hunt and Hess grade 2
    b. and mild one-sided weakness and confusion? Hunt and Hess grade 3
    c. deep coma and decerebrate rigidity?   Hunt and Hess grade 5

31. **Complete the World Federation of Neurologic Surgeons (WFNS) grading scale for SAH grade.**   Table 77.4
    a. Grade 0: _____   unruptured
    b. Grade 1 Glasgow Coma Scale (GCS): _____ GCS 15
    c. Grade 2 GCS: _____   GCS 13 to 14
    d. Grade 3 GCS: _____   GCS 13 to 14 and major focal deficit
    e. Grade 4 GCS: _____   GCS 7 to 12
    f. Grade 5 GCS: _____   GCS 3 to 6

■ Initial Management of SAH

32. **List nine potential complications of SAH.**   77.8.1
    (Hint: veraNdsah)
    a. v_____   vasospasm
    b. e_____   embolus—pulmonary
    c. r_____   rebleed
    d. a_____   arachnoid granulation blockage
    e. N_____   Na metabolism
    f. d_____   deep vein thrombosis
    g. s_____   seizures
    h. a_____   acute hydrocephalus
    i. h_____   hyponatremia

33. **Complete the orders for SAH patient.**   77.8.3
    a. intravenous (IV) fluids?   normal saline (NS) and 20 milliequivalents (mEq) KCl
    b. rate?   2 mL/kg/hour
    c. blood pressure parameters?   SBP 120-160
    d. calcium channel blocker?   yes-Nimodipine
    e. dose?   60 mg PO/NG every 4 hours

77

34. **True or False. During the post-SAH period, with the aneurysm unclipped, phenothiazines should be avoided because**

77.8.3

a. they may be overly sedating and obscure neurological assessment.   false

b. they may lower seizure threshold.   true

c. they cause elevation of systolic blood pressure.   false

d. their metabolites may hasten vasospasm,   false

e. instead use _____.   Zofran

35. **True or False. The following is the most reliable parameter to differentiate syndrome of inappropriate diuretic hormone (SIADH) from cerebral salt wasting syndrome:**

77.8.5

a. serum atrial natriuretic factor (ANF) and brain natriuretic factor (BNF)   false

b. urine Na+ and osmolarity   false

c. serum Na+ and osmolarity   false

d. extracellular fluid volume   true

e. 24-hour urine output   false

36. **Complete the following:**

77.8.5

a. True or False. Cerebral salt wasting (CSW) is best differentiated from SIADH by measuring the:

  i.   serum sodium   false

  ii. intravascular volume   false

  iii. urine osmolarity   false

  iv. extracellular fluid volume   true

b. Keeping serum Na levels normal is important because hyponatremic patients have three times the rate of d_____ c_____ i_____ as do normal natremic patients.   delayed cerebral infarction

37. **Cerebral salt wasting is**

77.8.5

a. more common after SAH than _____.   SIADH

b. Treat with _____ _____.   normal saline

c. Use caution regarding the rate of treatment because you risk producing _____ _____ _____.   central pontine myelinolysis

77

■ Rebleeding

38. **True or False. Regarding rebleeding.**   77.9.1
    a. The maximum frequency of rebleeding   false (4% on day 1)
       from SAH is on day 7.
    b. Approximately 50% of ruptured   true
       aneurysms will rebleed within 6 months.
    c. Epsilon-aminocaproic acid may decrease   true
       the risk of rebleeding.

39. **Complete the following:**   77.9.1
    a. Maximum frequency of rebleeding is on   first
       the _____ day
    b. at a rate of _____%   4%
    c. then at _____%   1.5%
    d. for _____ days.   13
    e. Total of rebleed in 2 weeks = _____% 15 to 20%
    f. _____% in 6 months   50%
    g. Thereafter rebleed rate is ___% per year. 3%
    h. Time period of the highest risk of   first 6 hours
       rebleeding is the _____.

■ Pregnancy and Intracranial Hemorrhage

40. **True or False. Intracranial hemorrhage**   77.10.1
    during pregnancy is more commonly
    caused by:
    a. AVM   false, 23%
    b. aneurysms   true, 77%

41. **True or False. The following is a**   77.10.2
    correct recommendation for pregnant
    patients with SAH:
    a. Do not perform CT or angiogram.   false (They are okay if the
                                                 fetus is shielded.)
    b. Mannitol, Nipride, and nimodipine can   false (They are not to be used
       be used as usual.   in pregnancy.)
    c. Delay surgery until pregnancy has come   false (Clipping is
       to term.   recommended in the
                                                 pregnant patient.)
    d. Deliver by C-section.   false (There is no different
                                                 fetal or maternal outcome by
                                                 C-section or vaginal delivery.)
    e. MRI is safe in pregnancy.   true
    f. Gadolinium is safe in pregnancy.   not yet studied
    g. Angiographic contrast is safe.   true
    h. Treatment recommendation is surgical   true
       clipping.

77

■ Hydrocephalus after SAH

42. Complete the following about acute post-SAH hydrocephalus: 77.11.2

a. Frequency of hydrocephalus in SAH is ___ - ___%.

    15-20

b. Hydrocephalus is more frequently associated with aneurysms in what location?

    posterior circulation aneurysms

c. What aneurysm has a low incidence of hydrocephalus?

    MCA aneurysms

d. The proper treatment is placement of a _____ _____.

    ventriculostomy drain

e. It is recommended to keep the ICP in the range of ___ - ___ mm Hg.

    15-25

f. This reduces the tendency to _____.

    rebleed

43. Complete the following about chronic post-SAH hydrocephalus: 77.11.3

a. Approximately _____% of patients with acute post-SAH hydrocephalus need permanent cerebrospinal fluid diversion.

    50

b. _____ _____ and _____ _____ are associated with shunt dependency.

    Intraventricular blood; Fisher grade

c. There was _____ difference in the rate of shunt placement between patients who underwent rapid versus gradual weaning of the ventriculostomy drain.

    no

77

78

Critical Care of Aneurysm Patients

■ Neurogenic Stress Cardiomyopathy (NSC)

1. Neurogenic stress cardiomyopathy: 78.1.1
a. Is impaired cardiac function not   coronary artery disease
attributable to _____.
b. May be _____.   reversible
c. Is distinguished from acute myocardial   lower than expected
ischemia by _____ _____
_____ cardiac enzymes.
d. Is treated by increasing _____ using cardiac output;
these two medications: _____ or   Milrinone;
_____.   Dobutamine

2. EKG changes that can occur after SAH: 78.1.2
a. T waves may be i_____.   inverted
b. QT may be p_____.   prolonged
c.
   i. ST segments may be e_____   elevated
   ii. or d_____.   depressed

3. The mechanism for the EKG changes is   78.1.3
thought to be due to
a. h_____ i_____,   hypothalamic ischemia
b. which causes increased _____ tone,   sympathetic tone
c. which releases a surge of c_____,   catecholamines
d. which produces s_____ ischemia,   subendocardial
e. or c_____ a_____ vasospasm.   coronary artery

4. Complete the following about cardiac
problems and SAH:
a. EKG changes occur in _____%.   50   78.1.2
b. The mechanism is (Hint: hics)   78.1.3
   i. h_____ i_____   hypothalamic ischemia
   ii. i_____ s_____ t_____ increased sympathetic tone
   iii. c_____ s_____   catecholamine surge
   iv. s_____ i_____   subendocardial ischemia

■ Vasospasm

5. **Complete the following about vasospasm:**
   a. also known as _____ _____ | delayed ischemic neurologic | 78.3.2
      _____ _____ | deficit
   b. True or False. Higher incidence occurs in: | | 78.3.3
      i.   ACA distribution | true
      ii. MCA distribution | false

6. **Complete the following regarding cerebral vasospasms:** | | 78.3.3
   a. The incidence of radiographic cerebral vasospasm is ____ - ____% | 20-100
   b. as measured on day _____. | 7
   c. The incidence of symptomatic cerebral vasospasm is _____%. | 30
   d. Produces infarction in _____%. | 60
   e. Produces mortality in _____%. | 7
   f. Onset almost never before day _____. | 3
   g. Resolved by day _____. | 12
   h. Radiographically resolves over ___ - ___ weeks | 3-4

7. **Complete the following:** | | 78.3.3
   a. Spasmogenic region on ACA and MCA is the _____. | proximal 9 cm
   b. True or False. There is more vasospasm with:
      i.   cigarette smoking | true
      ii. lower Hunt and Hess grade | false
      iii. amount of blood on CT | true
      iv. advancing age of patient | true
      v.   presence of intraventricular hemorrhage | false
      vi. presence of intraparenchymal hemorrhage | false

8. **Complete the following about Fisher grade:** | | Table 78.2
   a. Describe the Fisher grading system.
      i.   Grade 1 | no blood
      ii. Grade 2 | slight—less than 1 mm
      iii. Grade 3 | localized clot—more than 1 mm
      iv. Grade 4 | intracerebral or intraventricular clot
   b. Clinical vasospasm is essentially limited to Fisher grade _____. | 3

9. **What chemicals have been identified as critical mediators of vasospasm?** | | 78.3.4
   a. decreased production of _____ and _____ | nitrous oxide; prostacyclins
   b. overproduction of _____ | endothelin-1

78

10. **What transcranial Doppler (TCD)**   Table 78.5
    values are consistent with vasospasm?
    a. Velocity at MCA of more than _____.   120 cm/sec
    b. _____ ratio of more than _____   Lindegaard, 3
       between
    c. the _____ and the _____   MCA, ICA
       indicates vasospasm.
    d. Velocity < than _____ and ratio   120, 3
       <_____ is normal.
    e. Velocity between _____ and   120, 200
       _____ is mild vasospasm.
    f. Velocity above _____ is severe   200
       vasospasm.
    g. Ratio between _____ and _____   3 and 6
       is mild vasospasm.
    h. Ratio above _____ is severe   6
       vasospasm.

11. **Complete the following:**   78.3.6
    a. Describe the treatment for vasospasm
       i.   avoid h_____, a_____, and   hypovolemia, anemia, and
            h_____   hypotension
       ii. surgery?   do early
       iii. remove c_____   clots
       iv. drug?   calcium channel blocker-
                                                  nimodipine
       v.   catheter?   dilatation
       vi. drain?   bloody CSF
       vii. obtain hematocrit of ____ - ____%   30-35
    b. Angioplasty produces clinical   60-80
       improvement in ____ - ____%.
    c. Intra-arterial drugs
       i.   The primary drug used is _____   Verapamil; hypotension
            but watch for _____.
       ii. N_____ restores vessel diameter   Nicardipine; 60
            to at least _____%.
       iii. Other drugs used include P_____   Papaverine and Nitroglycerin
            and N_____.

12. **Complete the following:**   78.3.7
    a. What is "triple H" therapy?
       i.   h_____v_____   hypervolemia
       ii. h_____t_____   hypertension
       iii. h_____d_____   hemodilution
    b. The fluid to use is _____ _____.   normal saline
    c. Maximum systolic blood pressure for an   160mm Hg
       untreated aneurysm is _____.
    d. Maximum systolic blood pressure for a   220mm Hg
       treated aneurysm is _____.
    e. What do you do if triple H does not   endovascular techniques
       work?
    f. Hemodilution is used to lower   30-35%
       hematocrit to ____ - ____

13. **Triple H therapy may cause pulmonary**   17   78.3.7
    edema in _____% of patients.

■ Post-Op Orders for Aneurysm Clipping

14. **Complete the following about dose for**   78.4
    calcium channel blocker:

    a. What is the name of antivasospasm   nimodipine
       medication/drug?

    b. dose: _____ mg every _____   60 mg every 4 hours
       hours

    c. route: _____   by mouth or nasogastric tube
    d. duration: _____   21 days
    e. unless _____   patient going home intact—if
                                                   so, may stop the calcium
                                                   channel blocker

78

79

SAH from Cerebral Aneurysm Rupture

■ Etiology of Cerebral Aneurysms

1. Matching. What are ideas regarding the etiology of aneurysms? Match the lettered term with the numbered description.

79.2

Description:
① less elastic; ② less muscle; ③ more prominent; ④ less supportive connective tissue

Term: (a-d) below

a. tunica media — ②
b. adventitia — ①
c. internal elastic lamina — ③
d. location—occur — ④

■ Location of Cerebral Aneurysms

2. Give the % incidence of cerebral aneurysm for each of the following:

79.3

a. A-comm — 30%
b. P-comm — 25%
c. MCA — 20%
d. posterior circulation — 15%
e. basilar — 10%
f. multiple — 20 to 30%

■ Presentation of Cerebral Aneurysms

3. Complete the following about intraventricular hemorrhage:

79.4.2

a. General
  i. True or False. It does not affect morbidity-mortality. — false
  ii. It has a mortality of _____%. — 64%
b. A-comm aneurysms rupture into the ventricle through the _____ _____. — lamina terminalis

c. Distal basilar artery aneurysms rupture through the _____ of the _____ _____.   floor of the third ventricle

d. PICA aneurysm may rupture through the
   i. _____ of _____   foramen of Luschka
   ii. and into the _____ _____.   fourth ventricle

4. Third nerve palsy can occur with   79.4.3
a. _____ or   aneurysm
b. _____.   diabetes
c. One can differentiate by examining the _____.   pupils

   i. Pupil dilated in _____.   aneurysm
   ii. Pupil not dilated in _____.   diabetic
d. The mnemonic is "_____"   "diabetes deletes the pupil"
   from the third nerve palsy syndrome.
e. Aneurysms _____ the pupil.   include
f. NPSTN means _____ palsy.   non-pupil-sparing third nerve

■ Conditions Associated with Aneurysms

5. True or False. All of the following conditions may be associated with SAH: 79.5.1
a. hypertension   true
b. Osler-Weber-Rendu syndrome   true
c. diabetes mellitus   false (Diabetes insipidus can be associated.)
d. renal fibromuscular dysplasia   true
e. Ehlers-Danlos type IV   true

6. The following conditions are associated with an increased incidence of aneurysm: 79.5.1
a. a_____ d_____ p_____   autosomal dominant polycystic kidney disease—
   k_____ d_____   15%
b. a_____ m_____   arteriorvenous malformation
c. a _____   atherosclerosis
d. b_____ e_____   bacterial endocarditis
e. c_____ of the a_____   coarctation of the aorta
f. c_____ t_____ d_____   connective tissue disorders
g. Eh_____-Da_____   Ehlers-Danlos type IV
h. fib_____ d_____ r_____   fibromuscular dysplasia renal
   d_____   disease—7%
i. f_____ o_____   familial occurrences
j. M_____ s_____   Marfan syndrome
k. m_____ d_____   moyamoya disease
l. O_____-W_____-R_____   Osler-Weber-Rendu
   s_____   syndrome
m. p_____ e_____   pseudoxanthoma elasticum

79

7. **Complete the following about aneurysms and polycystic kidney disease:**   79.5.2
    a. ADPKD stands for _____ _____ _____ _____.   adult polycystic kidney disease
    b. Incidence is 1 in _____ autopsies.   500
    c. Prevalence of aneurysms in patients with ADPKD is ____ - ____%.   10 to 30%—15% a reasonable estimate
    d. Risk of SAH in a person with ADPKD is ___ to ___ times the general population.   10 to 20 times
    e. Screening protocol in a patient with ADPKD with a prior aneurysm or a kindred with aneurysm is to perform _____ every ___ to ___ years.   MRA every 2 to 3

■ Treatment Options for Aneurysms

8. **Complete the following:**   79.6.3
    a. In trapping an aneurysm is it better to tie off the common carotid artery or the internal carotid artery?   common carotid occlusion is better
    b. It reduces the incidence of _____ _____.   thromboembolic phenomenon

9. **True or False. Regarding treatment options for aneurysms.**   79.6.3
    a. The following procedures offer protection if the aneurysm can't be clipped or coiled:
        i.   wrapping with muscle   false
        ii.   wrapping with cotton   false
        iii. wrapping with muslin   false
        iv.   coating with plastic resin   false
        v.   coating with polymer   false
        vi.   coating with Teflon   false
        vii. coating with fibrin glue   false
    b. In such cases you could consider trapping or bypass or carotid ligation.   true

10. **True or False. Coils are not ideal for**   79.6.5
    a. very small aneurysms   true
    b. very large aneurysms   true
    c. aneurysms with wide necks   true
    d. If after coiling residual filling is noted you should "recoil."   false (Proceed with surgery.)

11. **Data for Guglielmi detachable coils indicate**   79.6.5
    a. morbidity: _____%   4%
    b. mortality: _____%   1%
    c. complete obliteration of aneurysm: _____%   40%
    d. subsequently required open surgical repair: _____%   20%

79

■ Timing of Aneurysm Surgery

12. **Complete the following about timing for aneurysm surgery:**   79.7.1
   a. The definition of early surgery is less than _____ to _____ hours.   48 to 96 hours
   b. Late surgery is after ____ to ____ days.   10 to 14 days
   c. More likely to delay surgery when _____.   treating a basilar artery aneurysm because you want a lax brain during the surgical approach
   d. Avoid doing surgery between days _____ and _____ because that is considered a _____ _____.   4 and 10; vasospastic interval

13. **Complete the following regarding vasospasm treatment:**   79.7.1
   a. It peaks in incidence between _____ and _____ days.   6 and 8 days
   b. It never occurs before day _____.   3
   c. Vasospastic interval during which surgery should be avoided is days _____ to _____.   4 to 10

■ General Technical Considerations of Aneurysm Surgery

14. **Complete the following regarding aneurysmal rest.**   79.8.2
   a. What is an aneurysmal rest?   residual unclipped part of aneurysm
   b. Why are they dangerous?   they may bleed
   c. What is the incidence of rebleeding?   3.7%
   d. There is a risk per year of ____ to ____%.   0.4 to 0.8%
   e. How should they be handled?   serial angiography
   f. If they increase in size, treat with _____ or _____ _____.   surgery or endovascular coiling

15. **Answer the following about CSF drainage during craniotomy:**   79.8.3
   a. True or False. CSF should be drained before opening the dura.   false (This is associated with an increased incidence of rebleeding.)
   b. True or False. CSF should be drained after opening the dura.   true
   c. What is the rate of rebleeding with CSF drainage?   0.3%

16. **Complete the following regarding cerebral protection during surgery:**   79.8.3
   a. O_2 consumption by the neuron is for two functions:
      i. to maintain _____ _____   cell integrity
      ii. for conduction of _____   electrical impulse

79

b. If there is occlusion of a vessel it produces _____   ischemia

c. due to _____ _____.   oxygen deficiency

d. This precludes
  i. a_____ g_____ and   aerobic glycolysis
  ii. o_____ p_____   oxidative phosphorylation
e. What happens to adenosine triphosphate (ATP) production?   it declines
f. What happens to the cell?   cell death occurs

17. **What can be done to protect against ischemia?**   79.8.3
a. Tactics to reduce injury by ischemia include
  i. n_____   nimodipine—calcium channel blockers
  ii. b_____   barbiturates—free radical scavengers
  iii. m_____   mannitol
b. Tactics to reduce the cerebral metabolic rate of oxygen consumption ($CMRO_2$) required include
  i. reducing electrical activity of the neuron with _____.   barbiturates-etomidate
  ii. reducing maintenance energy of the neuron with _____.   hypothermia

18. **Answer the following about temporary clipping during aneurysm surgery:**   79.8.3
a. True or False. Under 5 minutes occlusion is well tolerated.   true
b. If occluded 10 to 15 minutes, must add _____.   dose and drip titrated to burst suppression
c. If occluded more than 20 minutes, _____ _____.   not tolerated

19. **Answer the following about post-op angiography after aneurysm or AVM surgery:**   79.8.4
a. True or False. It is not needed.   false
b. _____% showed unexpected findings.   19%
c. True or False. It is the standard of care.   false
d. True or False. It is recommended.   true

20. **Complete the following regarding drugs useful in aneurysm surgery:**   79.8.5
a. What special medications should be used during temporary clipping of an aneurysm?   etomidate or propofol
b. What do they do?   suppress neuronal activity by reducing neuronal metabolism
c. By how much?   50%

d. What is the side effect of etomidate? lowers seizure threshold
e. Guard against this side effect by using preoperative
_____. antiepileptic drugs

21. Complete the following about intraoperative aneurysm rupture (IAR):   79.8.6

a. True or False. Intraoperative aneurysm rupture increases the morbidity and mortality of surgery threefold. true

b. True or False. Techniques to decrease the probability of intraoperative rupture include
   i. preventing hypertension true
   ii. minimizing brain retraction true
   iii. sharp vs. blunt dissection true
   iv. radical removal of sphenoid wing true

c. List the three general stages of aneurysm surgery during which intraoperative rupture is most likely to occur. stage 1 = initial exposure, stage 2 = dissection of the aneurysm, and stage 3 = clip application

d. During which of these three stages is intraoperative rupture most likely to occur? dissection of aneurysm (stage 2)

22. True or False. During intraoperative rupture by clip application, bleeding reduces as clip blades approximate. false   79.8.6

23. Complete the following about aneurysm recurrence after treatment: 79.8.7

a. Can an incompletely clipped aneurysm bleed? yes—0.4 to 0.8% per year

b. Can an incompletely coiled aneurysm bleed? yes—0.16% per year

c. Can an aneurysm that has been completely obliterated recur and bleed? yes—0.37% per year

80

Aneurysm Type by Location

■ Anterior Communicating Artery Aneurysms

1. Complete the following: 80.1.1
a. The most common site of ruptured   A-commA
   aneurysms is _____.
b. Diabetes insipidus and/or hypothalamic   A-commA
   dysfunction can be the presenting
   symptoms of an aneurysm of the
   _____.

2. Complete the following about   80.1.2
   aneurysm type by location:
a. The single most common site for an   A-commA
   aneurysm is _____.
b. Subarachnoid hemorrhage from an A-   63%
   comm aneurysm rupture is associated
   with an intracerebral hematoma in what
   percentage of cases?
c. The most common site for subarachnoid   anterior interhemispheric
   blood on a CT associated with A-comm   fissure
   aneurysm rupture is _____ _____
   _____.
d. In what percentage of cases?   virtually 100%

3. Complete the following: 80.1.2
a. Vasospasm from A-comm aneurysm   apathy and abulia
   rupture can cause bilateral ACA infarcts
   in the frontal lobes and result in the
   symptoms of _____ and _____.
b. Frontal lobe infarcts occur in _____% 20%
   of cases of A-comm aneurysm rupture.
c. This results in a virtual _____-like   prefrontal
   lobotomy.

4. True or False. Regarding A-comm   80.1.4
   aneurysms:
a. It is unnecessary to assess the side from false
   which an A-comm aneurysm fills by
   angiography because all A-comm
   aneurysms should be approached from
   the right side.

b. Surgical approaches to an A-comm aneurysm include
    i.   pterional approach   true
    ii. anterior interhemispheric approach   true
    iii. transcallosal approach   true
    iv. subfrontal approach   true

c. The two most common sites for distal ACA aneurysms are
    i.   terminal pericallosal artery   false
    ii. terminal callosomarginal artery   false
    iii. frontopolar artery origin   true
    iv. bifurcation of pericallosal and callosomarginal arteries above the splenium of the corpus callosum   true

5. **There are three indications for left pterional craniotomy for A-comm aneurysm.**   80.1.4

a. pointing to _____   the right
b. feeder from _____   the left ACA
c. multiple _____   additional left-sided aneurysm(s)

■ Distal Anterior Cerebral Artery Aneurysms

6. **Pericallosal aneurysms are anatomically close to which part of the corpus callosum?**   genu   80.2.1

7. **True or False. Regarding ACA and A-commA aneurysms and approaches.**

a.
    i.   The more distally located ACA aneurysms are generally due to posttraumatic, infectious, or embolic etiologies.   true   80.2.1
    ii. Aneurysms up to 1 cm from the A-commA may be approached through a standard pterional craniotomy.   true   80.2.2
    iii. Aneurysms > 1 cm distal to the A-commA may also be easily approached through a pterional craniotomy with partial gyrus rectus resection.   false
    iv. ACA aneurysms distal to the genu of the corpus callosum may be approached via an interhemispheric route.   true

b. Prolonged retraction of the cingulate gyrus during an interhemispheric approach may result in a foot drop that is usually temporary.   false

80

8. **Which approach should be used for aneurysms > 1 cm distal to A-comm?**   basal frontal interhemispheric approach, right side preferred   80.2.2

■ Posterior Communicating Artery Aneurysms

9. **Complete the following:**   80.3.1
   a. Which aneurysm presents with a third nerve palsy?   posterior communicating artery
   b. What is the status of the pupil?   dilated
   c. What position does the eye have at rest?   "down and out"
   d. If due to P-comm, the pupil is _____   not spared
   e. because pupillary fibers run on the _____ of the third nerve.   surface
   f. If due to diabetes, the pupil is _____   spared
   g. because motor fibers run in the _____ part of the third nerve and are affected by pathology of the _____ _____.   deeper; vasa nervorum

10. **True or False. Regarding P-comm aneurysms.**   80.3.1
    a. Third nerve palsies associated with P-comm aneurysms are not pupil sparing in 99% of cases.   true
    b. P-comm aneurysms most commonly occur at the junction of the P-comm with the PCA.   false
    c. Before clipping a P-comm aneurysm, the origin of the anterior choroidal artery must be identified and excluded from the clip.   true
    d. Most P-comm aneurysms project laterally, inferiorly, and posteriorly.   true

11. **What congenital anomaly must be discovered on angiogram prior to surgery for P-comm aneurysm?**   fetal origin of the PCA   80.3.2

■ Supraclinoid Aneurysms

12. **What is the name of the dural constriction around the carotid artery**   80.6.1
    a. as it exits the cavernous sinus?   proximal carotid ring
    b. as it enters the subarachnoid space?   distal carotid ring or clinoidal ring

13. **List the supraclinoid branches of the ICA.**   80.6.1
    (Hint: ospa)
    a. o_____   ophthalmic
    b. s_____ h_____   superior hypophyseal
    c. p_____ c_____   posterior communicating
    d. a_____ c_____   anterior choroidal

14. Ophthalmic artery aneurysms 80.6.2
  a. arise just distal to the origin of the   ophthalmic artery
     _____ _____ and
  b. project _____.   dorsomedially

15. Name two major presentations of 80.6.2
    ophthalmic artery aneurysms.
  a. S_____   SAH (45%)
  b. v_____ _____ _____   visual field defect (45%)
    i. True or False. A superior nasal   false
        homonymous quadrantanopsia
        usually means impingement on the
        lateral portion of the optic nerve.
    ii. True or False. An ipsilateral   true
        monocular inferior nasal field cut
        may result from compression of the
        optic nerve against the falciform
        ligament.

16. Complete the following: 80.6.2
  a. List the two variants of superior
     hypophyseal artery aneurysms.
    i. p_____   paraclinoid
    ii. s_____   suprasellar
  b. Which variant of superior hypophyseal   suprasellar variant
     artery aneurysm can mimic pituitary
     tumor clinically and on CT?
  c. Under what circumstances?   when it is a giant aneurysm
  d. It may present clinically with _____   hypopituitarism
  e. and visual symptoms of _____   bitemporal hemianopsia
     _____.

17. Complete the following: 80.6.2
  a. On angiogram, a notch in a giant   optic nerve
     ophthalmic artery aneurysm is due to
     the _____ _____.
  b. The notch, if present, is located in the   anterior-superior-medial
     _____-_____-_____ aspect.

18. Complete the following: 80.6.3
  a. What happens if you occlude the   It is tolerated without loss of
     ophthalmic artery?   vision in most patients.
  b. True or False. A contralateral ophthalmic   false
     aneurysm is rare.
  c. If present, can both be clipped at the   yes
     same surgery?

19. Answer the following: 80.6.3
  a. Can you sacrifice a superior hypophyseal   Yes, the pituitary receives
     artery?   bilateral blood supply.
  b. Can you clip a contralateral superior   No, this is not technically
     hypophyseal aneurysm?   feasible.

80

■ Posterior Circulation Aneurysms

20. **Matching. Match the frequency of posterior circulation aneurysms compared with anterior circulation aneurysms to the lettered conditions.**
   ① same frequency; ② posterior is more frequent
   a. clinical syndrome of SAH   ①   80.7.1
   b. respiratory arrest   ②
   c. neurogenic pulmonary edema   ②
   d. midbrain syndrome from vasospasm ②
   e. hydrocephalus   ②   80.7.2

21. **True or False. 20% of patients with a**   true   80.7.2
   posterior fossa SAH will require
   permanent ventricular shunting.

22. **Regarding vertebral artery aneurysms.**   80.7.3
   a. The preoperative angiogram should   contralateral vertebral artery
       assess the patency of the _____
       _____ _____ in the event that
       trapping is necessary.
   b. The Allcock test involves vertebral   carotid compression
       angiography with _____ _____ to
       assess the patency of the circle of Willis.
   c. Vertebral artery (VA) aneurysms most   VA; PICA
       commonly occur at the junction of the
       _____ with the _____.
   d. True or False. Nontraumatic VA   false
       aneurysms are more common than
       dissecting, traumatic VA aneurysms.

23. **Complete the following regarding**   80.7.3
   PICA aneurysms:
   a. They represent _____% of cerebral   3%
       aneurysms.
   b. The most common site is at _____   VA-PICA
       junction.
   c. Aneurysms far more distal on PICA tend   fragile;
       to be _____ and therefore should be promptly
       treated _____.
   d. Blood from rupture is predominantly in   fourth ventricle
       the _____ _____.

24. **Complete the following:**   80.7.6
   a. The most common site for a posterior   basilar tip
       circulation aneurysm is the _____
       _____.

80

b. True or False. Regarding basilar tip
    aneurysms.

    i.   Surgical treatment is associated with   true
         a 5% overall mortality rate.
    ii. Surgical approaches include   false
         pterional and supracerebellar
         infratentorial routes.
    iii. Because of the technical difficulties   true
         associated with clipping basilar
         aneurysms many still recommend
         waiting up to 1 week prior to
         surgery.
    iv. The morbidity rate of 12% is mostly   true
         due to perforating vessel injury.

25. **On angiography the following**   80.7.6
    characteristics should be noted about
    basilar artery aneurysms:

    a. Direction dome points?   usually superiorly
    b. P-comm characteristics
        i.   P-comm _____   flow
        ii. may need _____ _____.   Allcock test
    c. Bifurcation characteristics:
        i.   Assess position of _____   bifurcation
        ii. in relation to _____.   dorsum sella
        iii. If high, use _____ _____   pterional transsylvian
             _____.   approach
        iv. If low, use _____ _____.   subtemporal approach

26. **Matching. Match the numbered**   80.7.6
    approaches to the conditions for the
    basilar artery aneurysm surgical
    approach.
    Approach: ① subtemporal approach;
    ② pterional approach
    Conditions: (a-h) below

    a. bifurcation is high   ②
    b. aneurysm projects   ①
        posteriorly/posteriorly inferiorly
    c. low bifurcation   ①
    d. concomitant anterior circulation   ②
        aneurysms
    e. for better visualization of P1 and   ②
        thalamoperforating vessels
    f. for less temporal lobe retraction   ②
    g. for shorter distance (by 1 cm)   ①
    h. produces a risk to third nerve (mild and ②
        temporary)

27. **What is the % risk of oculomotor palsy**   30%   80.7.6
    by the pterional approach?

28. **Complete the following about basilar**   80.7.6
    artery aneurysms:
    a. Mortality is _____%.   5%
    b. Morbidity is _____%.   12%

80

Special Aneurysms and Non-Aneurysmal SAH

■ Unruptured Aneurysms

1. **Complete the following about unruptured aneurysms:**

a. Estimated prevalence of incidental aneurysms is ___ - ___% of the population.

5-10%

81.1.1

b. Annual risk of rupture of aneurysms <10 mm estimated by ISUIA is _____, but other studies suggest the risk is closer to _____.

0.05%/year; 1%/year

81.1.3

2. **Complete the following about surgical management of unruptured aneurysms:**

81.1.4

a. Surgical morbidity is estimated to be _____% and mortality _____%.

2%; 6%

b. 3 factors used to determine whether to treat are s_____, p_____ a_____, and l_____.

size, patient age; location

c. Treatment should also be recommended for patients with h_____ of a_____ S_____, s_____ f_____ h_____, s_____ a_____, and e_____ or c_____ in a_____ c_____.

history of aneurysmal SAH, strong family history, symptomatic aneurysms; enlargement or change in aneurysm configuration

3. **Cavernous carotid artery aneurysms:**

81.1.4

a. Most develop on the h_____ segment of the artery.

horizontal

b. Usually present with h_____ or c_____ s_____ s_____.

headache; cavernous sinus syndrome

c. Cavernous sinus syndrome produces d_____ and t_____ n_____ p_____ that is pupil-s_____.

diplopia; third nerve palsy; sparing

d. When these aneurysms rupture, they usually produce a c____-c_____ f____.

a carotid-cavernous fistula

4. **Indications for treatment of cavernous carotid artery aneurysms:**
(Hint: gees)

81.1.4

a. g_____

giant aneurysm

b. e_____

enlarging aneurysm

c.   e_____   before endarterectomy
d.   s_____   symptomatic

5.   **Treatment options for cavernous**   81.1.4
     carotid artery aneurysms:
a.   Preferred treatment technique is   endovascular
     e_____.
b.   o_____ s_____ t_____ is rarely   open surgical treatment
     appropriate.

■ Multiple Aneurysms

6.   **Complete the following about**   81.2
     multiple aneurysms:
a.   Present in ___ - _____% of SAH cases.   15-33.5%
b.   When a patient presents with SAH and is
     found to have multiple aneurysms, the
     following clues can be used to determine
     the source of SAH: (Hint: evil)
     i.   e_____   epicenter of blood
     ii.   v_____   vasospasm on angiogram
     iii. i_____   irregularities in shape
     iv.   l_____   largest aneurysm

■ Familial Aneurysms

7.   **Complete the following about familial**   81.3.1
     aneurysms:
a.   In patients with SAH, _____% have a   9.4%;
     1st-degree relative with SAH or   14%
     aneurysm and _____% have a 2nd-
     degree relative.
b.   Most common relative to also have an   sibling
     aneurysm is a s_____.
c.   Aneurysms in siblings occur at i_____   identical;
     or m_____ i_____ location.   mirror image
d.   Familial aneurysms tend to rupture at a   smaller;
     s_____ size and at a y_____ age.   younger

8.   **Screening recommendations for**   81.3.3
     familial aneurysms:
a.   Recommended for f_____-d_____   first-degree;
     relatives of affected family members   2
     when _____ or more family
     members have an aneurysm or history of
     SAH.
b.   Also recommended in patients with   coarctation of the aorta;
     c_____ of the a_____ or with   ADPKD
     A_____.
c.   Screen using M_____ or C_____   MRA; CTA
     scans.
d.   To confirm findings, use D_____.   DSA

81

■ Traumatic Aneurysms

9. **Complete the following about traumatic aneurysms:**   81.4.1
   a. Represent _____% of aneurysms.   <1%
   b. They are not really aneurysms but are   pseudoaneurysms
      p_____.
   c. Mechanisms of injury resulting in   penetrating trauma,
      traumatic aneurysms include   closed head injury;
      p_____ t_____, c_____   iatrogenic
      h_____ i_____, and i_____.

■ Mycotic Aneurysms

10. **Complete the following about mycotic aneurysms:**
    a. The etiology for these aneurysms is   infectious   81.5.1
       i_____.
    b. Represent _____% of aneurysms.   4%   81.5.2
    c. Most common location is d_____   distal MCA branches
       M_____ b_____.
    d. Often associated with subacute bacterial   endocarditis
       e_____.
    e. Infectious work-up includes b_____   blood cultures, lumbar   81.5.3
       c_____, l_____ p_____, and   puncture; echo
       e_____.
    f. F_____ morphology makes surgical   Fusiform;   81.5.4
       treatment difficult and/or risky, and so   4-6 weeks
       treated acutely with ____ - ____ weeks
       of antibiotics.
    g. Delayed clipping indicated in patients   SAH;
       with S_____ and with f_____   failed
       response to antibiotics.

■ Giant Aneurysms

11. **Complete the following about giant aneurysms:**
    a. Defined as an aneurysm >_____ cm.   2.5   81.6.1
    b. Represent ____ - ____% of aneurysms.   3-5%
    c. Present with h_____, T_____,   hemorrhage, TIA;
       or m_____ e_____.   mass effect
    d. DSA often u_____ size of aneurysm   underestimates;   81.6.2
       due to t_____ parts that do not fill   thrombosed
       with contrast.
    e. Direct surgical clipping is possible in only   50%   81.6.3
       _____% of cases.
    f. Other surgical treatment options include   bypass; clipping,
       b_____ followed by c_____,   trapping, ligation;
       t_____, l_____, or   wrapping
       w_____.

■ SAH of Unknown Etiology

12. SAH of unknown etiology:

a. "Angiogram-negative SAH" occurs in ___   7-10%   81.8.1
- ___% of cases.

b. Causes

   i.   i_____ angiography. Must see   inadequate;
        both P_____ origins and   PICA;
        A_____.   AComm

   ii. Aneurysm obscured by h_____.   hemorrhage

   iii. t_____ of aneurysm.   thrombosis

   iv. Aneurysms too s_____ to be   small
        seen.

   v.   Lack of filling due to v_____ of   vasospasm
        parent vessel.

   vi. Repeat angiogram is recommended   10-14   81.8.3
        after ___ - ___ days.

   vii. If the first 2 angiograms are   3-6;
        negative, a third angiogram is   1%
        recommended after ___ - ___
        months and has a _____%
        chance of revealing a source of SAH.

■ Pretruncal Nonaneurysmal SAH (PNSAH)

13. SAH of unknown etiology:

a. Also known as p_____ S_____,   perimesencephalic SAH   81.9.1
   which is a misnomer since

b. hemorrhage is located in front of the   brainstem;
   b_____ centered in front of the   pons
   p_____.

c. Perimesencephalic cisterns include:
   (Hint: Iraq)

   i.   i_____   interpenduncular

   ii. r_____   crural

   iii. a_____   ambient

   iv. q_____   quadrigeminal

d. Considered to be a b_____ condition benign;
   with g_____ outcome, l_____   good; less;
   risk of rebleeding, and l_____ risk of   less;
   v_____ compared to patients with   vasospasm
   SAH of unknown etiology.

e. Represent ____ - ____% of angiogram-   20-68%   81.9.3
   negative SAH.

f. Repeat angiography is n_____   not   81.9.6
   indicated.

g. Management does not include   hyperdynamic therapy;   81.9.7
   h_____ t_____ or c_____   calcium channel blockers
   c_____ b_____ given low risk
   of vasospasm.

h. Hydrocephalus requiring shunting occurs 1%
   in _____%.

82

Vascular Malformations

■ General Information and Classification

1. **Complete the following about vascular malformations:**   82.1
   a. 4 classic types include A_____, c_____, c_____, D_____.
      AVM, cavernoma, capillary telangiectasia, DVA
   b. A_____ is the most prevalent type, accounting for ___ - ___% of vascular malformations.
      AVM; 44-60%
   c. A direct fistula is also known as A_____ and includes V_____ of G_____ m_____, d_____ A_____, and C_____.
      AVF; Vein of Galen malformation, dural AVF; CCF

■ Arteriovenous Malformation (AVM)

2. **Complete the following about AVMs:**   82.2.1
   a. Arterial blood flows directly from a_____ to v_____ without normal interposed c_____ b_____ but with n_____ instead.
      arteries; veins; capillary beds; nidus
   b. C_____ rather than acquired.
      Congenital
   c. Associated with the hereditary syndrome O_____-W_____-R_____, also known as h_____ h_____ t_____.
      Osler-Weber-Rendu; hereditary hemorrhagic telangiectasia

3. **AVM presentation:**
   a. Average age of patients diagnosed with AVMs is _____.
      33 years-old   82.2.4
   b. AVMs most commonly present with h_____.
      hemorrhage   82.2.5
   c. Another common presentation is s_____.
      seizures

4. **AVMs and hemorrhage**   82.2.5
   a. Peak age for hemorrhage is ___ - ___.
      15-20 years-old
   b. Mortality for each bleed is _____%.
      10%
   c. Morbidity for each bleed is ___ - ___%.
      30-50%

d. Most common site for hemorrhage is
i_____, present in _____% of
cases.

intraparenchymal;
82%

e. Other sites include I_____,
S_____, and s_____ h_____.

IVH, SAH;
subdural hematoma

5. Risk factors related to AVM rupture: 82.2.5

a. Small AVMs present more often as
h_____, whereas large AVMs present
with s_____.

hemorrhage;
seizures

b. D_____ venous drainage and prior
h_____ are also associated with AVM
rupture.

Deep;
hemorrhage

6. Risk of AVM rupture: 82.2.5

a. Average risk of hemorrhage from an
AVM is ___ - ___% per year.

2-4%

b. What is the risk of bleeding (at least
once) from an AVM during the lifetime of
a 35 year-old healthy male, assuming a
3% annual bleeding risk?

73%

7. AVMs and aneurysms: 82.2.5

a. _____% of patients with AVMs have
aneurysms.

7%

b. Aneurysms associated with AVMs usually
arise from a f_____ artery.

feeder

c. If it is not clear which bled, the AVM or
the aneurysm, it is usually the
a_____.

aneurysm

d. Do aneurysms regress after AVM
removal?

yes (66%)

8. MRI characteristics of AVMs: 82.2.6

a. F_____ v_____ on T1- or T2-
weighted imaging.

Flow voids

b. Presence of e_____ can help
differentiate AVM from t_____.

edema;
tumor

c. A complete hemosiderin ring suggests
AVM over t_____.

tumor

d. What sequence best shows
hemosiderin?

gradient echo

9. Spetzler-Martin grading of AVMs: 82.2.7

a. Grade ranges from _____ to
_____.

1 to 5

b. Graded features of an AVM include
s_____, e_____ of _____,
and p_____ of _____ _____.

size, eloquence of adjacent
brain; pattern of venous
drainage

c. The Spetzler-Martin grade of a 4 cm AVM
that drains into the vein of Galen and is
located in the visual cortex is _____.

4

d. This AVM has a major surgical morbidity
of _____% and a minor surgical
morbidity of _____%.

7%;
20%

10. **Complete the following about AVM treatment:**   82.2.8
   a. The treatment of choice for AVMs is s_____.   surgery
   b. Surgery eliminates the risk of bleeding almost i_____.   immediately
   c. Conventional radiation is effective in less than _____% of cases.   20%
   d. SRS takes ___ - ___ years to work.   1-3
   e. Endovascular embolization:
      i. Does not permanently o_____ AVMs.   obliterate
      ii. Does f_____ surgery.   facilitate
      iii. Induces acute h_____ changes.   hemodynamic
      iv. May require m_____ procedures.   multiple
   f. What pretreatment can be used to reduce the incidence of normal perfusion pressure breakthrough?   propranolol 20 mg four times a day for 3 days

■ Venous Angiomas

11. **Complete the following about venous angiomas:**
   a. Also known as d_____ v_____ a_____.   developmental venous anomaly (DVA)   82.3.1
   b. Demonstrable on angiography as a s_____ pattern.   starburst
   c. Seizures are r_____.   rare
   d. Hemorrhage is r_____.   rare
   e. L_____-flow, l_____-pressure lesions.   Low; low
   f. What is the treatment of choice?   no treatment needed   82.3.3

■ Angiographically Occult Vascular Malformations

12. **Angiographically occult vascular malformation (AOVM) presentation:**
   a. The incidence of angiographically occult vascular malformations is _____%.   10%   82.4.2
   b. They most often present with s_____ or h_____, rather than h_____.   seizures or headache; hemorrhage   82.4.3
   c. The most common angiographically occult vascular malformation is A_____.   AVM

■ Osler-Weber-Rendu Syndrome

13. **Capillary telangiectasias:**   82.5.1
   a. Usually found i_____ without c_____ significance.   incidentally; clinical
   b. Usually s_____ but may be m_____ when seen as part of a syndrome.   solitary; multiple

c. Syndromes include O_____-W_____-   Osler-Weber-Rendu (aka
     R_____, L_____-B_____, M_____-   hereditary hemorrhagic
     M_____, S_____-W_____   telangiectasia), Louis-Barr
         (aka ataxia telangiectasia),
         Myburn-Mason, Sturge-
         Weber

82

■ Cavernous Malformation

14. Cavernous malformations:
   a. Most often present with s_____.   seizures   82.6.1
   b. They are angiographically o_____.   occult
   c. Account for ___ - ___% of all CNS   5-13%   82.6.3
      vascular malformations.
   d. Present with   82.6.5
      i. s_____ in 60%.   seizures
      ii. p_____ n_____ deficit in   progressive neurological
         50%.
      iii. h_____ in 20%.   hemorrhage
      iv. i_____ finding in 50%.   incidental

15. Cavernous malformation genetics: 82.6.4
   a. Cavernous malformations can occur   sporadically;
      s_____ or in a h_____ form.   hereditary
   b. M_____ lesions are more common in   Multiple;
      the h_____ form.   hereditary
   c. There are _____ genetic subtypes.   3
   d. CCM1 subtype is more common in   Hispanics
      H_____.
   e. Genetic subtypes are inherited in an   autosomal dominant;
      a_____ d_____ pattern with   variable
      v_____ expressivity.
   f. DVA may be seen adjacent to s_____   solitary
      cavernous malformations.
   g. F_____-d_____ relatives of patients   First-degree;
      with more than one family member   screening;
      having a cavernous malformation should   genetic
      have MRI s_____ and appropriate
      g_____ counseling.

16. Cavernous malformation bleeding   82.6.5
      risk:
   a. Risk of significant bleeding is ___ - ___%   2-3%
      per year.
   b. Bleeding risk is higher in f_____.   females
   c. P_____ h_____, p_____, and   Prior hemorrhage, pregnancy;
      p_____ are not clearly risk factors for   parturition
      hemorrhage. (Hint: 3Ps)

82

17. **Radiographic evaluation of cavernous malformations:**   82.6.6
    a. The most sensitive test is M_____.   MRI
    b. The most sensitive sequence is G_____-e_____ T_____.   Gradient-echo T2WI
    c. Display a pathognomonic p_____ pattern.   popcorn

18. **Management of cavernous malformations:**   82.6.7
    a. Three treatment options include o_____, s_____, or S_____.   observation, surgery; SRS
    b. New onset seizures may be an indication for s_____ because removal before k_____ may reduce future seizures.   surgery; kindling
    c. S_____ should not be considered as an alternative to s_____.   SRS; surgery

■ Dural Arteriovenous Fistulae (DAVF)

19. **Complete the following about dural arteriovenous fistulae:**
    a. Arteriovenous shunt is contained within the d_____.   dura   82.7.1
    b. Most common location is t_____/s_____ _____.   transverse/sigmoid sinus
    c. Considered to be a_____ rather than c_____ lesions.   acquired; congenital
    d. Primary etiology is v_____ s_____ t_____.   venous sinus thrombosis   82.7.2
    e. Most common presenting symptom is p_____ t_____.   pulsatile tinnitus   82.7.4
    f. C_____ v_____ d_____ with v_____ h_____ is the most common cause of morbidity and mortality, and thus is the strongest indication for t_____.   Cortical venous drainage with venous hypertension; treatment
    g. D_____ is required to establish the diagnosis.   DSA   82.7.5

■ Vein of Galen Malformation

20. **Vein of Galen malformation:**
    a. Feeders are primarily from c_____ a_____.   choroidal arteries   82.8.1
    b. Drainage is into the m_____ v_____ of the p_____.   medial vein of the prosencephalon
    c. Trigger symptoms by causing h_____ and c_____ h_____ f_____.   hydrocephalus; congestive heart failure   82.8.2
    d. If untreated mortality is ___ - ___%.   60-100%   82.8.4

■ Carotid-Cavernous Fistula

21. **Complete the following about carotid-cavernous fistulae:**

a. Classified as d_____ and i_____ types.

direct; indirect   82.9.1

b. Type A: h_____-flow shunt between l_____ and c_____ s_____.

high; ICA; cavernous sinus

c. Type B: l_____-flow shunt with feeders from m_____ b_____ of l_____.

low; meningeal branches of ICA

d. Type C: l_____-flow shunt with feeders from m_____ b_____ of E_____.

low; meningeal branches of ECA

e. Type D: l_____-flow shunt with feeders from b_____ of l_____ and E_____.

low; branches of ICA and ECA

f. Direct CCF occurs in _____% of head trauma patients.

0.2%

g. ___ - ___% of low-flow CCF spontaneously t_____.

20-50%; thrombose   82.9.4

h. U_____ t_____ is usually indicated for h_____-flow CCF.

Urgent treatment; high

i. Preservation of v_____ is another critical indication for treatment.

vision

j. E_____ e_____ is the treatment of choice.

Endovascular embolization

82

83

General Information and Stroke Physiology

■ Definitions

1. **Types of cerebral infarction:**   83.1
   a. TIA = t_____ neuronal dysfunction   transient;
      without p_____ acute infarction.   permanent
   b. Ischemic infarction = p_____ death   permanent;
      of neurons caused by inadequate   perfusion
      p_____.
   c. Watershed infarct = infarction located in   bordering
      two b_____ arterial distributions.

■ Cerebrovascular Hemodynamics

2. **Cerebrovascular hemodynamics:**
   a. Cerebral blood flow _____ is   <20;   83.2.1
      associated with i_____ and if   ischemia;
      prolonged will produce c____ d_____.   cell death
   b. Types of responses of cerebral blood   acetazolamide   83.2.4
      flow to vasodilator challenge with
      a_____:
      i.   Type 1 = n_____ baseline CBF   normal;
           with ___ - ___% i_____.   30-60% increase
      ii. Type 2 = d_____ baseline CBF   decreased;
           with _____% i_____.   <10% increase
      iii. Type 3 = d_____ baseline CBF   decreased;
           with d_____, suggesting   decrease;
           s_____ phenomenon.   steal

■ Collateral Circulation

3. **Collateral circulation:**   83.3.1
   a. Flow through C_____ of W_____   Circle of Willis
   b. via a_____ c_____ artery and   anterior communicating;
      p_____ c_____ artery.   posterior communicating
   c. Also r_____ flow through o_____ retrograde; ophthalmic
      artery.
   d. Also d_____-l_____   dural-leptomeningeal
      anastomoses.

■ "Occlusion" Syndromes

4. "Occlusion" syndromes   83.4.1

a. Overall annual ischemic stroke risk in symptomatic ICA occlusion is _____%.   7%

b. A_____ syndrome and B_____ syndrome are caused by occlusion of p_____ c_____ a_____.   Anton; Balint; posterior cerebral artery

c. Bilateral thalamic and mesencephalic infarctions are caused by occlusion of artery of P_____.   Percheron

d. Eponym for lateral medullary syndrome is W_____ s_____.   Wallenberg's syndrome

e. This syndrome is classically attributed to P_____ occlusion but in ___ - ___% of cases involves the v_____ a_____.   PICA; 80-85%; vertebral artery

f. This syndrome also produces only s_____ loss and no m_____ function loss.   sensory; motor

g. Small infarcts in deep cerebrum or brainstem are called l_____ strokes.   lacunar

h. Pure sensory loss indicates lacunar stroke in p_____ t_____.   posteroventral thalamus

i. Pure hemiparesis indicates lacunar stroke in p_____ l_____ of i_____ c_____.   posterior limb; internal capsule

83

■ Stroke in Young Adults

5. Stroke in young adults:

a. Only _____% of ischemic strokes occur in patients who are _____ years-old.   3%; <40 years-old   83.5.1

b. Most common cause is t_____, _____%.   trauma, 22%   83.5.2

c. Other causes include a_____, e_____, v_____, h_____ s_____, and p_____.   atherosclerosis, embolism, vasculopathy, hypercoagulable state; peripartum

■ Atherosclerotic Carotid Artery Disease

6. Atherosclerotic carotid artery disease:

a. Carotid artery lesions are considered symptomatic if there is o_____ or m_____ ischemic episodes in the d_____ of the vessel.   one; more; distribution   83.6.2

b. They are considered asymptomatic if the patient only has non-specific v_____ complaints, d_____, or s_____ not associated with TIA or stroke.   visual; dizziness; syncope

83

c. ____% of atherosclerotic carotid strokes occur without warning symptoms.   80%

d. Asymptomatic carotid stenosis is usually discovered as a c_____ b_____.   carotid bruit

e. Accuracy of a bruit predicting carotid stenosis is ___ - ___%.   50-83%

f. Screening for carotid stenosis may be considered for patients who are o_____ than _____ years old and have multiple c_____ risk factors.   older than 55 years old; cardiovascular   83.6.3

g. The gold standard test to evaluate carotid stenosis is D_____.   DSA

h. Percent stenosis by NASCET criteria is _____ (formula), where N is measured at maximal n_____ and D is measured d_____ to the c_____ b_____.   [1-(N/D)]x100%; narrowing; distal; carotid bulb

i. Percent stenosis by ECST criteria is _____ (formula), where N is measured at maximal n_____ and B is measured at the c_____ b_____.   [1-(N/B)]x100%; narrowing; carotid bulb

j. Doppler ultrasound sensitivity _____% and specificity _____%.   88%; 76%

k. MRA sensitivity _____% and specificity _____%.   91%; 88%

l. CTA sensitivity _____% and specificity _____%.   85%; 93%

7. Medical treatment for carotid stenosis: 83.6.4

a. Includes anti-p_____, anti-h_____, anti-c_____, anti-l_____, anti-d_____, and anti-s_____.   anti-platelet, -hypertensive, -coagulation, -lipid, -diabetic, -smoking

b. Aspirin irreversibly inhibits c_____.   cyclooxygenase

c. Optimal dose of Aspirin for cerebrovascular ischemia is d_____.   debated

d. Aspirin reduces risk of stroke following TIA by ___ - ___%.   25-30%

e. Daily doses of 81 or 325 mg were b_____ than higher doses.   better

f. Plavix inhibits A_____-induced platelet fibrinogen binding   ADP

8. Asymptomatic carotid stenosis: 83.6.4

a. Stroke rate is ____% per year.   2%

b. ___% of these strokes are not d_____.   50%; disabling

c. Carotid endarterectomy may be better than medical management if stenosis _____%.   >60%

d. 2 main studies comparing surgical vs. medical management of asymptomatic carotid stenosis are A_____ and A_____.   ACST, ACAS

84

Evaluation and Treatment for Stroke

■ Rationale for Acute Stroke Treatment

1. **Penumbra:**
   84.1.1
   a. Tissue at r_____ that retains v_____ for a period of t_____ through suboptimal perfusion from c_____ is called the p_____. — risk; viability; time; collaterals; penumbra
   b. The goal of stroke treatments is p_____ of this s_____ neuronal injury. — prevention; secondary

■ Evaluation

2. **Key components of history:**
   84.2.1
   a. Time last seen n_____. — normal
   b. N_____ s_____ s_____ s_____. — NIH Stroke Scale score

3. **Role of CT scan:**
   84.2.2
   a. Used mainly to rule-out h_____. — hemorrhage
   b. H_____ a_____ sign can be seen on CT _____ hours after stroke, but it has low s_____. — Hyperdense artery; <6 hours; sensitivity
   c. At 24 hours, stroke identified as l_____ density on CT. — low
   d. M_____ effect reaches a maximum ___ - ___ days after the stroke. — Mass; 2-4 days
   e. CT enhancement in stroke: (Hint: rule of 2's) _____% enhance at _____ days, _____% enhance at _____ months. — 2%; 2; 2%; 2

4. **Other imaging studies:**
   a. CTA is used to identify location and extent of v_____ o_____. — vascular occlusion
   84.2.3
   b. CT perfusion identifies salvageable p_____. — penumbra
   84.2.4
   c. Infarcted core has d_____ CBF within region of d_____ CBV. — decreased; decreased

d. Penumbra has d_____ CBV   decreased;
w_____ d_____ CBF; m_____   without decreased;
between CBF and CBV.   mismatch

e. MRI is more s_____ than CT,   sensitive;   84.2.1
particularly in first _____ hours after   24 hours
stroke.

5. NIH stroke scale score: 84.2.8
a. Higher score correlates with more   proximal
p_____ vessel occlusion.
b. Complete hemianopia adds _____   2
points.
c. Severe aphasia adds _____ points.   2
d. Performance of all commands adds   0
_____ points.

■ Management of TIA or Stroke

6. Management of ischemic stroke   84.3.1
a. Within 4.5 hours of symptom onset,   IV tPA
patient may be a candidate for I_____
t_____.
b. 4.5-6 hours after onset, may use   IA tPA;
I_____t_____ or m_____   mechanical thrombectomy
t_____.
c. 6-8 hours after onset, may perform   mechanical thrombectomy;
m_____ t_____ after checking   perfusion
p_____ scan.
d. P_____ circulation strokes may be   Posterior;
treated more a_____.   aggressively

7. Tissue plasminogen activator: 84.3.2
a. Alteplase = t_____.   tPA
b. IV tPA contraindications include:
    i. i_____   intracerebral hemorrhage
    ii. known _____ or _____   aneurysm or AVM
    iii. active _____   internal bleeding
    iv. anti_____   anticoagulation
    v. platelet count _____   <100K
    vi. h_____ t_____, s_____, or   head trauma, stroke, brain
       b_____ s_____ within past   surgery; 3 months
       _____ months
    vii. SBP > _____   185 mmHg
c. After administering tPA, anticoagulation   24 hours
and antiplatelets are held for _____
hours.
d. There is increased risk for s_____   symptomatic intracerebral
i_____ h_____ with use of tPA,   hemorrhage; mortality
but no increased risk of m_____.

84

8. **Blood pressure guidelines:**   84.3.4
    a. If no prior history of hypertension, do   160-170;
        not lower SBP below ___ - ___ and DBP   95-105
        below ___ - ___.
    b. If prior history of hypertension, do not   180-185;
        lower SBP below ___ - ___ and DBP   105-110
        below ___ - ___.

9. **Anticoagulation in ischemic stroke:**   84.3.4
    a. American Heart Association   preference
        recommended the use of heparin
        remains a matter of p_____ by the
        treating physician.
    b. Effectiveness of heparin is unproven   cardioembolic
        except with c_____ stroke.
    c. Stop warfarin after _____ months.   6
    d. A_____ should be administered to   Aspirin 325 mg
        most patients.

84

■ Carotid Endarterectomy

10. **Symptomatic carotid stenosis:**
    a. NASCET stands for N_____ A_____   North American Symptomatic   84.4.1
        S_____ C_____ E_____   Carotid Endarterectomy Trial
        T_____.
    b. Carotid endarterectomy (CEA) for   >70%; 17%; 7%
        symptomatic carotid stenosis
        _____% reduces strokes by
        _____% at 18 months and reduces
        death by _____% at 18 months.
    c. Only need to wait _____ days after   7 days   84.4.2
        acute stroke to perform CEA.

11. **CEA surgery complications:**   84.4.4
    a. _____ days before surgery patient   5;
        should be started on a_____, which   aspirin 325 mg;
        should be c_____ the day of surgery.   continued
    b. Aspirin should be h_____ 24-48 hours   held
        postop.
    c. Morbidity absolute upper limit is   3%
        _____%.
    d. In-hospital mortality is _____%.   1%
    e. List postop complications:
        (Hint: ch$_4$arm$_2$s$_2$)
        i.   c_____ n_____ i_____   cranial nerve injury
        ii.   h_____   headache
        iii. h_____   hoarseness
        iv.   h_____   hyperperfusion
        v.   h_____   hypertension
        vi.   a_____ d_____   arteriotomy disruption
        vii. r_____   restenosis
        viii. m_____   morbidity
        ix.   m_____   mortality
        x.   s_____   seizures
        xi.   s_____   stroke

f. Incidence of hypoglossal nerve injury is   1%
    _____%.
g. Tongue deviates t_____ the i_____.   towards the injury
h. Hoarseness is most commonly caused by   edema;
    e_____ and not n_____   nerve injury
    i_____.
i. Unilateral vocal cord paralysis is due to   vagus;
    v_____ or r_____ l_____ nerve   recurrent laryngeal
    injury.
j. Lip asymmetry is due to m_____   mandibular branch of facial
    b_____ of f_____ nerve injury.
k. Hypertension may occur as a result of   carotid sinus baroreceptor
    loss of the c_____ s_____
    b_____ reflex.
l. Intracerebral hemorrhage occurs in   0.6%;
    _____% and is related to c_____   cerebral hyperperfusion
    h_____.
m. Incidence of post-op ischemic stroke is   5%
    _____%.
n. Post-op TIAs are usually due to c_____   carotid occlusion;
    o_____ but may also be due to   microemboli
    m_____.
o. Late restenosis occurs in ___% at _____;   25% at 1 year;
    within 2 years postop it is due to   fibrous hyperplasia;
    f_____ h_____ and after 2 years it   atherosclerosis
    is due to a_____.
p. If TIAs occur in recovery room, then   CT
    obtain C_____.
q. If fixed deficit occurs in recovery room,   do not;
    then d_____ n_____ obtain CT;   reexploration
    instead r_____ indicated.
r. If arteriotomy closure is disrupted, then   open wound;
    o_____ w_____ first to e_____   evacuate;
    clot, then have anesthesia i_____   intubate;
    patient, and finally revise   OR
    endarterectomy in O_____.

12. CEA surgery technique: 84.4.5
a. There is n_____ d_____ between   no difference;
    the use of l_____ and g_____   local; general
    anesthesia.
b. Use a shunt if there is h_____   hemodynamic intolerance;
    i_____ to clamping or if s_____   stump;
    pressure is _____.   <25 mmHg
c. C_____ f_____ vein crosses over the   Common facial
    carotid bifurcation.
d. H_____ nerve is in vicinity of   Hypoglossal;
    f_____ v_____.   facial vein
e. S_____ t_____ artery is first   Superior thyroid artery;
    branch of E_____ and helps   ECA;
    differentiate E_____ from I_____.   ECA; ICA
f. Place temporary clip on s_____   superior thyroid artery
    t_____ a_____.
g. Order of occlusion of vessels is I_____   ICA, CCA, ECA
    C_____ E_____ (Hint: ICE).

h. P_____ g_____ may reduce risk of   Patch graft
    perioperative occlusion and restenosis.
i. Order of releasing the vessels is   ECA, CCA, ICA
    E_____ C_____ I_____.

■ Carotid Angioplasty/Stenting

13. **Carotid angioplasty/stenting:**   84.5.2
    a. Should be considered instead of CEA in   cardiovascular
        patients with severe c_____ disease.
    b. Also in patients with:
        i.   contralateral c_____   comorbidities
        ii. l_____ n_____ p_____ to   laryngeal nerve palsy
             neck
        iii. previous CEA with r_____   radiation treatment,
             t_____, r_____   restenosis
        iv. h_____ carotid bifurcation   high
        v.   s_____ t_____ lesions   severe tandem
        vi. age _____   >80 years-old

84

85

Special Conditions

■ Totally Occluded Internal Carotid Artery

1. **Totally occluded internal carotid artery:**

   a. ___ - ___% of patients with carotid territory stroke or TIA have ipsilateral carotid occlusion.

   10-15%

   85.1.1

   b. Patients with mild deficit have stroke rate of ___ - ___% per year related to the occluded carotid.

   3-5%

   85.1.3

   c. ___ - ___% of patients with acute occlusion and profound deficit make a good recovery.

   2-12%

   d. C_____-occluded carotid has p_____ patency rate and l_____ gain from re-opening.

   Chronically; poor; little

   85.1.5

   e. R_____ filling of ICA to pretrous or cavernous segment from ECA or from contralateral ICA is a g_____ sign of operability.

   Retrograde; good

■ Cerebellar Infarction

2. **Cerebellar infarction:**

   a. _____% of patients developing signs of b_____ c_____ will die within hours to days.

   80%; brainstem compression

   85.2.1

   b. Symptoms generally increase within ___ - ___ hours following onset.

   12-96 hours

   c. Operation of choice is s_____ d_____.

   suboccipital decompression

   85.2.3

   d. Avoid using v_____ d_____ alone as this may cause u_____ h_____ and does not relieve b_____ c_____.

   ventricular drainage; upward herniation; brainstem compression

   85.2.6

■ Malignant Middle Cerebral Artery Territory Infarction

3. Malignant middle cerebral artery territory infarction:

a. Occurs in up to _____% of stroke patients.
   10%
   85.3.1

b. Carries a mortality of up to _____%.
   80%

c. T_____ herniation occurs within _____ days of stroke.
   Transtentorial; 2-4 days

d. H_____ can reduce mortality to _____% among all comers.
   Hemicraniectomy; 37%
   85.3.2

e. Better results if surgery performed b_____ any signs of herniation.
   before

f. 3 r_____ c_____ t_____ found that hemicraniectomy with _____ hours of stroke onset decreased m_____ and increased favorable f_____ o_____.
   randomized controlled trials; 48 hours; mortality; functional outcome

85

■ Cardiogenic Brain Embolism

4. Cardiogenic brain embolism:

a. _____ stroke in _____ is cardioembolic.
   1 in 6
   85.4.1

b. _____% of patients will have a stroke within ___ - ___ weeks of an acute MI, and the risk is higher with a_____ wall MI.
   2.5%; 1-2; anterior
   85.4.2

c. Patients with A-fib have a _____% rate of stroke per year without treatment.
   4.5%
   85.4.3

d. Ischemic stroke rate per year for patients with mechanical heart valves who are on anticoagulation is _____% per year for mitral and _____% per year for aortic valves.
   3% per year; 1.5% per year
   85.4.4

e. P_____ embolism can occur with a p_____ f_____ o_____, which is present in ___ - ___% of the general population.
   Paradoxical; patent foramen ovale; 10-18%
   85.4.5

■ Vertebrobasilar Insufficiency

5. Vertebrobasilar insufficiency:

a. Six of the symptoms of VBI begin with the letter "d." They are:
   85.5.2

   i.   dr_____ _____
   drop attack

   ii.   di_____
   diplopia

   iii.   dy_____
   dysarthria

   iv.   de_____ _____ _____
   defect in vision

   v.   diz_____
   dizziness

   vi.   de_____ b_____
   deficit bilaterally

b. Clinical diagnosis of VBI requires _____ or more of the symptoms listed above.   2

c. The most common cause of VBI is h_____ i_____.   hemodynamic insufficiency   85.5.3

d. S_____ s_____ causes r_____ flow in the v_____ artery due to p_____ stenosis of the s_____ artery.   Subclavian steal; reversed; vertebral; proximal; subclavian

e. Stroke rate is ___ - ___% per year.   4.5-7%   85.5.4

f. A_____ is the mainstay of medical management.   Anticoagulation   85.5.6

85 ■ Bow Hunter's Stroke

6. Bow hunter's stroke:

a. Bow hunter's stroke is caused by occlusion of the v_____ artery resulting from h_____ r_____.   vertebral; head rotation   85.6.1

b. The vessel occluded is c_____ to the direction of head rotation.   contralateral

c. It is more likely in patients with incompetent p_____ c_____ arteries.   posterior communicating

d. An appropriate test for this condition is d_____ c_____ a_____.   dynamic cerebral angiography   85.6.3

e. The treatment of choice is d_____ of the v_____ artery at C_____.   decompression; vertebral; C1-2   85.6.4

f. If symptoms persist, then perform C_____ f_____.   C1-2 fusion

■ Cerebrovascular Venous Thrombosis

7. Cerebrovascular venous thrombosis:

a. Hypercoagulable states include: (Hint: a^2p^4rs)   85.7.2

   i. a_____ III deficiency   antithrombin

   ii. a_____ antibodies   antiphospholipid

   iii. p_____ C deficiency   protein

   iv. p_____ S deficiency   protein

   v. p_____ n_____ hemoglobinuria   paroxysmal nocturnal

   vi. p_____ deficiency   plasminogen

   vii. r_____ to activated protein C   resistance

   viii. s_____ lupus erythematosis   systemic

b. Occurs in mothers with incidence of _____, and the highest risk is f_____ _____ weeks post-partum.   1/10,000 births; first 2 weeks

c. Frequency of dural sinus involvement: 85.7.3

   i. _____% superior sagittal sinus   70%

   ii. _____% left transverse sinus   70%

   iii. _____% multiple sinuses   71%

d. Clinical symptoms associated with   85.7.5
    superior sagittal sinus thrombosis:
    i.   Anterior 1/3 n_____ s_____   no symptoms
    ii. m_____ 1/3 increased muscle   middle
         tone
    iii. p_____ 1/3 cortical blindness or   posterior
         edema/death
e. Jugular bulb thrombosis may produce
    the following symptoms:
    (Hint: bash)
    i.   b_____   breathlessness
    ii. a_____   aphonia
    iii. s_____ d_____   swallowing difficulty
    iv. h_____   hoarseness
f. The best way to diagnose venous sinus   MRI;
    thrombosis is by M_____ or   DSA
    D_____.
g. CT findings: 85.7.6
    i.   May be normal in ___ - ___%.   10-20%
    ii. H_____ sinuses and veins,   Hyperdense;
         dubbed the c_____ sign, is   cord
         pathognomonic.
    iii. Petechial "flame" h_____.   hemorrhages
    iv. Small ventricles in _____%.   50%
    v.   E_____ d_____ sign seen   Empty delta; contrast
         on CT scan with c_____.
    vi. White matter e_____.   edema
    vii. Above findings occur b_____.   bilaterally
h. H_____ is the treatment of choice for   Heparin;   85.7.7
    venous sinus thrombosis, even when   intracerebral hemorrhage
    associated with i_____ h_____.
i. Must not treat with s_____ because   steroids;
    they reduce f_____ and thereby   fibrinolysis;
    increase t_____.   thrombosis
j. Should also correct u_____   underlying abnormality;
    a_____ and control h_____.   hypertension
k. Continue anticoagulation for ___ - ___   3-6 months
    months.
l. If medical management fails, can   decompressive craniectomy,
    perform d_____ c_____,   direct surgical treatment;
    d_____ s_____ t_____, or   endovascular clot retrieval
    e_____ c_____ r_____.
m. Mortality is approximately _____%.   30%
n. Poor prognosticators are e_____   extremes of age, coma, rapid   85.7.8
    o_____ a_____, c_____,   neurological deterioration;
    r_____ n_____ d_____,   deep venous
    and d_____ v_____
    involvement.

■ Moyamoya Disease

8. **Moyamoya disease:**

a. Characterized by p_____ s_____ occlusion of o_____ or usually b_____ ICAs and their major b_____, with secondary formation of collaterals that have a p_____ o_____ s_____ appearance.
progressive spontaneous; one; both; branches; puff of smoke
85.8.1

b. The 2 types are p_____ or s_____.
primary; secondary

c. Primary moyamoya is neither a_____ nor i_____ in origin.
atherosclerotic; inflammatory
85.8.2

d. Can be associated with a_____ in 3 locations (C_____ of W_____, c_____, M_____ v_____), and with increased frequency of v_____ aneurysms.
aneurysms; Circle of Willis, choroidals, Moyamoya vessels; vertebrobasilar

e. 2 age peaks: j_____ or a_____, _____ decades.
juvenile; adult, 3rd/4th decades
85.8.3

f. Presentation in children is with i_____ attacks and in adults with h_____.
ischemic; hemorrhage
85.8.4

g. Prognosis is p_____ with _____% rate of major deficit or death within _____ years of diagnosis.
poor; 73%; 2 years
85.8.5

h. Diagnose with M_____ and D_____.
MRI/A; DSA
85.8.6

i. Medical treatment has n_____ proven benefit.
no

j. Surgical treatment includes d_____ or i_____ revascularization.
direct; indirect
85.8.7

k. The direct revascularization treatment of choice is S_____-M_____ b_____.
STA-MCA bypass

l. Indirect revascularization is reserved for y_____ patients and include EMS (_____), EDAS (_____), and OPT (_____).
younger; encephalomyosynangiosis; encephaloduroarteriosynangiosis; omental pedicle transposition

m. With surgical treatment, the prognosis is g_____ in 58%.
good

n. Guidelines for management of asymptomatic moyamoya have n_____ been established.
not

■ Extracranial-Intracranial (EC/IC) Bypass

9. EC/IC bypass: 85.9.1

a. EC/IC bypass study was published in _____.   1985

b. Study critics highlight study's failure to distinguish between h_____ vs. t_____ causes of stroke.   hemodynamic; thromboembolic

c. Imaging technologies introduced since the study can now identify f_____-d_____ ischemia.   flow-dependent

d. Misery perfusion = o_____ e_____ f_____ increases when a_____ unable to maintain adequate c_____ b_____ f_____ to meet m_____ d_____.   oxygen extraction fraction; autoregulation; cerebral blood flow; metabolic demands

e. Current indications for EC/IC bypass include patients with m_____ p_____, certain a_____, t_____, and m_____ disease.   misery perfusion; aneurysms, tumors; moyamoya

f. Bypass grafts:

  i. Pedicled arterial grafts include: S_____ and o_____ arteries that are considered l_____ flow.   STA; occipital; low

  ii. R_____ artery graft that is m_____ to h_____ flow.   Radial; moderate to high

  iii. S_____ vein graft that is h_____ flow and associated with l_____ graft patency rates.   Saphenous; high; lowest

85

86

Cerebral Arterial Dissections

■ General Information

1. **Key concepts:**   86.1
   a. Hemorrhage between i_____ and   intima;
      m_____ layers of vessel wall.   media
   b. Can present with p_____,   pain, Horner's syndrome,
      H_____, T_____, or   TIA/stroke;
      S_____.   SAH
   c. Causes include s_____, t_____,   spontaneous, trauma;
      or i_____.   iatrogenic
   d. Extracranial dissections usually treated   medically
      m_____.
   e. Intracranial dissections with S_____   SAH;
      are treated with s_____.   surgery

■ Sites of Dissection

2. **Sites of dissection:**   86.5
   a. Most common site is v_____   vertebral artery, 60%
      a_____, _____%.
   b. Basilar/ICA/MCA _____%.   30%
   c. ACA/PCA/PICA _____%.   10%

■ Evaluation

3. **Imaging:**   86.7
   a. CTA may obviate need for D_____.   DSA
   b. D_____ is the definitive diagnostic   DSA
      study.
   c. Pathognomonic sign on DSA is d_____   double lumen sign
      l_____ s_____.
   d. Most helpful MRI sequence is T_____   T1WI with fat suppression
      with f_____ s_____.

■ Overall Outcome

4. Outcomes: 86.8

a. Overall mortality is _____%.   26%

b. _____% have a favorable outcome.   70%

c. Mortality is higher in I_____ lesions   ICA (49%);
(_____%) than in v_____ lesions   vertebral (22%)
(_____%).

■ Vessel Specific Information

5. Complete the following about carotid   86.9.1
dissections:

a. Most commonly caused by t_____.   trauma

b. The most common initial symptom is   ipsilateral headache
i_____ h_____.

c. May also present with H_____   Horner's
syndrome.

6. Complete the following about   86.9.2
vertebral dissections:

a. Most commonly caused by t_____,   trauma;
and so most commonly located within   extracranial
e_____ portion of vertebral artery.

b. Intracranial dissection can present with   SAH
S_____.

c. Treatment is generally medical with   anticoagulation
a_____.

d. A_____ are equally effective.   Antiplatelets

e. E_____ or s_____ treatment is   Endovascular; surgical;
recommended for i_____   intracranial
dissections.

f. Endovascular treatment is indicated   medical therapy;
when m_____ t_____ is   contraindicated;
ineffective, medical therapy is   symptomatic flow-limiting
c_____, or when there is s_____   stenosis
f_____-l_____ s_____.

86

87

Intracerebral Hemorrhage

■ Intracerebral Hemorrhage in Adults

1. **Intracerebral hemorrhage key concepts:**   87.2
   a. Accounts for ___ - ___% of strokes.   15-30%
   b. Presentation differs from ischemic infarct because it includes h_____, v_____, and a_____.   headache, vomiting; altered consciousness
   c. Hematoma v_____ correlates with morbidity and mortality.   volume
   d. Hematoma enlarges in at least _____% of cases within first _____ hours of onset.   33%; 3
   e. Angiography is recommended except in patients older than _____ years old with preexisting h_____ and hematoma in t_____, p_____, or p_____ f_____.   45; hypertension; thalamus, putamen; posterior fossa

---

■ Epidemiology

2. **Risk factors:**   87.3.2
   a. Incidence increases significantly after age _____ and d_____ with each decade of age until age 80.   55; doubles
   b. Preventable risk factors include a_____ c_____, c_____, d_____.   alcohol consumption, cigarettes, drugs

■ Locations of Hemorrhage within the Brain

3. **Locations of intracerebral hemorrhage:**

   a. Hypertensive hemorrhage sites of predilection are: 87.4.1

      i.   b_____ g_____; ; basal ganglia; 50%
           _____%

      ii. t_____; _____%   thalamus; 15%

      iii. p_____; ___ - ___%   pons; 10-15%

      iv. c_____; _____%   cerebellum; 10%

      v.   c_____ w_____   cerebral white matter; 10-
           m_____; ___ - ___%   20%

      vi. b_____; ___ - ___%   brainstem; 1-6%

   b. Most common location for deep   putamen; lenticulostriate
      hematoma is p_____ and is due to   arteries
      rupture of l_____ a_____.

   c. Incidence of lobar hemorrhages is ___ -   10-30%   87.4.2
      ___%

   d. Compared with deep hemorrhages,   better
      lobar hemorrhages have a b_____
      prognosis.

87

■ Etiologies

4. **List the causes of lobar hemorrhage:**   87.5.2
   (Hint: teach it)

   a. t_____   tumor

   b. e_____ of d_____ l_____   extension of deep ICH

   c. a_____ a_____   amyloid angiopathy

   d. c_____ m_____   cerebrovascular
                                          malformation

   e. h_____ c_____   hemorrhagic conversion

   f. i_____   idiopathic

   g. t_____   trauma

5. **Hemorrhagic transformation of an ischemic infarct:**   87.5.2

   a. Estimated to occur in _____%   43%

   b. within the first m_____   month

   c. and may occur within _____ hours.   24

6. **Coagulation disorders and intracerebral hemorrhage:**   87.5.2

   a. Incidence of symptomatic ICH within 36   2-4%
      hours of treatment with rtPA is ___ -
      ___%.

   b. Aspirin is associated with increased risk   less than 1%
      of ICH at a rate of l_____ than
      _____% per year.

7. Infection and intracerebral hemorrhage: 87.5.2

a. 3 types of infection that predispose to ICH:

   i.   f_____   fungal
   ii. g_____   granulomas
   iii. h_____ s_____   herpes simplex

8. Hypertension and intracerebral hemorrhage:

a. Hypertension is a risk factor for   pons; cerebellum   87.5.4
   hemorrhage in what 2 locations?

b. It is not a risk factor for at least   35%
   _____% of basal ganglia
   hemorrhages.

c. C_____-B_____ a_____   Charcot-Bouchard aneurysms   87.5.5
   are the source of some hypertensive
   hemorrhages.

9. Amyloid angiopathy: 87.5.6

a. Present in _____% of patients over 50%;
   _____ years old, but most do not   70;
   h_____.   hemorrhage

b. Accounts for _____% of ICH cases.   10%

c. Should be suspected in patients with   recurrent;
   r_____ hemorrhages in the   lobar
   l_____ location.

d. Associated with deposition of b_____ beta amyloid;
   a_____ that appears on polarized   birefringent apple green
   light as b_____ a_____ g_____.

e. Genetic link is a_____ E.   Apolipoprotein E

f. Is not associated with s_____   systemic amyloidosis
   a_____.

10. Hemorrhagic brain tumors: 87.5.7

a. Primary brain tumors associated with   glioblastoma multiforme;
   ICH include g_____ m_____ and   lymphoma
   l_____.

b. Metastatic tumors associated with ICH   lung, choriocarcinoma,
   include l_____, c_____,   melanoma;
   m_____, and r_____ c_____.   renal cell

11. Anticoagulation and intracerebral hemorrhage: 87.5.8

a. Incidence of bleeding complications in   10%
   patients on anticoagulation is
   _____% per year.

b. Incidence of intracerebral hemorrhage is 0.3-1.8%
   ___ - ___% per year.

c. Mortality in the intracerebral   65%
   hemorrhage group is _____%.

87

■ Clinical

12. **Clinical presentation of intracerebral hemorrhage:**
    a. Unlike embolic/ischemic stroke, the neurological deficit with ICH has p_____ onset over m_____ to h_____.
       progressive; minutes; hours   87.6.1

    b. Thalamic ICH is usually associated with h_____ loss, m_____ loss if i_____ c_____ is compressed, and e_____ signs with upper b_____ extension.
       hemisensory; motor; internal capsule; eye; brainstem   87.6.3

    c. Thalamic ICH >_____ cm has high mortality.
       3.3

    d. Cerebellar ICH produces c_____ before h_____ due to b_____ compression.
       coma; hemiparesis; brainstem

13. **Rebleeding:**   87.6.4
    a. Rebleeding is more common with b_____ g_____ ICH than l_____ ICH.
       basal ganglia; lobar

    b. Incidence d_____ with time.
       decreases

    c. ___ - ___% in first 1-3 hours.
       33-38%

    d. _____% in 3-6 hours.
       16%

    e. S_____ sign on CTA correlated with increased risk of ICH expansion.
       Spot

    f. Incidence of late rebleeding is ___ - ___%.
       1.8-5.3%

14. **Edema and intracerebral hemorrhage:**   87.6.4
    a. Edema can cause delayed d_____ after ICH.
       deterioration

    b. The component that is released by clot and presumed to be the most likely cause of surrounding delayed edema is t_____.
       thrombinin

■ Evaluation

15. **Evaluation of intracerebral hemorrhage:**
    a. ICH volume is approximated by the e_____ method.
       ellipsoid   87.7.1

    b. Formula is _____.
       (AP x LAT x HT)/2

    c. On average, clot size decreases _____mm/day
       0.75

    d. Density decreases _____ Hounsfield units/day
       2

87

e. With l_____ change for the first   little;
    _____ weeks.   2

f. List the sequence of hemoglobin   Table 87.4
    evolution after ICH: (Hint: On days my
    mom's home)
    i.   o_____ 0 to 1 day   oxyhemoglobin
    ii.   d_____ 1 to 3 days   deoxyhemoglobin
    iii. m_____ 3 to 7 days   methemoglobin
    iv.   m_____ 7 to 14 days   methemoglobin
    v.   h_____ 14 plus days   hemosiderin

16. **ICH score:**
a. Give the number of points for the   Table 87.5
    following factors:
    i.   GCS 3-4: _____ points   2
    ii.   GCS 5-12: _____ points   1
    iii. GCS 13-15: _____ points   0
    iv.   Age > 80: _____ points   1
    v.   Age < 80: _____ points   0
    vi.   Infratentorial location: _____   1
          points
    vii. Supratentorial location: _____   0
          points
    viii. Volume > 30 cc: _____ points   1
    ix.   Volume < 30 cc: _____ points   0
    x.   IVH present: _____ points   1

b. Give the 30-day mortality based on ICH   Table 87.6
    score:
    i.   0 points _____%   0%
    ii.   1 points _____%   13%
    iii. 2 points _____%   26%
    iv.   3 points _____%   72%
    v.   4 points _____%   97%
    vi.   5 points _____%   100%
    vii. 6 points _____%   100%

■ Initial Management of ICH

17. **Medical management:**
a. Reduce MAP to pre-morbid level if   20%   87.8.1
    known or by _____% if unknown.
b. Suggested target BP is _____.   140/90   87.8.2
c. Platelet goal is >_____.   100K
d. Most studies suggest that resumption of   safe   87.8.4
    anticoagulation after ICH is s_____.
e. Probability of ischemic stroke 30 days
    following cessation of warfarin for 10
    days:
    i.   _____% for those treated for   2.9%
          prosthetic heart valve
    ii.   _____% for AFibb   2.6%
    iii. _____% for cardioembolic   4.8%
          stroke

87

■ Surgical Treatment

18. Surgical management: 87.9.2
a. Indications for surgery:
   i. ICH with significant m_____   mass effect
      e_____
   ii. ICH with s_____   symptoms
   iii. ICH volume _____   10-30 cc
   iv. l_____ and c_____   lobar, cerebellar
      locations
   v. y_____ age   young
b. Surgery is recommended for cerebellar ICH if GCS is _____, size is _____ and h_____ present.   13 or less; 4 cm or more, hydrocephalus

■ ICH in Young Adults

19. Name the top 5 causes of nontraumatic ICH in young adults (other than "undetermined" which accounts for ~1/4):   Table 87.7
Hint: AHadt
a. A_____, _____%   AVM, 30%
b. H_____, _____%   HTN, 15%
c. a_____, _____%   aneurysm, 10%
d. d_____, _____%   drugs, 7%
e. t_____, _____%   tumor, 4%

87

■ Intracerebral Hemorrhage in the Newborn

20. ICH in the newborn:
a. G_____ m_____ progressively i_____ until _____ weeks gestational age.   Germinal matrix; involutes; 36   87.12.2
b. Matrix may persist in p_____ infants and cause hemorrhage.   premature
c. Site of hemorrhage depends on a_____.   age
d. Between 24-28 weeks, ICH located in b_____ of c_____.   body of caudate
e. 29 weeks or more, ICH located in h_____ of c_____.   head of caudate   87.12.4
f. List the risk factors: (Hint: vespacc)
   i. v_____ e_____   volume expansion
   ii. E_____   ECMO
   iii. s_____   seizures
   iv. p_____   pneumothorax
   v. a_____   asphyxia
   vi. c_____ h_____ d_____   cyanotic heart disease
   vii. c_____ a_____ by m_____   cocaine abuse by mother

g. Grading system of P_____.   Papile   Table 87.8
    i.   Grade I = s_____.   subependymal
    ii. Grade II = I_____ without   IVH; ventricle dilation
         v_____ d_____.
    iii. Grade III = I_____ with v_____   IVH; ventricle dilation
         d_____.
    iv. Grade IV = I_____ with p_____   IVH; parenchymal ICH
         I_____.

h. Hydrocephalus develops in ___ - ___%   20-50%;   87.12.7
    about ___ - ___ weeks after ICH.   1-3 weeks

i. Diagnosed using u_____ imaging.   ultrasound   87.12.9

j. Medical treatments are n_____   not   87.12.10
    effective.

k. Surgical options include serial   lumbar puncture, ventricular
    l_____ p_____, v_____   tap, temporary ventricular
    t_____, t_____ v_____   access device, shunt
    a_____ d_____, s_____.

l. Prerequisites before shunt insertion   2000 grams or more;
    include infant weight of _____ and   less than 100 mg/dl
    CSF protein of _____.

m. Outcomes:
    i.   Mortality ___ - ___% with severe   50-65%   Table 87.9
         ICH.
    ii. Hydrocephalus ___ - ___% with   65-100%
         severe ICH.
    iii. _____% ambulatory with grade   100%   87.12.11
         II ICH.
    iv. _____% IQ normal range with   75%
         grade II ICH.

87

88

Outcome Assessment

■ Cancer. Head Injury. Cerebrovascular Events. Spinal Cord Injury

1. **Matching. Match the following outcome scores with the condition they are designed to assess.**
   Outcome scores: ① Karnofsky; ② Rancho Los Amigos; ③ Glasgow Outcome; ④ Modified Rankin; ⑤ Barthel; ⑥ Functional Independence Measure; ⑦ WHO performance score

a.	cerebrovascular	④, ⑤	88.3.1
b.	spinal cord	⑥	88.4
c.	cancer	①, ⑦	88.1
d.	head injury	②, ③	88.2

2. **True or False. A higher number indicates better function.**

a.	Karnofsky scale	true	88.1
b.	WHO Performance Scale	false	
c.	Rancho Los Amigos scale	true	88.2
d.	Glasgow Outcome scale	true	
e.	Modified Rankin scale	false	88.3
f.	Barthel scale	true	
g.	Functional Independence Measure	true	88.4

3. **On the Karnofsky scale, which score represents the transition from being able to engage in normal activity to only caring for self?**

   a. 80%
   b. 85%
   c. 75%
   d. 70%

   d. 70%. *Table 88.1*
   There are no 75 or 85 scores. 70 cares for self, unable to carry on normal activity or work; 50 requires considerable care; and 40 is disabled.

89

Differential Diagnosis by Location or Radiographic Finding – Intracranial

■ Posterior Fossa Lesions

1. **If a solitary intraparenchymal lesion in the p-fossa in an adult is seen, a m_____ must be ruled out.**
   metastasis (from an extracranial primary malignancy) — 89.2.1

2. **The most common primary intra-axial p-fossa tumor in adults is h_____.**
   hemangioblastoma — 89.2.1

3. **Complete the following about hemangioblastomas:** — 89.2.1
   a. Account for ___-___% of p-fossa tumors. 7-12%
   b. Usually see s_____ v_____ on MRI. signal voids (serpentine appearance)

4. **Besides embolism and thrombosis of a plaque, 2 other etiologies for a cerebellar stroke are:** — 89.2.1
   a. v_____ a_____ vertebral artery dissection
      d_____
   b. v_____ h_____ vertebrobasilar hypoplasia

5. **Multiple lesions in the cerebellum can be suggestive of:** — 89.2.1
   a. m_____ metastases
   b. h_____ associated with hemangioblastomas; VHL
      V____
   c. a_____ abscesses
   d. c_____ m_____ cavernous malformations

6. **As a group, a_____ are the most common pediatric brain tumors in the p-fossa.**
   astrocytomas — 89.2.1

7. **The following 3 types of tumors account for the majority of infratentorial tumors in patients less than 18 years of age:**   89.2.1
   a. P_____ including m_____: ___% (of infratentorial tumors)   PNET; medulloblastoma: 27%
   b. a_____ including p_____ a_____: ___%   astrocytomas; pilocytic astrocytoma: 27%
   c. b_____ g_____: ___%   brainstem gliomas: 28%

8. **The following facts help differentiate medulloblastomas and ependymomas:**   89.2.1
   a. "Banana sign" is seen with _____.   medulloblastoma
   b. Grow from anterior aspect of 4th ventricle _____.   medulloblastoma
   c. Tend to grow from floor of 4th ventricle.   ependymomas
   d. Tend to be inhomogeneous on T1WI MRI.   ependymomas
   e. Calcification is common.   ependymomas

9. **Complete the following about CPA lesions:**   89.2.2
   a. Acoustic neuromas are more accurately known as v_____ s_____ and occur in ___ to ___% of CPA lesions.   vestibular schwannomas; 80-90%
   b. Meningioma occurs in ___ to ___% of CPA lesions.   5-10%
   c. Epidermoid occurs in ___ to ___% of CPA lesions.   5-7%

89

10. **Match the tumor with the characteristic finding:**   89.2.2
    ① vestibular schwannoma;
    ② meningioma
    Characteristic: (a-f) below
    a. Hearing loss occurs early.   ①
    b. Facial weakness occurs early.   ②
    c. Internal auditory canal is enlarged.   ①
    d. Calcifications seen more commonly.   ②
    e. Represents 90% of CPA tumors.   ①
    f. Homogeneous signal and enhancement.   ②

11. **Match the cystic lesions of the CPA which its characteristic findings:**   89.2.2
    ① arachnoid cyst; ② epidermoid cyst; ③ dermoid cyst; ④ cholesterol granuloma
    Characteristic: (a-d) below
    a. High signal on T1WI and high signal on T2WI and associated with bone destruction.   ④
    b. Cystic component has same intensity as CSF.   ①

    c.   High signal on DWMRI differentiates this ②
from arachnoid cyst.

    d.   T1WI intensity similar to fat and usually ③
midline.

12. **What are some differentiating**   89.2.2
features that distinguish neuromas of
the V, VII, and VIII cranial nerves?

    a.   Neuromas of CN ___ can pass through   CN VIII
the tentorial hiatus medially.

    b.   Neuromas of CN ___ can cross into the   CN V
middle fossa via the petrous apex.

    c.   Neuromas of CN ___ can cross the   CN VII
midpetrosal bone.

13. **Complete the following about**   89.2.4
foramen magnum lesions:

    a.   Most are _____ (extra-axial vs.   extra-axial
intra-axial.)

    b.   A mass behind the dens compressing the chordoma
spinal cord is a c_____ until proven
otherwise.

    c.   The second most common site of origin   anterior lip
of posterior fossa meningiomas is the
a_____ l___ of the foramen magnum

    d.   C_____ p_____ is usually an   Craniocervical pain
early symptoms of lesions in this
location.

89

■ Multiple Intracranial Lesions on CT or MRI

14. **Infectious causes of multiple**   89.3
intracranial lesions on imaging
include:

    a.   t_____   toxoplasmosis

    b.   fungal etiologies including:

        i.   a_____   aspergillosis

        ii.   c_____   coccidiomycosis

        iii. c_____   cryptococcus

        iv. c_____   candidiasis

    c.   Parasitic etiologies including:

        i.   e_____   echinococcus

        ii.   s_____   schistosomiasis

        iii. p_____   paragonimiasis

15. **Complete the following about**   89.3
multiple intracranial lesions on
imaging:

    a.   What percentage of gliomas are   6%
multicentric?

    b.   HSV usually occurs in the t_____ temporal
lobe.

    c.   MS lesions are located in the   periventricular
p_____ area.

d. Dural sinus thrombosis can cause multiple v_____ i_____   venous infarcts

e. Multiple "hypertensive" hemorrhages is likely due to a_____ a_____   amyloid angiopathy

■ Ring-Enhancing Lesions on CT/MRI

16. **What are the classic etiologies for ring-enhancing lesions on imaging?** (hint: MAGIC DR. L)   89.4.3

   a. M_____   Metastases
   b. A_____   Abscess
   c. G_____   GBM
   d. I_____   Infarction
   e. C_____   Contusion
   f. D_____   Demyelination
   g. R_____   Radiation
   h. L_____   Lymphoma (primary vs. metastatic)

■ White Matter Lesions

17. **List conditions that can affect the corpus callosum:**   89.5.2

   a. m_____ _____   multiple sclerosis
   b. G_____   GBM
   c. l_____   lymphoma
   d. l_____   lipoma
   e. d_____ a_____ i_____   diffuse axonal injury

89

■ Sellar, Suprasellar and Parasellar Lesions

18. **The most common enhancing pituitary lesion in adults is a p_____ a_____.**   pituitary adenoma   89.6.1

19. **The most common sellar and parasellar lesions in children are c_____ and g_____.**   craniopharyngiomas and germinomas   89.6.1

20. **Regarding pituitary tumors.**   89.6.2

   a. Adenohypophyseal tumors include pituitary a_____ and c_____.   adenomas, carcinomas

   b. Neurohypophyseal tumors include m_____, p_____, and a_____   metastases, pituicytomas, and astrocytomas

   c. What is the most common tumor found in the posterior pituitary?   metastases (most common primaries are lung and breast)

21. The pituitary gland can normally be slightly enlarged in w_____ of c_____ age.

women of childbearing age

89.6.2

22. Complete the following about pituitary hyperplasia:

89.6.2

a. Thyrotroph hyperplasia is most likely due to _____ _____.

primary hypothyroidism

b. Gonadotroph hyperplasia is most likely due to _____ _____.

primary hypogonadism

c. Somatotroph hyperplasia is most likely due to _____ ___-___ _____.

ectopic GH-RH secretion

d. Lactotroph hyperplasia is most likely due to _____.

pregnancy

23. Suprasellar germ cell tumors are:

89.6.2

a. more common in _____ (men vs. women)

women (pineal region more common in men)

b. triad of d_____ i_____, p_____, and v_____ d_____

diabetes insipidus, panhypopituitarism; visual deficits

24. Complete the following about juxtasellar masses:

89.6.2

a. Craniopharyngiomas account for ___% of tumors in this region in adults and ___% in children.

20%; 54%

b. To differentiate meningiomas from pituitary adenomas, use g_____.

gadolinium

c. On imaging, meningiomas demonstrate:

i. Enhancement?

bright homogenous enhancement

ii. Epicenter is s_____.

suprasellar

iii. May see d_____ t_____.

dural tail

iv. Is sellar enlarged or not enlarged?

Usually not enlarged

v. Tend to encase _____ _____.

carotid arteries

25. Pituitary hypophysitis and adenomas can be distinguished by the following: (hypophysitis vs. adenoma)

a. Symmetric enlargement is most often seen with _____.

hypophysitis

Table 89.2

b. Sellar floor may be eroded with _____.

adenoma

c. Enhancement more intense with _____.

hypophysitis

d. Pituitary stalk thickened with _____.

hypophysitis

e. Associated with pregnancy

hypophysitis

89.6.4

26. True or False regarding lymphocytic hypophysitis:

89.6.6

a. May cause hypopituitarism.

true

b. Most cases are seen in men.

false - in women in late pregnancy or early post-partum period

c. Requires surgery for treatment.

false - treatment with steroids

d. May produce diabetes insipidus.

true

■ Intracranial Cysts

27. **Complete the following about arachnoid cyst:**   89.7.1
    a. aka l_____ c_____   leptomeningeal cyst
    b. Due to a d_____ of the a_____.   duplication; arachnoid
    c. Reach maximum size in __ month(s).   1 month
    d. Need surgery in about ___% of cases.   30%

28. **Complete the following about cavum septum pellucidum:**
    a. Present in all p_____ b_____   premature babies;   Table 89.3
       and 97% of n_____.   newborns
    b. Present in ___% of adults.   10%
    c. What is it?   Variable slit-like fluid-filled   89.7.3
                                                space between the leaflets of
                                                the left and right septum
                                                pellucidum.
    d. Seen in _____ suffering from   boxers;
       c_____ t_____   chronic traumatic
       e_____   encephalopathy

29. **Cavum vergae is located posterior to**   cavum septum pellucidum   Table 89.3
    and communicates with c_____   (CSP)
    s_____ p_____.

30. **Complete the following about cavum**   Table 89.3
    velum interpositum:
    a. Due to separation of the c_____ of the crura;
       f_____   fornix
    b. between the t_____ and the   thalami;
       t_____ v_____.   third ventricle
    c. Present in ___% of children less than 1 60%
       year of age.
    d. Present in ____% of children between   30%
       1 and 10 years old

89

■ Orbital Lesions

31. **The most common benign primary**   cavernous hemangioma;   89.8.2
    intraorbital neoplasm is   melanoma
    c_____ h_____. The most
    common primary intraocular
    malignancy in adults is m_____.

32. **Complete the following about orbital**   89.8.3
    and ocular lesions:
    a. The most common orbital lesion in   dermoid cyst
       children is a d_____ c_____
    b. The most common malignant tumor of   rhabdomyosarcoma
       the orbit in this age group is
       r_____.
    c. The most common primary intraocular   retinoblastoma
       malignancy in children is r_____.

33. **Match the orbital lesions with their characteristics. (multiple answers may be correct for a given characteristic)**
    ① capillary hemangioma;
    ② lymphangioma; ③ lymphoma;
    ④ thyroid ophthalmoplegia
    Characteristic: (a-e) below

    89.8.2

    a. infantile proptosis   ①, ②
    b. regress spontaneously   ①
    c. do not regress   ②
    d. painless proptosis   ③, ④
    e. bilateral 80% of the time   ④

■ Skull Lesions

34. **Complete the following about skull lesions:**

    89.10.1

    a. The most common benign tumors of the skull are o_____ and h_____.   osteomas, hemangiomas
    b. The most common malignancy of the skull is o_____ s_____.   osteogenic sarcoma

35. **Complete the following about characteristics of skull lesions:**

    89.10.1

    a. Multiplicity suggests m_____.   malignancy
    b. Expansion of diploe suggests a b_____ lesion.   benign
    c. Peripheral sclerosis suggests a b_____ lesion.   benign
    d. Full-thickness lesions suggest m_____.   malignancy
    e. Multiple sharply demarcated and punched-out defects suggest m_____ m_____.   multiple myeloma
    f. Presence of peripheral vascular channels is highly suggestive of _____ lesions.   benign

36. **Complete the following:**

    89.10.1

    a. Which skull lesion demonstrates a
       i.   trabecular pattern?   hemangioma
       ii. sunburst pattern?   hemangioma
       iii. islands of bone pattern?   fibrous dysplasia
       iv. tenderness to palpation?   Langerhans cell histiocytosis lesion
    b. Eosinophilic granuloma is the mildest form of L_____ c_____ h_____.   Langerhans cell histiocytosis

37. **The following can cause diffuse demineralization or destruction of the skull:**

    89.10.3

    a. h_____   hyperparathyroidism
    b. m_____   metastases
    c. m_____ m_____   multiple myeloma
    d. o_____   osteoporosis

38. The following can cause diffuse or generalized increased skull density: 89.10.5

a. a_____   anemia
b. f_____ d_____   fibrous dysplasia
c. h_____ i_____   hyperostosis interna
   g_____   generalisata
d. o_____ m_____   osteoblastic metastases
                                              (prostate and breast)
e. P_____ d_____   Paget's disease

39. A pneumocele is an enlargement of an   air sinus; has; air sinus; does   89.10.9
a____ s_____ that _____ (has   not have
vs. does not have) bone erosion.
Pneumosinus dilatans is an
enlargement of an a___ s_____
that _____ (has vs. does not have)
bone erosion.

■ Combined Intracranial/Extracranial Lesions

40. Can intra-axial lesions grow out of the   Typically, no. However, a   89.11
skull?   fungating malignant glioma
                                              may do this.

■ Intracranial Hyperdensities

41. What can cause an intra-axial   89.12
structure to appear hyperdense with
respect to normal brain tissue on a
non-contrast CT?

a. a_____ b_____   acute blood
b. c_____   calcium
c. l___ f_____ v_____   low flow vessels
d. m_____   melanoma (melanin can
                                              appear hyperdense)

■ Intracranial Calcifications

42. The following are physiologic causes   89.13.1
of localized intracranial calcifications:

a. c_____ p_____   choroid plexus
b. a_____ g_____   arachnoid granulation
c. d_____ s_____   diaphragma sellae
d. d_____   dura
e. p_____ g_____   pineal gland

43. Choroid plexus calcifications have the   89.13.2
following features:

a. ___% of patients by 5th decade of life   75%
demonstrate calcifications.
b. Calcifications are rare under age ___.   age 3

89

c. If calcifications present under age 10,   choroid plexus papilloma
    consider c_____ p_____
    p_____.
d. If calcified, choroid plexus in the   neurofibromatosis
    temporal horn, then consider
    n_____.

44. **Complete the following about basal**   89.13.2
    ganglia calcifications:
a. Common in e_____   elderly
b. Causes include:
    i.   h_____   hyperparathyroidism
    ii. a_____ use   anticonvulsant use
    iii. F_____ disease   Fahr's disease
c. Correlated with psychiatric diseases if >   0.5 cm
    ____ cm.

45. **Fahr's disease involves progressive**   calcification;   89.13.2
    idiopathic c_____ of the   basal ganglia (medial
    b_____ g_____, s_____   portions), sulcal depths;
    d_____ of cerebral cortex, and   dentate nuclei
    d_____ n_____.

■ Intraventricular Lesions

46. **Complete the following about**   89.14.2
    intraventricular lesions:
a. What is the most common lesion?   astrocytoma
b. Lesion at the foramen of Monro?   colloid cyst
c. 3rd ventricle lesion with punctate   craniopharyngioma
    calcifications?
d. Fills the 4th ventricle with "banana   medulloblastoma
    sign"?
e. Most common low density 4th ventricle   epidermoid
    lesion?
f. Free-floating fat in ventricles?   dermoid with cyst rupture
g. Has fat and calcifications?   teratoma
h. At the septum pellucidum?   central neurocytoma
i. Densely enhancing with calcifications?   meningioma

47. **Intraventricular meningiomas are:**   89.14.2
a. Usually arterial supply from a_____   anterior choroidal artery
    c_____ artery
b. Less common arterial supply from   medial posterior choroidal
    m_____ p_____   artery, lateral posterior
    c_____ artery and l_____   choroidal artery
    p_____ c_____ artery.
c. Tumor thought to arise from   arachnoid cap cells
    _____ _____ cells.

89

48. **Match the tumor that is found most often in the following ventricles:**
    ① astrocytoma; ② medulloblastoma;
    ③ meningioma; ④ ependymoma;
    ⑤ colloid cyst; ⑥ epidermoid;
    ⑦ dermoid; ⑧ teratoma
    Ventricle: (a-e) below

    Table 89.4

   a. 3rd ventricle   ⑤
   b. 4th ventricle   ②
   c. atrium of lateral ventricle   ③
   d. frontal horn of lateral ventricle   ①
   e. body of lateral ventricle   ④

49. **The following are lesions that can be found in the posterior of the 3rd ventricle:**

    89.14.3

   a. p_____   pinealoma
   b. m_____   meningioma
   c. a_____ c_____   arachnoid cyst
   d. a_____ of v_____ of G_____   aneurysm of vein of Galen

50. **Which masses within the lateral ventricles do not enhance?**

    89.14.3

   a. c_____   cysts
   b. d_____   dermoids
   c. e_____   epidermoids
   d. s_____   subependymomas

■ Periventricular Lesions

89

51. **What is the differential for a periventricular solid enhancing lesion?**

    89.15.1

   a. l_____   lymphoma
   b. e_____   ependymoma
   c. m_____   metastases
   d. m_____ in child   medulloblastoma
   e. p_____ t_____ pineal tumor
   f. G_____   GBM

52. **What are some etiologies of low-density periventricular lesions?**

    89.15.2

   a. t_____ e_____   transependymal edema
   b. m_____ s_____   multiple sclerosis
   c. s_____ a_____   subacute arteriosclerotic
      e_____   encephalopathy (aka
                               Binswanger's disease)
   d. l_____   leukoaraiosis

■ Ependymal and Subependymal Enhancement

53. **What is the differential for ependymal**   89.17
   and subependymal enhancement?
   (Hint: some overlap with periventricular
   lesions)
   a.   v_____   ventriculitis
   b.   c_____ m_____   carcinomatous meningitis
                                     (would see meningeal
                                     enhancement as well)
   c.   m_____ s_____   multiple sclerosis
   d.   t_____ s_____   tuberous sclerosis
                                     (supependymal hamartomas)

54. **In immunocompromised patients,**   89.17
   what do the following patterns
   suggest?
   a.   thin linear enhancement   viral infection (CMV, varicella-
                                     zoster)
   b.   nodular enhancement   CNS lymphoma

■ Intraventricular Hemorrhage

55. **Complete the following about**   89.18
   intraventricular hemorrhage:
   a.   Most occur as a result of   extension of
        _____ of _____ intraparenchymal
        _____.   hemorrhage
        i.   In the adult, this may originate in   thalamus, putamen
             the t_____ or p_____.
        ii. In a newborn, this may originate in   subependymal region
             the s_____.
   b.   Aneurysms account for about ___% of   25%
        IVH in adults.
   c.   What are the typical locations of an   a-comm, distal basilar artery,
        involved aneurysm?   carotid terminus, vertebral
                                     artery, distal PICA

■ Medial Temporal Lobe Lesions

56. **The most common medial temporal**   89.19
   lobe lesions are:
   a.   h_____   hamartoma
   b.   m_____ t_____   mesial temporal sclerosis
        s_____
   c.   g_____   glioma

89

■ Intranasal/Intracranial Lesions

57. **Complete the following about**   89.22
    intranasal/intracranial lesions:

    a. M_____ is a fungal infection   Mucormycosis
        seen primarily in diabetics or
        immunocompromised patients.

    b. Nasopharyngeal carcinomas are   EBV
        associated with _____ infection.

    c. A s_____ u_____   sinonasal undifferentiated
        c_____ (aka _____) is an   carcinoma; SNUC
        aggressive carcinoma that may invade
        into the frontal fossa and cavernous
        sinus.

    d. E_____ arises from crest   Esthesioneuroblastoma;
        cells of the nasal vault and often   epistaxis;
        demonstrates intracranial invasion.   nasal obstruction
        Typically presents with e_____ or
        n_____ o_____.

    e. A nasal polypoid mass in a newborn   encephalocele;
        should be considered an   pulsatile;
        e_____ until proven   swells
        otherwise. It can be distinguished by a
        nasal glioma because it is often
        p_____ and s_____ with the
        Valsalva maneuver.

89

90

Differential Diagnosis by Location or Radiographic Finding – Spine

■ Atlantoaxial Subluxation

1. **What are the disease processes causing atlantoaxial subluxation?**   90.2
   a. incompetence of the _____ _____ ligament | transverse atlantal ligament
      i.   r_____ a_____ | rheumatoid arthritis
      ii. t_____ | trauma
      iii. c_____ l_____ | congenital laxity (esp. with Down syndrome)
      iv. chronic _____ use | steroid
      v.   chronic _____ infections | retropharyngeal
   b. incompetence of the _____ _____ | odontoid process
      i.   f_____ | fracture
      ii.   o_ o_____ | os odontoideum
      iii. r_____ a_____ | rheumatoid arthritis
      iv.   erosion by t_____ | tumor
      v.   M_____ syndrome | Morquio syndrome (hypoplasia of dens)
      vi.   c_____ d_____ | congenital dysplasia
      vii. i_____ | infection

2. **Complete the following about atlantoaxial subluxation:**   90.2
   a. Incompetence of the _____ _____ ligament | transverse atlantal
   b. results in increased _____ interval. | atlantodental

3. **Complete the following regarding differential diagnosis by location:**   90.2
   a. Morquio syndrome is hypoplasia of the _____ | dens
   b. due to a m_____. | mucopolysaccharidosis
   c. It may result in _____ subluxation. | atlantoaxial

■ Abnormalities in Vertebral Bodies

4. **What are 8 malignancies that have a tendency to metastasize to the vertebral bodies?**

   prostate, breast, lung, renal cell, thyroid, lymphoma, melanoma, and multiple myeloma

   90.3

5. **General differential for vertebral body lesions:**

   90.3

   a. n_____   neoplasm (metastatic vs. primary)

   b. i_____   infection (osteomyelitis vs. discitis)

   c. f_____ i_____   fatty infiltration

   d. d_____ changes   degenerative changes

   e. m_____ diseases including P_____ disease, o_____, and a_____ s_____   metabolic; Paget's disease, osteoporosis, ankylosing spondylitis

■ Pathologic Fractures of the Spine

6. **What are the 6 criteria for vertebra plana? What are 3 etiologies that may lead to this phenomenon?**

   90.5.3

   a. Criteria:

   1. uniform collapse of vertebral body into flat thin disc
   2. increased density of vertebra
   3. spares neural arches
   4. normal disc and intervertebral disc space
   5. intervertebral vacuum cleft sign (pathognomonic)
   6. no kyphosis

   b. Etiologies:

   1. Langerhans cell histiocytosis
   2. Calve-Kummel-Verneuil disease (avascular necrosis of the vertebral body)
   3. hemangioma

90

■ Destructive Lesions of the Spine

7. **If vertebral body destruction is associated with destruction of the disc space, what general etiology is this suggestive of?**

   infection (often involves at least two adjacent vertebral levels)

   90.7.2

■ Vertebral Hyperostosis

8. **What is the differential diagnosis of vertebral body hyperostosis?**   90.8

   a. P_____ _____   Paget's disease

   b. m_____ including l_____   Metastases (osteoblastic);
       as well as p_____ c_____ in men   lymphoma; prostate cancer;
       and b_____ c_____ in women   breast cancer

■ Sacral Lesions

9. **Complete the following about sacral agenesis:**   90.9

   a. Sacral agenesis is also known as _____   caudal regression syndrome
       _____ _____.

   b. __-__% have _____ mothers.   16-20%, diabetic mothers

   c. Increased incidence of _____   spinal
       abnormalities.

■ Enhancing Nerve Roots

10. **What is the differential for an enhancing nerve root?**   90.10

   a. t_____ such as m_____   tumor; meningeal
       c_____ or l_____   carcinomatosis; lymphoma

   b. i_____ especially if patient has   infection; AIDS (consider
       _____   CMV)

   c. i_____ including _____-   inflammatory; Guillain-Barré,
       _____ or _____   sarcoidosis

90

■ Intraspinal Cysts

11. **What is the differential for an intraspinal cyst?**   90.12

   a. s_____ m_____ c_____   spinal meningeal cysts
   b. c_____ n_____   cystic neurofibroma
   c. e_____   ependymoma
   d. s_____   syringomyelia
   e. dilated c_____ c_____   dilated central canal

91

Differential Diagnosis (DDx) by Signs and Symptoms – Primarily Intracranial

■ Syncope and Apoplexy

1. **Complete the following about the causes of syncope:**
   a. Prevalence of syncope is about ___% and is higher in the e_____.
      50%; elderly   91.3.1
   b. In about ___% of cases, no cause can be diagnosed.
      40%   91.3.2
   c. Cerebrovascular causes include:
     i. s_____   subarachnoid hemorrhage (most commonly aneurysmal)
        h_____
     ii. b_____ infarction   brainstem infarction
     iii. v_____   vertebrobasilar insufficiency
        i_____
     iv. p_____ a_____   pituitary apoplexy
   d. Disorder of AV node conduction leading to syncope with bradycardia is called _____.
      Stokes-Adams syndrome
   e. Syncope while wearing a tight collar or while shaving may be due to _____ _____ _____.
      carotid sinus syncope
   f. Micturition or cough causing syncope is called t_____ syncope and is usually associated with elevation in i_____ pressure.
      triggered; intrathoracic
   g. Orthostatic hypotension is defined as a drop in systolic BP of at least _____ mm Hg or diastolic BP of at least _____ mm Hg on standing.
      20; 10

2. **When are neurodiagnostic tests (EEG, CT scan, MRI, carotid Doppler) warranted in the setting of syncope?**
      seizures, altered mental status, Todd's paralysis, known history of cerebrovascular compromise, new focal deficits, new language deficits   91.3.3

■ Transient Neurologic Deficit

3. **Complete the following about**   91.4
   transient neurological deficits (TIA):
   a. By definition, lasts less than ___ hours.   24
   b. Symptoms will usually subside within   20 minutes
      ___ _____ (minutes vs. hours)
   c. They are a result of i_____.   ischemia
   d. Differential for a transient neurologic
      deficit includes:
      i.   t_____ i_____ a_____   transient ischemic attack
      ii. m_____   migraine
      iii. s_____ followed by   seizure;
           _____ _____   Todd's paralysis
      iv. c_____ s_____ h_____   chronic subdural hematoma
   e. TIA-like symptoms from cerebral   antiplatelet;
      amyloid angiopathy require avoidance of   anticoagulant
      a_____ or a_____ medications.

■ Diplopia

4. **Complete the following regarding the**   91.6
   etiology of diplopia secondary to VI
   nerve palsy:
   a. i_____ i_____   increased intracranial
      p_____   pressure
   b. s_____ s_____   sphenoid sinusitis
   c. t_____   tumor

5. **The differential for diplopia includes:**   91.6
   a. c_____ n_____ p_____   cranial nerve palsies
   b. i_____ m_____   intraorbital mass
   c. G_____ disease   Graves' disease
   d. m_____ g_____   myasthenia gravis
   e. g_____ c____ a_____   giant cell arteritis
   f. b_____   botulism
   g. secondary to t_____   trauma

■ Anosmia

6. **Complete the following about**   91.7
   anosmia:
   a. Most common cause is a severe u_____   upper respiratory infection
      r_____ i_____.
   b. Second most common cause is   head trauma;
      h_____ t_____ with a __-__%   7-15%
      occurrence in severe cases.
   c. Intracranial neoplasms such as   olfactory groove
      o_____ g_____   meningiomas
      m_____ can be a cause.
   d. Congenital anosmia is also known as   Kallmann syndrome
      K_____ syndrome.

91

■ Multiple Cranial Nerve Palsies (Cranial Neuropathies)

7. **Complete the following about cranial neuropathies:**

   a. Congenital facial diplegia is also known as M_____ s_____.
   Möbius syndrome — 91.8.1

   b. It affects which half of the face more?
   upper half

   c. Which other cranial nerves may be involved?
   CN VI, III, or XII

   d. Lyme disease can cause CN_____ palsy.
   CN VII (unilateral or bilateral)

   e. Affects which half of the face?
   lower half

   f. True or False. It may also involve other cranial nerves.
   False

   g. Tuberculous meningitis usually involves which cranial nerve first and most frequently?
   CN VI

   h. Weber's syndrome involves CN ___ and c_____ h_____.
   CN III and contralateral hemiparesis

   i. Millard-Gubler syndrome involves CN ___ and CN ____ as well as c_____ h_____.
   CN VI and VII; contralateral hemiparesis

   j. A mass in the ____ ventricle may compress the f_____ c_____ causing facial diplegia.
   4th ventricle; facial colliculus — 91.8.2

8. **Complete the following about cavernous sinus syndrome:** — 91.8.2

   a. Which cranial nerves can be involved with a lesion in the cavernous sinus?
   CN III, IV, V1, V2, and VI

   b. Clinical symptoms include d_____ due to o_____.
   diplopia; opthalmoplegia

   c. With CN ___ palsy in cavernous sinus syndrome, the pupil _____ (will vs. will not) be dilated.
   CN III; will not

9. **Complete the following about osteopetrosis:** — 91.8.2

   a. Also known as m_____ b_____.
   marble bone

   b. It is a g_____ disorder involving defective o_____ resorption of bone.
   genetic; osteoclastic

   c. Patients will have _____ (increased vs. decreased) bone density.
   increased

   d. Most common neurologic manifestation is b_____.
   blindness

   e. Treatment consists of bilateral o_____ n_____ decompression.
   optic nerve

91

■ Binocular Blindness

10. **What is the differential diagnosis for**   91.9
    new onset binocular blindness?
    a. bilateral o_____ l_____   occipital lobe;
        dysfunction secondary to either   trauma;
        t_____ or i_____   ischemia
    b. s_____   seizures (Epileptic blindness)
    c. m_____   migraines
    d. p_____ i_____ o_____   posterior ischemic optic
        n_____   neuropathy
    e. bilateral v_____ h_____   vitreous hemorrhage
    f. f_____ such as _____   functional; conversion
        disorder

■ Monocular Blindness

11. **Complete the following about**   91.10
    temporal arteritis:
    a. Also known as g_____ c_____   giant cell arteritis
        a_____
    b. Usually due to ischemia of the:
        i.   o_____ n_____   optic nerve
        ii. o_____ t_____   optic tract
        iii. c_____ r_____ a_____   central retinal artery
             (less likely)

■ Exophthalmos

12. **Complete the following about**
    exophthalmos:
    a. Also known as p_____.   proptosis   91.11.1
    b. If history of trauma, differential should   carotid cavernous fistula   91.11.2
        include c_____ c_____ f_____.
    c. If following frontal-orbital surgery,   orbital roof defect
        differential should include o_____
        r_____ defect.

13. **What is the differential of pulsatile**   91.11.2
    exophthalmos?
    a. c_____ c_____ f_____   carotid cavernous fistula
    b. o_____ r_____ d_____ with   orbital roof defect
        transmitted intracranial pulsations
    c. v_____ t_____   vascular tumor

■ Ptosis

14. What is the differential diagnosis for   91.12
etiologies causing ptosis?

a. c_____   congenital (often autosomal
                                                    dominant inheritance)
b. t_____ to eyelid   trauma
c. CN _____ palsy or seen in H_____   CN III; Horner's syndrome
    syndrome
d. m_____ g_____   myasthenia gravis
e. b_____   botulism
f. mechanical obstruction secondary to   tumor;
    t_____ or extension of m_____   mucocele
    from frontal sinus
g. d_____ induced   drug (alcohol, opium, etc.)

■ Tinnitus

15. Complete the following about   91.15.2
pulsatile tinnitus:

a. Most cases of pulsatile tinnitus are due   vascular
    to v_____ lesions.
b. Workup includes: M_____ and   MRI (with and without
    a_____.   enhancement); angiogram

16. What is the differential for non-   91.15.3
pulsatile tinnitus?

a. occlusion of e_____ e_____   external ear
b. o_____ m_____   otitis media
c. M_____ d_____   Meniere's disease
d. l_____   labyrinthitis
e. e_____ _____ tumors   endolymphatic sac
f. Drugs such as s_____,   salicylates, quinine;
    q_____, and a_____   aminoglycosides

91

■ Language Disturbance

17. Complete the following about   91.17
language disturbances:

a. Wernicke's aphasia is a f_____   fluent
    aphasia.
b. Conduction aphasia is associated with   fluent;
    f_____ speech and p_____.   paraphasias;
    Patients _____ (are vs. are not) aware   are not
    of their deficits.
c. Bilateral frontal lobe dysfunction is   akinetic mutism
    associated with a_____
    m_____.

92

Differential Diagnosis (DDx) by Signs and Symptoms – Primarily Spine and Other

■ Myelopathy

1. **True or False. The following are potential causes of myelopathy:**   92.2
    a. cervical or thoracic spinal stenosis   true
    b. chronic anemia   true
    c. Cushing's disease   true
    d. Lyme disease   true
    e. acquired immunodeficiency syndrome (AIDS)   true

2. **How does anemia produce myelopathy?**   92.2
    a. Chronic anemia can lead to b_____ m_____ hypertrophy and c_____ c_____.   bone marrow; cord compression
    b. Pernicious anemia can lead to s_____ c_____ d_____.   subacute combined degeneration

3. **E_____ l_____ is seen in Cushing's disease and can produce myelopathy.**   Epidural lipomatosis   92.2

4. **Order the following location of neoplastic masses causing myelopathy in order of most common to least common:**   92.2
    a. intramedullary   extradural,
    b. extradural   intradural extramedullary,
    c. intradural extramedullary   intramedullary

5. **What are the frequencies of spinal cord tumors in the following locations?**   92.2
    a. extradural: __%   55%
    b. intradural extramedullary: __%   40%
    c. intradural intramedullary: __%   5%

6. **Complete the following about spinal cord infarction:**
   92.2
   a. Although uncommon, spinal cord infarction most often occurs in the territory of the a_____ s_____ artery and most commonly at the level of ____.

   anterior spinal artery; T4

   b. This occurs because this region is a w_____ area.

   watershed

   c. This spares the p_____ c_____.

   posterior columns

   d. Causes of infarction include:
      i. h_____
      ii. a_____
      iii. e_____
      iv. a_____ d_____
      v. s_____ s_____

   hypotension
   atherosclerosis
   embolization
   aortic dissection
   spinal stenosis

7. **Necrotizing myelopathy associated with spontaneous thrombosis of a spinal cord AVM that presents as spastic to flaccid paraplegia with ascending sensory level is called F_____-A_____.**

   Foix-Alajouanine disease   92.2

8. **Regarding acute (idiopathic) transverse myelitis:**
   92.2
   a. True or False. Clinical onset is indistinguishable from acute spinal cord compression.

   true

   b. _____ (Abnormal vs. Normal) imaging is expected on CT, myelogram and MRI.

   Normal

   c. Cerebrospinal fluid (CSF) analysis shows p_____ and h_____.

   pleocytosis and hyperproteinemia

   d. The t_____ region is the most common level.

   thoracic

   e. True or False. The most common onset is 20 to 40 years of age.

   false - most common during first 2 decades of life

   f. True or False. Usually results in a diagnosis of multiple sclerosis.

   false - MS is diagnosed in only 7%

9. **Abdominal cutaneous reflexes are almost always absent in m_____ s_____.**

   multiple sclerosis   92.2

10. **Regarding Devic's syndrome:**
    92.2
    a. Characterized by acute bilateral o_____ n_____ and m_____.

    optic neuritis; myelopathy

    b. True or False. The transverse myelitis can be a cause of complete block on myelography.

    true

    c. True or False. More common in Asia than in the United States.

    true

    d. True or False. It is a variant of multiple sclerosis.

    true

92

11. N_____ o_____ is another
     name for Devic's syndrome.   Neuromyelitis optica   92.2

12. The following are part of the   92.2
     mechanism responsible for pernicious
     anemia:
     a. malabsorption of B12 in the   distal ileum
         d_____ i_____
     b. lack of secretion of intrinsic factor by   gastric parietal cells
         g_____ p_____ c_____

13. Complete the following about viral   92.2
     causes of myelopathy:
     a. Herpes varicella-zoster can rarely cause   necrotizing myelopathy
         n_____ m_____.
     b. HSV type 2 may cause a_____   ascending myelitis
         m_____.
     c. CMV may cause t_____   transverse myelitis
         m_____.

14. AIDS can produce myelopathy via   vacuolization   92.2
     v_____ of the spinal
     cord.

15. Match the disease with the important   92.2
     feature:
     ① pernicious anemia; ② Guillain-Barré;
     ③ ALS
     Features: (a-m) below
     a. ascending weakness   ②
     b. atrophic weakness of hands   ③
     c. symmetrical paresthesias   ①
     d. posterior column involvement   ①
     e. normal sensation   ②
     f. dementia   ①
     g. areflexia   ②
     h. serum b12 levels   ①
     i. fasciculations   ③
     j. Shilling test   ①
     k. preserved sphincter control   ③
     l. treatment with b12   ①
     m. proprioception difficulty   ①

16. What are symptoms of ALS?   92.2
     a. s_____   spasticity
     b. a_____ of h_____ and   atrophy of hands and
         f_____   forearms
     c. f_____   fasciculations
     d. usually preserved s_____   sphincter control
         c_____

92

■ Sciatica

17. **Complete the following about sciatica:**

  a. The sciatic nerve contains roots from L___ to L___.   L4 to S3   92.3.1

  b. The nerve passes out of the pelvis through the g_____ s_____ f_____.   greater sciatic foramen

  c. In the lower third of the thigh, it divides into the t_____ and the c_____ p_____ nerves.   tibial; common peroneal

  d. Most common cause is r_____ due to h_____ l_____ d_____   radiculopathy; herniated lumbar disc   92.3.2

18. **Complete the following about herpes zoster:**   92.3.2

  a. May rarely cause r_____.   radiculopathy

  b. Lumbosacral dermatomas are involved in ___-___%   10-15%

  c. Typically, skin lesions follow pain in ___-___ days.   3-5 days

  d. True or False. Motor weakness can occur.   true

  e. True or False. Urinary retention can occur.   true

19. **Complete the following about piriformis syndrome:**   92.3.2

  a. What are the major symptoms of piriformis syndrome?   pain in the sciatic nerve distribution with weakness of external rotation and abduction of the hip

  b. Friedberg test consists of force i_____ r_____ of the high and thigh e_____.   internal rotation; extension

20. **Complete the following about extraspinal tumors causing sciatica:**   92.3.3

  a. What characterizes the pain?

    i. i_____   insidious

    ii. c_____   constant

    iii. p_____   progressive

    iv. positional vs. non-positional?   non-positional

    v. worse in morning or at night?   night

  b. About ___% will have a previous history of a tumor.   20%

21. **Femoral neuropathy is often mistakenly identified as a radiculopathy at the L___ level.**   L4   92.3.4

92

22. **Does femoral neuropathy or L4 radiculopathy lead to the following symptoms?**   92.3.4

    a. weak quadriceps   both femoral neuropathy and L4 radiculopathy

    b. sensory loss occurring along the anterior thigh.   femoral neuropathy

    c. Iliopsoas is weak in_____ _____.   femoral neuropathy

    d. Thigh adductors may be weak in____ _____.   L4 radiculopathy

23. **A peroneal nerve palsy may be mistaken for radiculopathy at what level?**   L5   92.3.4

■ Acute Paraplegia or Quadriplegia

24. **Signs of spinal cord compression include:**   92.4.1

    a. -p_____ or -p_____   -plegia or -paresis (para/quadri)

    b. u_____ _____   urinary retention

    c. s_____ l_____   sensory level

    d. possible positive B_____   Babinski

    e. altered r_____   reflexes (hypo vs. hyper)

25. **Complete the following about para/quadriplegia in infancy:**   92.4.2

    a. Congenital degeneration of anterior horn cells leading to weakness, areflexia, tongue fasciculations, with normal sensation is s_____ m_____ a_____.   spinal muscular atrophy (Werdnig-Hoffmann disease is most severe form.)

    b. This is also known as f_____ b_____ syndrome.   "floppy baby syndrome"

    c. If ileus, hypotonia, weakness, and mydriasis, suspect c_____ b_____ bacterial infection.   clostridium botulinum

26. **Complete the following about para/quadriplegia:**   92.4.2

    a. Classic ascending paralysis is seen with G_____-B_____ syndrome   Guillain-Barré syndrome

    b. If post-viral, paraplegia may be secondary to t_____ m_____.   transverse myelitis

    c. Rapid correction of hyponatremia may lead to c_____ p_____ m_____.   central pontine myelinolysis

    d. A lesion in the p_____ area may involve both motor strips.   parasagittal

92

Hemiparesis or Hemiplegia

27. The most common etiology for pure motor hemiplegia without sensory loss is a l_____ i_____ of the contralateral i_____ c_____.

lacunar infarct; internal capsule

92.5.2

28. What are the different locations in which a lesion can cause hemiplegia?

92.5.2

  a. c_____ h_____

cerebral hemisphere (motor strip)

  b. i_____ c_____

internal capsule

  c. b_____

brainstem

  d. c_____ j_____

cervicomedullary junction

  e. unilateral s_____ c_____

spinal cord

  f. While not a lesion, h_____ may be associated with hemiparesis

hypoglycemia

Low Back Pain

29. Complete the following about back pain:

92.6.2

  a. If a patient is writhing in pain, consider a_____ or v_____ etiology such as an a_____ d_____.

abdominal; vascular; aortic dissection

  b. If constant pain at bed rest, consider a s_____ t_____

spinal tumor

  c. If nocturnal back pain relieved by aspirin, consider o_____ o_____ or a benign o_____.

osteoid osteoma; osteoblastoma

  d. Morning back stiffness, hip pain, hip swelling, no relief with rest, and improvement with exercise is suggestive of s_____ or e_____ a_____ s_____.

sacroiliitis; early ankylosing spondylitis

30. What are 3 major symptoms of cauda equina syndrome?

Perineal (aka saddle) anesthesia, progressive weakness, urinary incontinence

92.6.2

31. Complete the following about cauda equine syndrome:

92.6.2

  a. What are 4 treatable etiologies?

Etiologies include epidural abscess, epidural hematoma, tumor (intradural or extradural), massive central disc herniation.

  b. It requires _____ (non-emergent or emergent) diagnostic evaluation.

emergent

92

32. **Complete the following about annular tears:**   92.6.2
    a. Asymptomatic in ___% of 50-60 year old patients.   40%
    b. Asymptomatic in ___% of 60-70 year old patients.   75%

33. **Two medications that are associated with acute back pain are:**   92.6.2
    a. s_____   statins
    b. p_____ i_____   phosphodiesterase inhibitors
                                                      such as tadalafil

34. **Disc herniation through the cartilaginous end-plate into the vertebral body is called a S_____ n_____.**   Schmorl's node   92.6.3

35. **Complete the following about chronic low back pain:**   92.6.3
    a. After 3 months, about ___% of patients with low back pain will have persistent symptoms. A structural diagnosis is found in about ___% of these patients.   5%; 50%
    b. Erosive changes adjacent to sacroiliac joint and positive HLA-B27 suggests a_____ s_____.   ankylosing spondylitis

---

■ Foot Drop

36. **Which exam findings help differentiate common peroneal nerve palsy from L4/L5 radiculopathy?**   92.7.1
    a. strength of p_____ t_____ with foot i_____   posterior tibialis; foot inversion (should be involved with radiculopathy but spared in peroneal nerve palsy)
    b. strength of g_____ m_____ with i_____ r_____ and f_____ of hip   gluteus medius; internal rotation and flexion (should be involve with radiculopathy but spared in peroneal nerve palsy)

37. **Complete the following about foot drop:**
    a. Due to weakness of a_____ t_____.   anterior tibialis   92.7.1
    b. This typically involves cord levels L___ and L___.   L4, L5
    c. Often accompanied by weak e_____ d_____ l_____ and e_____ h_____ l_____, which are innervated by the d_____ p_____ nerve.   extensor digitorum longus; extensor hallucis longus; deep peroneal nerve

92

d. "Flail foot" may be caused by s_____ nerve dysfunction.

sciatic nerve

92.7.2

e. Which division of the sciatic nerve is more sensitive to injury (peroneal vs. tibial)?

peroneal division more sensitive to injury

38. What are the neurologic etiologies for a foot drop?

92.7.3

a. p_____ nerve injury

peroneal (deep vs. common)

b. L___ or L___ radiculopathy

L5; L4

c. l_____ p_____ injury

lumbar plexus

d. _____ nerve injury

sciatic

e. A____

ALS

f. C_____-M_____-T_____

Charcot-Marie-Tooth

g. h_____ m_____ p_____

heavy metal poisoning

h. p_____ lesion

parasagittal lesion

i. s_____ c_____ injury

spinal cord

39. What are the muscles and nerve roots that produce the following movements?

a. thigh adduction

adductors, L2-3

Fig. 92.1

b. knee extension

quadriceps, L2-4

c. internal rotation at hip

gluteus medius, L4-5, S1

d. hip extension

gluteus maximus, L5, S1-2

e. knee flexion

biceps femoris, L5, S1-2

Table 92.3

f. foot plantar flexion

gastrocnemius, S1-2

g. foot inversion

tibialis posterior, L4-5

h. foot eversion

peroneus longus and brevis, L5, S1

i. ankle dorsiflexion

anterior tibialis, L4-5

40. Thigh adduction involves:

Fig. 92.1

a. muscles

adductors

b. nerve

obturator

c. roots

L2,3

41. Knee extension involves:

Fig. 92.1

a. muscles

quadriceps

b. nerve

femoral

c. roots

L2-4

42. Internal rotation of the thigh involves:

Fig. 92.1

a. muscle

gluteus medius

b. nerve

superior gluteal

c. roots

L4-5, S1

d. If weak, means lesion is very p_____

proximal

43. Digging heels into bed involves:

Fig. 92.1

a. muscle

gluteus maximus

b. nerve

inferior gluteal

c. roots

L5, S1-2

d. If weak, means lesion is very p_____.

proximal

92

44. Knee flexion with thigh flexed involves:
a. muscles   lateral hamstrings
b. nerve   sciatic
c. roots   L5, S1-2

Fig. 92.1

45. Plantar flexion of foot involves:
a. muscle   gastrocnemius
b. nerve   sciatic
c. roots   S1-2

Table 92.3

46. Foot inversion involves:
a. muscle   posterior tibial
b. nerve   tibial
c. roots   L4-5
d. If strong but in the presence of a foot   common peroneal
   drop, it means that the injury is distal to
   the take-off of the c_____
   p_____ nerve.

Table 92.3

47. Foot eversion involves:
a. muscles   peroneus longus and brevis
b. nerve   superficial peroneal
c. roots   L5, S1
d. If strong but in the presence of a foot   deep peroneal
   drop, it means that the injury is in the
   d_____ p_____ nerve.

Table 92.3

48. What are the ways to distinguish foot drop from injury to the deep vs. common peroneal nerve?
a. Deep peroneal nerve:
   i.   major weakness symptom   foot drop
   ii. weak muscle   anterior tibial
   iii. sensory loss   web space
b. Common peroneal nerve:
   i.   major weakness symptom   foot drop and weak eversion
   ii. weak muscles   anterior tibial and peroneus
                                     longus and brevis
   iii. sensory loss   lateral leg and foot

Table 92.3

49. What distinguishes superficial peroneal nerve injury?
a. major weakness symptom   foot eversion
b. weak muscles   peroneus longus and brevis
c. presence of foot drop?   no
d. Sensory loss   lateral leg and foot

Table 92.3

50. Complete the following:
a. Painless foot drop is likely due to   peroneal nerve (palsy)
   p_____ n_____.
b. Painful foot drop is likely due to   radiculopathy
   r_____.

92.7.3

92

c. Painless foot drop without sensory loss could be due to a p_____ lesion, which would be associated with a B_____ reflex and _____ (hypo vs. hyperactive) reflexes.

parasagittal; Babinski; hyperactive

■ Weakness/Atrophy of the Hands/UEs

51. Complete the following regarding lesion location and findings in "cruciate paralysis":

92.8.1

a. Physical exam demonstrates bilateral u_____ e_____ weakness and h_____ a_____.

upper extremity; hand atrophy

b. This is due to pressure on the p_____ d_____.

pyramidal decussations

52. Atrophy of the first dorsal interosseous muscle is usually due to C__/T__ nerve root or u_____ nerve disease.

C8/T1; ulnar nerve

92.8.2

■ Radiculopathy, Upper Extremity (Cervical)

53. Myocardial infarction may present with symptoms similar to a radiculopathy at what level and side?

left C6

92.9

54. Complete the following:

92.9

a. The "empty can" test suggests _____ _____.

shoulder pathology

b. Interscapular pain suggests _____ _____.

referred pain with cervical radiculopathy or cholecystitis

55. Match the symptom with the position of the disc most likely to produce it:
① central cervical disc; ② lateral cervical disc
Symptom: (a-f) below

92.9, 92.10, 92.11

a. pain   ②
b. myelopathy   ①
c. bilateral symptoms   ①
d. upper extremity symptoms   ②
e. lower extremity symptoms   ①
f. numb-clumsy hand syndrome   ①

92

■ Burning Hands/Feet

56. **What are possible etiologies for a patient complaining of burning hands or feet?**   92.11

a. c_____ c_____ s_____   central cord syndrome
b. b_____ h_____ s_____   burning hands syndrome
c. n____-c_____ h_____ s_____   numb-clumsy hand syndrome
d. c_____ r_____ p_____   complex regional pain
   s_____   syndrome
e. p_____ n_____   peripheral neuropathy
f. e_____   erythermalgia (or
   erythromelalgia)
g. a_____ disease   arterial

■ Lhermitte's Sign

57. **Complete the following about Lhermitte's sign:**

a. What is the major symptom and what provokes it?   An electrical shock-like sensation radiating down the spine. Usually provoked by neck flexion.   92.13.1

b. Etiologies include: 92.13.2
   i.   m_____ s_____   multiple sclerosis
   ii.   c_____ s_____   cervical spondylosis
   iii. s_____ c_____   subacute combined
         d_____   degeneration
   iv.   tumor of the _____ _____   cervical cord
   v.   disc herniation in the _____   cervical
         region
   vi.   C_____ m_____   Chiari malformation
   vii. r_____ m_____   radiation myelopathy
   viii. c_____ c_____ s_____   central cord syndrome

■ Swallowing Difficulties

92

58. **Although swallowing difficulties are not uncommon after an A_____, this should prompt consideration for a post-op h_____.**   ACDF; hematoma   92.14

93

Procedures, Interventions, Operations: General Information

■ Intraoperative Dyes

1. Complete the following about intraoperative dyes:

93.2

a. _____ carries a small risk of seizure when administered intrathecally.

Fluorescein

b. _____ _____ is cytotoxic and should not be used at all.

Methylene blue

c. _____ can be used to demonstrate arteriovenous malformation (AVM) vessels intraoperatively and areas of blood brain barrier breakdown (e.g . tumors).

Fluorescein

d. _____ can be used to identify cerebrospinal fluid (CSF) leaks and is considered safe.

Fluorescein

e. _____ _____ used for intraoperative angiogram.

Indigocyanine green (ICG)

■ Operating Room Equipment

2. Complete the following about microscope setup

93.3.1

a. For spine cases the eyepiece is usually directly _____ the primary surgeon.

opposite

b. In contrast, for intracranial work, the observer's eyepiece is placed to the

_____.

right

c. The exceptions to this are:

   i. _____

   transphenoidial surgery

   ii. _____.

   right posterior fossa craniotomy in the lateral oblique position

3. **Complete the following on head-fixation**   93.3.2
   a. Alternatives to pinbased head fixation include
      i. _____   Horse-shoe head rest
      ii. _____   Doughnut fashioned out of
                              stockinette
      iii. _____   Prone-view
   b. Pin-stabilization is not recommended for   3
      use in children under the age of ___.
   c. These features of head-fixation should
      be considered depending on the type of
      case:
      i. radiolucent head holders for   vascular cases with
          _____   angiograms
      ii. attachment of _____   self-retaining retractor
          _____ _____ or   systems
      iii. _____ to the Mayfield system. image guidance systems

4. **Manufacture recommendations for**   93.3.2
   cranial pin placement include:
   a. Similar to a sweatband worn just about   orbits and pinna
      the _____ and _____.
   b. Avoid placing pins in the   squamous; frontal
      _____temporal bone or the _____
      sinuses.
   c. The single pin is placed _____ for   anteriorly;
      the supine position and on the _____ same
      side as the operation when doing prone
      posterior fossa cases.
   d. Adults should be placed in pins that have 60
      final resting tension between _____
      and 80 lbs.

■ Surgical Hemostasis

5. **Complete the following about surgical**
   hemostasis:
   a. Bone wax inhibits _____ formation.   bone   93.4.1
   b. True or False. The following chemical   93.4.2
      hemostatic agents exerts its effect by
      promoting platelet aggregation:
      i.   Gelfoam   false
      ii. Oxidized cellulose   false
      iii. Avitene   true (less so if platelets <10K)
      iv. Thrombin   false

6. **Match the surgical hemostasis**   93.4.2
   substance with its trade name:
   ① Thrombostat; ② Gelfoam; ③ Oxycel;
   ④ Surgicel; ⑤ Avitene
   a. gelatin sponge   ②
   b. oxidized cellulose   ③
   c. regenerated cellulose   ④

93

d. microfibrillar collagen   ⑤
e. thrombin   ①

■ Craniotomy General Information

7. **Complete the brain swelling**   93.5.3
    intraoperative checklist.
    (Hint: decompress)
    a. d_____ _____   drain CSF
    b. e_____ _____   elevate head
    c. c_____ (_____) CO_2 (hypercarbia)
    d. o_____ of _____ _____   obstruction of jugular veins
    e. m_____   mannitol
    f. p_____   hyperventilate
    g. r_____ _____   remove bone
    h. e_____ _____   excise brain (temporal or
                                              frontal lobes)

    i. (s)
    j. (s)

8. **Complete the following regarding the**   93.5.4
    risks of craniotomy:
    a. increased neurological deficit (tumor   10%
        case): _____%
    b. postop hemorrhage: _____%   1%
    c. infection: _____%   2%
    d. anesthetic complications: _____%   0.2%

9. **Complete the following regarding**   93.5.4
    anticonvulsants:
    a. True or False. Maintain their use if   true (use Keppra)
        cortical incision is anticipated.
    b. Describe the method of loading.   500 mg PO/IV q12 hours

10. **List the possible causes for acute post-**   93.5.5
    operative deterioration
    a. h_____   hematoma
    b. a_____ h_____   acute hydrocephalus
    c. c_____ i_____   cerebral infarction
    d. p_____   pneumosephalus
    e. e_____   edema
    f. v_____   vasospasm
    g. s_____   seizure
    h. p_____ a_____   persistent anesthetic

11. **If postoperative seizures occur,**   93.5.5
    consider the following:
    (Hint: abci)
    a. a_____ _____   anticonvulsant level—draw
                                              blood
    b. b_____   bolus—additional
                                              anticonvulsants

93

c. C_____ _____   CAT scan—to identify if any
                                          cause
d. i_____   intubate—to protect airway

12. **Complete the following regarding**   93.5.6
    postoperative headaches:
    a. "Syndrome of the trephined" can   2
        continue to improve out to ___ years in
        one series for posterior fossa
        craniotomies.
    b. It has been described to be similar to   post-concussive syndrome
        _____-_____ syndrome.

■ Intraoperative Cortical Mapping (Brain Mapping)

13. **Answer the following questions**   93.6.2
    regarding locating the primary
    sensory cortex:
    a. Intraoperative SSEP may localize the   phase reversal
        primary sensory cortex by _____
        _____ potentials across the central
        sulcus.
    b. This is done with a strip electrode   perpendicular
        oriented in the _____ direction to the
        anticipated orientation of the central
        sulcus.

14. **Answer the following questions**   93.6.3
    regarding awake craniotomies:
    a. Critically important to understand and   local and short acting
        manage the anesthetic agents which
        include _____ and
        _____ paralytics as to not
        obscure electrical stimulation.
    b. Pre-operative practice with the patient   reading glasses
        can be important to identify necessary
        aids in the OR, such as _____
        _____.
    c. Local anesthesia should be considered in
        4 regions:
        i.   s_____   supraorbital and
                                        supratrochlear
        ii. a_____   auriculotemporal
        iii. p_____   postrauricular
        iv. o_____   occipital
    d. Intracranial, the _____ is pain   dura
        sensitive while the brain is not.

■ Cranioplasty

15. **Answer the following about cranioplasty**
   a. Indications include _____, _____ _____ and _____.

   cosmetic, symptomatic relief, and protection   93.7.1

   b. Material options include the _____ _____ _____, _____, _____, _____ _____ or _____.

   patient's own bone, methylmethacrylate, mesh, pre-fabricated custom flap; split thickness calvaria   93.7.3

16. **Localizing levels in spine surgery. Name pitfalls**   93.7.3
   a. The count can be off if there are not ___ ribs and ___ lumbar vertebra.

   12; 5

   b. The transverse process can mimic a rib at ____ if it is large.

   L1

■ Bone Graft

17. **Answer the following regarding bone graft:**   93.8.1
   a. Autologous bone or rhBMP is recommended in the setting of an _____ in conjunction with a threaded titanium cage. This is based on level __ evidence.

   ALIF; 1

18. **Which of the flowing should not be used to assess for fusion?**   93.8.2
   a. static x-rays alone

   do not use

   b. Technetium-99 bone scan

   do not use

   c. flexion/extension films

   do not use in the absence of instrumentation

   d. The correlation between fusion and clinical outcome is _____.

   not strong, possibly unrelated

19. **For spine fusions, components of bone graft that are important for fusion:**   93.8.3
   a. _____

   osteoinduction (stimulate cells to develop)

   b. _____

   osteogensis (formation of new bone)

   c. _____

   osteoconduction (structure of graft so new bone can build upon)

   d. _____ _____

   mechanical stability

20. **For each of the above graft characteristics which material has a very strong effect in each.**   93.8.3
   a. osteoinduction

   BMP

   b. osteogensis

   cancellous autograft

   c. osteoconduction

   cancellous autograft

93

d. mechanical stability   cortical or vascularized
                                                  autograph
e. BMP is FDA approved only for use in   ALIF
   _____ procedures, other uses are off
   label.

21. **Common autograft donor sites include**   93.8.3
    a. _____ _____   iliac crest
    b. _____   rib
    c. _____   fibula
    d. _____   bone removed during
                                                  decompression

22. **Bone graft procurement**   93.8.4
    a. Anterior iliac bone should be obtained 3- ASIS;
       4 cm lateral to the _____, to avoid   lateral femoral cutaneous
       the _____.   nerve
    b. Posterior iliac crest bone grafts are taken   medial; superior cluneal
       from the _____ 6-8 cm of the iliac   nerves (which cross the
       crest to avoid _____. Injury here   posterior iliac crest at 8 cm);
       can result in a _____.   numb buttock or painful
                                                  neuromas
    c. When isolating the fibula, the _____   peroneal;
       nerve is to be avoided at the proximal   7
       head. At least _____ cm should be distally
       preserved to maintain ankle stability.

■ Stereotactic Surgery

23. **Stereotactic surgery indications**
    a. _____   biopsy   93.9.2
    b. _____ _____   catheter placement
    c. _____ _____   electrode placement
    d. _____ _____   lesion generation
    e. _____   SRS
    f. _____   experimental (laser,
                                                  transplantation, other)
    g. The ability to make a diagnosis in the   82-99%;   93.9.3
       setting of a stereotactic biopsy ranges   AIDS
       from _____ to _____ in a large series
       and was slightly lower in patients with
       _____.
    h. The yield rate is higher for lesions that enhance
       _____ on CT or MRI.
    i. The most frequent complication is   hemorrhage;
       _____, which was slightly worse in   AIDS
       patients with _____.
    j. In non-immunocompromised patients,   multifocal high grade gliomas
       the highest rate of complication
       occurred in _____ _____
       _____ _____.

93

94

Specific Craniotomies

■ Posterior Fossa (Suboccipital) Craniectomy

1. **True or False. The correct treatment for air embolism sustained during a craniotomy performed with the patient in a sitting position is**

   Table 94.1

   a. to find and occlude site of entry or rapidly pack wound with sopping wet sponges. — true

   b. bilateral or right-sided jugular venous compression. — true

   c. ventilation with 100% O_2. — true

   d. rotating the patient right side down. — false (Patient should be turned left side down to trap air in the right atrium.)

   e. aspirating air from central venous pressure (CVP) catheter. — true

   f. avoiding positive end-expiratory pressure (PEEP), which is ineffective and may worsen the risk of paradoxical air embolism. — true

2. **Complete the following about posterior fossa craniectomy and air embolism:**

   94.1.2

   a. Effect of air in right atrium is
      i. h_____ — hypotension (due to impaired venous return)
      ii. a_____ — arrhythmias

   b. Paradoxical air embolism may occur in the presence of
      i. p_____ f_____ o_____ — patent foramen ovale
      ii. or p_____ arteriovenous (AV) f_____. — pulmonary AV fistula

   c. Incidence in sitting position is _____%. — 7 to 25%

   d. Precautions require:
      i. D_____ _____ _____ — Doppler precordial ultrasound
      ii. C_____ in _____ _____ — CVP catheter in right atrium

   e. Earliest clue to occurrence is _____. — fall in end tidal pCO_2

94

3. How does air embolism cause problems?   94.1.2
a. Air becomes trapped in the _____ _____,   right atrium
b. impairs _____ _____, and   venous return
c. produces _____.   hypotension

4. Outline the intraoperative treatment for air embolism during a craniotomy.   Table 94.1
(Hint: occlude)
a. o_____   occlude entry site
b. c_____   cover with wet laps
c. c_____   compress jugular veins
d. l_____   left side down lower head
e. u_____   ventilate/increase volume
f. d_____   discontinue nitrous
g. e_____   evacuate air

5. Earliest clues to occurrence include: 94.1.2
a. fall in _____ _____ _____   end tidal pCO_2
b. sound on Doppler is _____ _____   machinery sound
c. blood pressure _____   hypotension

6. True or False. The following approach is most applicable for a vertebral endarterectomy: 94.1.2
a. midline suboccipital craniotomy   false
b. extreme lateral posterior fossa approach   false
c. paramedian suboccipital craniotomy   true (Paramedian suboccipital craniotomy gives decent access to the vertebral artery and to the posterior inferior cerebellar artery [PICA] and the vertebrobasilar junction.)
d. subtemporal craniotomy   false

7. Consider the concept of "5-5-5."   94.1.3
a.
i. This relates to the _____ incision   skin
ii. for a linear _____ incision   paramedian
iii. for access to the _____.   CPA
b.
i. The first number relates to the mm medial to the _____ _____.   mastoid notch
ii. The second number relates to the _____ _____ the notch.   cm above
iii. The third number relates to the _____ _____ the notch.   cm below

94

8. **Matching. Match the incision with the objective.**   94.1.3
   Incision:
   ① 5-6-4; ② 5-5-5; ③ 5-4-6
   Objective: approach for (a-e) below
   a. the fifth nerve   ①
   b. hemifacial spasm   ②
   c. glossopharyngeal neuralgia   ③
   d. microvascular trigeminal decompression   ①
   e. vestibular schwannoma   ②

9. **Location of the inferior margin of the transverse sinus can be estimated**   94.1.3
   a. to be _____ f_____ _____   two finger breadths
      above the
   b. m_____ n_____.   mastoid notch

10. **Describe the Frazier burr hole.**   94.1.3
    a. It is used
       i.   p_____   prophylactically
       ii. to relieve p_____ swelling   post-operative
       iii. due to h_____ or   hydrocephalus
       iv. e_____.   edema
    b. It is located
       i.   _____ to _____ cm from the   3 to 4
            midline.
       ii. _____ to _____ cm above   6 to 7
            the inion in adults.
       iii. _____ to _____ cm above   3 to 4
            the inion in children.

11. **Complete the following regarding posterior fossa post-op complications:**   94.1.7
    a. Respiratory: prevent by _____   keeping patient intubated
       _____ _____.
    b. Hypertension: maintain SBP below   160 with nitroprusside
       _____ with _____.
    c. Acute hydrocephalus: treat with   ventricular tap—external
       _____ _____.   ventricular drain (EVD)
    d. Meningitis: prevent by prompt repair of cerebrospinal fluid (CSF) leak
       any _____ _____ _____.

12. **Blood pressure above _____ is**   160 mm Hg systolic   94.1.7
    dangerous for the post-operative
    posterior fossa patient.

13. **Complete the following regarding the**   94.1.7
    posterior fossa:
    a. Increased pressure in the posterior fossa
       is heralded by changes in
       i. b_____ p_____   blood pressure (increase)
       ii. r_____ p_____   respiratory pattern
    b. not by
       i.   p_____ i_____   pupillary inequality
       ii. m_____ s_____   level mental status
       iii. l_____ c_____   ICP changes

94

14. **Considerations for post-operative posterior fossa emergency include:**   94.1.7
    a. clinically
       i.   blood pressure (BP) _____   high
       ii. respirations _____   labored
    b. recommended treatment
       i.   i_____   intubate
       ii. t_____ _____   tap ventricle
       iii. o_____ _____   open wound
    c. Should you
       i.   obtain a computed tomographic   no
            (CT) scan first?
       ii. wait for operating room availability? no

15. **Indicate whether increased pressure in the posterior fossa or supratentorial compartment produces a change in the following:**   94.1.7
    a. pupillary reflexes: _____ _____   supratentorial compartment
    b. level of consciousness: _____   supratentorial compartment
       _____
    c. increase in intracranial pressure (ICP):   supratentorial compartment
       _____ _____
    d. changes in respiration: _____ _____   posterior fossa
    e. rise in blood pressure: _____ _____   posterior fossa

■ Pterional Craniotomy

16. **Matching. Match the head position with the location of the aneurysm.**   Fig. 94.5
    Head position:
    ① angled 30 degrees; ② angled 45 degrees; ③ angled 60 degrees
    Location of aneurysm:
    a. ICA P-comm   ①
    b. carotid terminus   ①
    c. middle cerebral artery   ②
    d. basilar bifurcation   ①
    e. A-comm   ③

17. **Name the artery(ies) that cross the sylvian fissure.**   none cross   94.2.2

■ Temporal Craniotomy

94

18. **True or False. A temporal craniotomy can allow access to the following structures:**   94.3.1
    a. foramen ovale   true
    b. Meckel's cave   true
    c. labyrinthine and upper tympanic portion true
       of the facial nerve

19. **A temporal lobectomy**   94.3.4
   a. can safely resect ___ - ___ cm in the   4—5 (before injury to
      dominant hemisphere   Wernicke area)
   b. and ___ - ___ cm in the nondominant   6—7 (before injury to optic
      hemisphere.   radiations)

■ Frontal Craniotomy

20. **Complete the following regarding the**   94.4.2
    superior sagittal sinus (SSS):
    a. The risk in sacrifice of the SSS is   venous infarction

      _____ _____.

    b. True or False. It almost always occurs
       with sacrifice of
       i.   the posterior third   true
       ii. the middle third   true
       iii. the anterior third   false

■ Approaches to the Third Ventricle

21. **Study Chart.**   94.7.1
    a. t_____   transcortical
    b. t_____   transcallosal
       i.   a_____   anterior
       ii. p_____   posterior
    c. s_____   subfrontal
       i.   s_____   subchiasmatic
       ii. o_____   opticocarotid
       iii. l_____ t_____   lamina terminalis
       iv. t_____   transsphenoidal
    d. t_____   transsphenoidal
    e. s_____   subtemporal
    f. s_____   stereotactic

22. **What is the risk of post-operative**   5%   94.7.1
    seizures after a transcortical approach
    to the anterior third ventricle (e.g., for
    a colloid cyst)?

23. **What are the principles of tumor**   94.7.2
    removal?
    a. Veins must be preserved at all _____.   costs
    b. First remove the tumor from within the   capsule

       _____.

    c. If adhesions seem unyielding, the most   incomplete intracapsular
       likely cause is i_____ i_____
       evacuation.

94

24. **Complete the following:**   94.7.3
    a. True or False. A disconnection syndrome
       (split-brain syndrome) is common with
       i.   posterior callosotomy through   true (where more visual
            splenium.   information crosses)
       ii. anterior callosotomy.   false
       iii. callosotomy < 2.5 cm in length from   false
            a point 1 to 2 cm behind the tip of
            the genu.
    b. Which of the above approaches avoids   callosotomy < 2.5 cm in
       the disconnection syndrome best?   length from a point 1 to 2 cm
                                                    behind the tip of the genu

25. **Describe the transcallosal approach to**   94.7.3
    the third ventricle.
    a. The superior sagittal sinus (SSS) is often   right
       to the _____ of the sagittal suture.
    b. The cranial opening should be
       i.   _____ anterior to the coronal   two third
            suture
       ii. and _____ behind it.   one third
    c. The two cingulate gyri may be adherent   corpus callosum
       in the midline and can be mistaken for
       the c_____ c_____.
    d.
       i.   The corpus callosum has a distinct   white
            _____ color.
       ii. It is located beneath the paired   pericallosal
            _____ arteries.
    e. The opening is usually made between   paired pericallosal
       the p_____ p_____ arteries.
    f. The trajectory of dissection is from the
       i.   c_____ s_____   coronal suture
       ii. to the e_____ a_____   external auditory meatus
            m_____.
       iii. The f_____ of M_____ lies   foramen of Monro
            along this line.
    g.
       i.   It is helpful to fenestrate the   septum pellucidum
            s_____ p_____
       ii. to prevent it from b_____ into   bulging
            the ventricle
       iii. especially in a case of c_____   colloid cyst
            c_____.

26. **How can you tell which ventricle you**   94.7.3
    are in?
    a. The foramen of Monro is located   medially
       m_____.
    b. If the choroid plexus goes to the left to   right
       enter the foramen of Monro you are in
       the _____ ventricle.

94

c. If you see no choroid plexus and no veins you may be in a c_____ s_____ p_____.

cavum septum pellucidum

d. The safe way to enlarge the foramen of Monro is posteriorly between the _____ _____ and the _____.

choroid plexus; fornix

27. **Complete the following about approaches to the third ventricle:**

a. The interhemispheric approach runs risk of injury to _____ _____ _____

bilateral cingulate gyrus   94.7.3

b. which may produce _____ _____.

transient mutism

c. The anterior transcallosal approach runs risk of injury to _____ _____

bilateral fornices

d. which may produce problem with s_____-t_____ m_____ and n_____ l_____.

short-term memory and new learning

e. The transcortical approach is   94.7.4

   i. made through the _____ _____ gyrus.

   middle frontal

   ii. This is about the same spot used for e_____ v_____ d_____,

   external ventricular drain

   iii. called _____ point.

   Kocher's point

■ Decompressive Craniectomy

28. **Indications for decompressive craniectomy:**

a.   94.10.1

   i. m_____ m_____ cerebral artery occlusion

   malignant middle

   ii. primarily for the n_____-d_____ hemisphere

   non-dominant

b. p_____ i_____ hypertension

persistent intracranial

c. True or False. It is necessary to open the dura.

true   94.10.3

d. Skull reimplantation can be considered after _____ to _____ weeks.

6 to 12

e.

   i. A _____ opening is best,

   large

   ii. approximately _____ by _____ cm or larger.

   12 by 12

94

95

Spine, Cervical

■ Anterior Approaches to the Cervical Spine

1. **Complete the following regarding extrapharyngeal approaches to the cervical spine**   95.1
   a. Extrapharyngeal approaches use n_____ intubation.
      nasotracheal
   b. The head is slightly e_____ and is rotated _____ degrees to the contralateral side.
      extended; 15
   c. In the medial extrapharyngeal approach, the branches of the _____ artery, u_____ nerves, and h_____ nerve are encountered.
      branches of external carotid artery, upper laryngeal nerves, and hypoglossal nerve
   d. In the lateral retropharyngeal approach the s_____ _____ nerve is encountered.
      spinal accessory nerve

■ Transoral Approach to Anterior Craniocervical Junction

2. **Complete the following regarding the transoral approach to the craniocervical junction:**   95.2.1
   a. Primarily useful for midline e_____ lesions.
      extradural
   b. Approach to intradural lesions is limited because of difficulties obtaining w_____ closure and increased risk of m_____.
      watertight; meningitis

3. **Complete the following regarding transoral approach to anterior craniocervical junction:**   95.2.2
   a. _____% of patients need posterior fusion after a transoral odontoidectomy.
      75%
   b. The patient must be able to open the mouth at least _____ mm.
      25 mm
   c. The tubercle of the a_____ can be palpated through the posterior pharynx in order to locate the m_____.
      atlas; midline

d. If C1 ring sparing is not done, the central_____ cm of the _____ is removed.

3; atlas

e. There is about ____-____ mm of working distance between the two vertebral arteries where they enter the f_____ t_____ at the inferior aspect of the lateral mass of _____.

20-25; foramen transversarium; C2

■ Occipitocervical Fusion

4. What are the disadvantages of occipitocervical fusion?   95.3

a. Decreased r_____ o___ m_____ at the occipitocervical junction

range of motion

b. _____ _____ is higher than with C1-C2 fusion alone.

non-union rate

5. True or False. The following is an indication for occipitocervical fusion: 95.3

a. congenital absence of complete C1 arch   true

b. upward migration of the odontoid into the foramen magnum   true

c. congenital anomalies of occipitocervical joints   true

d. type II odontoid fracture   false

6. Complete the following regarding occipitocervical fusion:

a. Patient will lose about _____% of neck flexion.   30%   95.3

b. Keel plate must be placed at the _____ region of the _____ occipital bone.   thickest; midline

c. It is advisable to _____ the thickness of the occipital bone pre-operatively.   measure   95.3.1

7. True or False. After occipitocervical fusion, a halo is indicated in the following patients for 8-12 weeks;   95.3.4

a. patients with severe C1 fractures   true

b. elderly patients   true

c. unreliable patients   true

d. smokers   true

95

■ Anterior Odontoid Screw Fixation

8. **Complete the following regarding anterior odontoid screw fixation:**

a. C1-C2 complex is responsible for _____% of head rotation.
50%
95.4.1

b. Stability of the C1-2 joint depends on the integrity of the o_____ p_____ and the a_____ t_____ ligament.
odontoid process; atlantal transverse

c. Indicated in patients who have a type_____ odontoid fracture and an intact t_____ ligament.
II; transverse
95.4.3

d. Patients with type _____ fractures are also indicated when the fracture line is in the c_____ portion of the body of C2 in an elderly patient who may not fuse as well with immobilization as a younger patient.
III; cephalad

e. Contraindications to anterior odontoid screw fixation include if there is a fracture of the v_____ b_____ and if the fracture is less than _____ months old.
vertebral body; 6
95.4.4

f. Following fixation the immediate post-op strength is only _____% of the normal odontoid.
50 %
95.4.5

g. Therefore, a cervical brace is recommended for _____ weeks unless the patient has significant osteoporosis at which point a _____ brace is recommended.
6; halo

h. With fractures < 6 months old, the union rate was _____ %.
95%

i. Chronic nonunions > 6 months old have a bony union rate of _____ %, and _____ % rate of presumed fibrous union.
31%; 38%

■ Atlantoaxial Fusion (C1–2 Arthrodesis)

9. **Complete the following about atlantoaxial fusion (C1-C2 arthrodesis).**
95.5.1

a. The patient will lose about _____% of head rotation.
50%

b. Indications for atlantoaxial fusion include a_____ dislocation due to incompetence of the t_____ a_____ ligament.
atlantoaxial; transverse atlantal

95

c. Atlantoaxial fusion is further indicated in patients with incompetence of the odontoid process including in patients with type _____ fractures with > _____ mm of displacement or in patients with B_____ h_____ sign characterized by vertebrobasilar insufficiency with head turning.

II;
6mm;
Bow hunter's sign

10. Describe the wiring and fusion technique and differentiate.   95.5.2

a. Brooks fusion involves _____ to _____ sublaminar wires with _____ _____ bone grafts.

C1 to C2;
two wedge

b. Gallie fusion involves midline wire under the arch of _____ with an _____ bone graft.

C1;
"H"

c. Dickman and Sonntag fusion involves wire passed sublaminar to _____ with a single _____ graft wedged between C1 and C2.

C1;
bicortical

11. Complete the following about C1-2 transarticular facet screws: 95.5.3

a. A major risk of the procedure is _____ artery injury.

vertebral artery

b. May be used as an adjunct to Dickman and Sonntag technique to achieve _____ stabilization.

immediate

c. Requires pre-op t_____ c_____ C_____ scans from the o_____ c_____ through _____ with sagittal reconstruction through the C1–2 facet on both sides to look for the presence of a v_____ a_____ in the intended path of the screw.

thin cut CT;
occipital condyles;
C3;
vertebral artery

d. A fusion rate of _____% has been reported.

99%

12. Complete the following about C1-2 lateral mass screws: 95.5.3

a. Involves placement of polyaxial mini screws in C1 _____ _____ and C2 _____ with rod fixation.

lateral mass; pedicle

b. Decreased risk of _____ _____ injury as compared to transarticular facet screws.

vertebral artery

c. May be used in the presence of C1-2 _____.

subluxation

95

d. Preoperative _____ _____ _____ scan is required to assess the _____-_____ thickness of the _____ arch of _____ in case the arch needs to be drilled to facilitate screw placement; as well as to determine screw _____ and to estimate _____-_____ angle for screws.

thin cut CT; cranio-caudal; posterior; C1; length; medio-lateral

e. When placing C1 screws the _____ may be as close as _____mm to the ideal exit site of the screw.

ICA; 1mm

f. Post-operatively, a cervical collar (soft or rigid, as preferred) is used for _____-_____ weeks.

4-6

■ C2 Screws

13. **The following are the four types of C2 screws:**

95.6.1

a. P_____ screws, which are directed _____.

Pedicle; medially

b. L_____ _____ screws, which are directed _____. These screws are sized to fall short of _____ _____.

Lateral mass; laterally; foramen transversarium

c. C1–2 t_____ screws, associated with more risk of VA injury

transarticular

d. T_____ screws

Translaminar

14. **Complete the following about placement of C3-6 lateral mass screws:**

Table 95.1

a. In the An method the screw is placed _____mm medial to the midpoint in the medio-lateral direction and in the midpoint in the cranio-caudal direction with a trajectory of _____ degrees lateral and _____ degrees cephalad.

1mm; 30 degrees; 15 degrees

b. In the Magerl method the screw is placed _____mm medial to the midpoint in the medio-lateral direction and _____mm cranial to the midpoint in the cranio-caudal direction with a trajectory of _____-_____ degrees lateral and _____ to the facet joint.

2mm; 2mm; 20-25 degrees; parallel

c. In the Roy-Camille method the screw is placed at the midpoint in the medio-lateral direction and cranio-caudal direction with a trajectory of _____-_____ degrees lateral and _____ degrees cranio-caudal.

0-10 degrees; 0 degrees

95

96

Spine, Thoracic and Lumbar

■ Anterior Access to the Cervico-Thoracic Junction/Upper Thoracic Spine. Anterior Access to Mid and Lower Thoracic Spine

1. **Complete the following about anterior access to the cervico-thoracic junction, upper thoracic spine and lower thoracic spine:**

a. The s_____ s_____ procedure allows access to _____ and occasionally _____.

  sternal splitting;
  T3;
  T5

  96.1.1

b. In accessing the mid thoracic spine with a right sided thoracotomy, the h_____, m_____, and b_____ vein do not impede access.

  heart, mediastinum;
  brachiocephalic vein

  96.2.2

c. In accessing the mid thoracic spine with a left sided thoracotomy, the a_____ is easier to mobilize and retract.

  aorta

d. In accessing the lower thoracic spine, a _____ sided thoracotomy is preferred as it is easier to mobilize the _____.

  left;
  aorta

  96.2.3

e. At T10, the attachment of the _____ increases the difficulty of the approach.

  diaphragm

■ Thoracic Pedicle Screws

2. **Complete the following about thoracic pedicle screws:**

a. Due to the dense bone of the shoulders, the thoracic spine is usually difficult to image from _____ to _____ on lateral fluoroscopy.

  T1 to T4

  96.3.1

b. With regards to the craniocaudal direction use the _____ of the transverse process as an entry point for thoracic levels T1, T2, T3 & T12.

  middle (mnemonic: T1–2-3 "mid tp")

  96.3.3

c. With regards to the craniocaudal direction, use the _____ of the transverse process as an entry point for thoracic levels T7, T8 T9.

top (mnemonic: T7–8-9 "top of the line")

d. When freehanding using landmarks, the screw is inserted _____ to the surface of the superior articular facet while "aiming" at the contralateral _____.

perpendicular, pedicle

e. Typical thoracic screw length is _____ –_____ mm.

35-40mm

f. Screw diameter should be approximately _____% of the pedicle diameter.

80%

■ Anterior Access to Thoracolumbar Junction. Anterior Access to the Lumbar Spine

3. **Complete the following about anterior access to the thoracolumbar junction and lumbar spine:**

a. A _____ sided approach is preferred because the _____ is easier to retract than the liver, and the _____ is easier to mobilize than the inferior vena cava.

left; spleen; aorta

96.4.1

b. It is important to flex the ipsilateral leg to relax the _____ muscle, permitting safer retraction of the ipsilateral lumbosacral plexus.

psoas

c. The anterior lumbar interbody fusion (ALIF) is relatively contraindicated in males because of risk of _____ _____ in 1–2% (as high as 45% in some reviews).

retrograde ejaculation

96.5.1

d. The bifurcation of the great vessels occurs just above to just below the _____ –_____ disc space, thus the ALIF is best suited for access to _____ –_____.

L4-5; L5-S1

e. At L5-S1, the _____ _____ _____ runs down the _____ of the VB and has to be sacrificed to do an ALIF.

anterior sacral artery; midline

96

■ Instrumentation/Fusion Pearls for the Lumbar and Lumbosacral Spine. Lumbosacral Pedicle Screws

4. **Complete the following regarding surgical fusion of lumbar and lumbosacral spine:**

a. A lumbar fusion that includes L1 should not be terminated at _____ or _____.

    L1 or T12   96.6

b. Pedicle screws should be _____ to _____ % of pedicle diameter and have a minor diameter ≥_____mm in the adult lumbar spine and be long enough to penetrate _____ to _____ % of the vertebral body.

    70 to 80%;   96.7.1
    5.5;
    70 to 80%

c. With open lumbar pedicle screw placement, the entry point is at the _____ of the transverse process, at the intersection of the center of the transverse process and the sagittal plane through the lateral aspect of the _____ _____.

    base;   96.7.3
    superior facet

d. Medial angles for lumbar pedicle screws:
  i.   L1 level—medial angle should be_____ degrees.   5 degrees
  ii. L2 level—medial angle should be_____ degrees.   10 degrees
  iii. L3 level—medial angle should be_____ degrees.   15 degrees
  iv. L4 level—medial angle should be_____ degrees.   20 degrees
  v.   L5 level—medial angle should be_____ degrees.   25 degrees (Each angle equals the VB level x 5.)
  vi. S1 level—medial angle should be_____ degrees.   25 degrees
  vii. S2 level—medial angle should be_____-_____ degrees laterally.   40-45 degrees

e. Each screw should cross _____ _____ of the vertebral body.   two thirds

f. On AP view, if screw tip crosses the midline, there is a_____ breach.   medial

g. Posterior lumbar interbody fusion (PLIF and TLIF) is relatively contraindicated with well-preserved _____-_____ height; and is usually supplemented with _____ _____ to prevent progressive _____.

    disc-space;   96.7.8
    pedicle screws;
    spondylolisthesis

h. Benefits of TLIF over PLIF include less _____ _____ retraction and avoidance of _____ _____ in reoperations.

    nerve root;
    scar tissue

96

■ Minimally Invasive Lateral Retroperitoneal Transpsoas Interbody Fusion

5. **Complete the following regarding minimally invasive lateral retroperitoneal transpsoas interbody fusion:**

a. Access is best from _____-_____; however, a similar retropleural approach can be employed in the thoracic spine up to _____.

   L1-L5; T4

   96.8.1

b. With thoracic lateral interbody fusions one cannot _____the contralateral _____.

   penetrate; anulus

c. LLIF is particularly useful in cases of a_____ s_____ f_____ because it obviates dealing with _____ or _____ from previous surgery which reduces the risk of _____.

   adjacent segment failure; scar tissue; hardware; durotomy

   96.8.2

d. LLIF, when combined with release of the a_____ l_____ l_____, can be used to correct _____ and to _____ lumbar lordosis.

   anterior longitudinal ligament; scoliosis; increase

e. LLIF is contraindicated in cases requiring d_____ d_____, disc space height > _____mm, or in cases with pathology at the _____-_____ space secondary to interference from the _____.

   direct decompression; 12mm; L5-S1; ilium

   96.8.3

f. A standalone cage should not be placed in patients with o_____, pre-operative i_____, or if the _____ _____ ligament is disrupted during placement.

   osteoporosis; instability; anterior longitudinal

   96.8.5

g. Common transient complications include thigh numbness in _____-_____% of cases due to injury to the _____ nerve and thigh flexion weakness dye to injury to the _____ muscle.

   10-12%; genitofemoral; psoas

   96.8.6

h. Fusion rates following LLIF range from _____-_____%.

   91-100%

   96.8.8

96

97

Miscellaneous Surgical Procedures

■ Lumbar Puncture. C1–2 Puncture and Cisternal Tap

1. **Complete the following about spinal punctures:**

a. Contraindications to lumbar punctures include patients with platelet count <_____ or patients with n_____ hydrocephalus .

50,000; non-communicating

97.3.1

b. In patients with SAH, a LP can increase the t_____ pressure and precipitate aneurysmal rupture.

transmural

c. A LP in patients with spinal block may produce deterioration in as many as __%.

14%

d. The conus medullaris is located between T12 and L1 in ___% of patients, between L1 and L2 in _____%, and between L2 and L3 in ___% of patients.

30%; 51-68%; 10%

97.3.2

e. The intercristal line connects the superior border of the i_____ c_____ and occurs in most adults between the spinous processes of _____ and_____.

iliac crests; L4 and L5

f. When performing a LP the needle is always advanced with the _____ in place in order to prevent introduction of _____ cells which could produce an iatrogenic e_____ t_____.

stylet; epidermal; epidermoid tumor

g. The Queckenstedt is a test for _____ block in which the j_____ v_____ is compressed, first on one side then on both while measuring ICP; if there is no block, the pressure will rise to ___-___ cm of fluid, and will drop to the original level within _____ seconds of release.

subarachnoid; jugular vein; 10-20; 10

h. In non-anemic patients there should be ___-___ WBCs for every _____ RBCs.

1-2; 1000

97.3.4

i. A RBC count > _____ that changes little as CSF drains and an elevated ratio of _____ to _____ distinguished SAH from _____ _____.

100,000; WBC to RBC; traumatic tap

j. Incidence of severe postpuncture headache (lasting longer than _____ days) is _____%.

7;
0.1 to 0.5%,

k. A CN _____ palsy can occur delayed _____-_____days post-LP and usually recovers after _____-_____weeks.

CN VI (usually unilateral);
5-14 days;
4-6 weeks

l. Epidural b_____ p_____ is a treatment for refractory post LP headache.

blood patch

m. The C1-2 puncture is contraindicated in patients with C_____ m_____due to risk of low lying c_____ t_____ and medullary k_____.

Chiari malformation;
cerebellar tonsils;
kink

97.5.1

■ Lumbar Catheter CSF Drainage

2. **Complete the following about lumbar catheter CSF drainage:**

a. Indications for drainage include reducing CSF pressure on a site of CSF _____/_____, reducing intracranial pressure in cases of _____ hydrocephalus or reducing CSF pressure to attempt to increase perfusion of the _____ _____.

leak/fistula;
communicating;
spinal cord

97.4.2

b. If the catheter does not thread into the spinal canal, the catheter must be withdrawn _____ with the needle to prevent _____ off the catheter tip.

together;
shearing

97.4.4

■ CSF Diversionary Procedures. Ventricular Access Device

3. **Complete the following regarding ventricular catheterization:**

97.6.1

a. Kocher's point is used as an entry point to place a catheter into the _____ _____ of the lateral ventricle and can be found _____-_____cm from midline and _____cm anterior to coronal suture which is approximately _____cm up from the nasion; the trajectory is _____ to surface of brain, which can be approximated by aiming towards m_____ c_____ of ipsilateral eye and the E_____.

frontal horn;
2-3cm (mid pupillary line);
1 cm;
11 cm;
perpendicular;
medial canthus;
EAM

b. Keen's point is about _____-_____cm superior to and posterior to the pinna and results in catheter placement into the_____.

2.5-3 cm;
trigone

c. Dandy's point is _____cm from midline, and _____cm above inion.

2 cm;
3 cm

d. Occipital-parietal approach is frequently used for shunting; a common entry point is _____ cm above and posterior to the top of the pinna; the catheter is initially inserted _____ to skull base towards the _____ of the forehead or ipsilateral _____ _____.

3 cm, parallel; middle; medial canthus

4. **Complete the following about ventricular shunts:**

a. List the layers to traverse in open placement of the peritoneal catheter. (Hint: samp^3)

97.6.3

   i.   s_____ _____

subcutaneous fat

   ii. a_____ _____ _____

anterior rectus sheath

   iii. m_____

muscle

   iv. p_____ _____ _____

posterior rectus sheath

   v.   p_____ _____

preperitoneal fat

   vi. p_____

peritoneum

b. If a connector must be used near the clavicle, place it _____ the clavicle to decrease the risk of _____.

above; disconnection

c. A ventriculoatrial shunt should be revised when the catheter tip is above_____.

T4

d. During third ventriculostomy the opening is made_____ to the mammillary bodies which is _____ to the tip of the basilar artery; after puncturing the floor be certain that the _____ of _____ is also perforated.

anterior; anterior; membrane of Liliequist

97.6.4

e. The needle to be used in an ommaya reservoir puncture is a _____ gauge or smaller _____ needle.

25; butterfly

97.7.4

■ Sural Nerve Biopsy

5. **Complete the following about sural nerve biopsies:**

a. The following are indications for sural nerve biopsy:

97.8.2

   i.   a_____

amyloidosis

   ii. C_____-M_____-T_____

Charcot-Marie-Tooth

   iii. d_____ a_____

diabetic amyotrophy

   iv. H_____ d_____

Hansen's disease

   v.   m_____ l_____

metachromatic leukodystrophy

   vi. v_____

vasculitis

b. At the level of the ankle the sural nerve lies between the _____ tendon and the _____ malleolus.

achilles; lateral

97.8.4

c. A tourniquet is used to distend the l_____ s_____ vein.

lesser saphenous

97.8.5

d. _____ loss is expected but does not persist for more than _____ weeks.

Sensory; several

97.8.3

98

Functional Neurosurgery

■ Deep Brain Stimulation

1. Characterize Parkinson's disease.
98.1
a. Best target is the _____ _____   subthalamic nucleus
b. It has similar efficacy to _____   levodopa
c. with fewer _____ _____.   side effects
d. Ablative surgery is giving way to _____.   DBS (deep brain stimulators)

2. Match the following conditions with their stimulation target sites.
98.1
Conditions:
① Tourette's syndrome; ② obsessive compulsive disorder; ③ depression
a. anterior capsule   ②, ③
b. thalamic   ①
c. STN   ②
d. subgenual   ③
e. cingulate gyrus   ③
f. pallidal   ①

■ Surgical Treatment of Parkinson's Disease

3. Matching. Regarding surgical ablative treatment of Parkinson's disease and its historical background, match the listed procedures with the appropriate phrase(s) and benefits.
Abandoned because:
① unpredictable results; ② tremor did not improve; ③ bradykinesia did not improve; ④ rigidity did not improve; ⑤ ipsilateral tremor persists; ⑥ side effects/resistance; ⑦ only modest benefits
Procedure: (a-e) below
a. anterior choroidal artery ligation   ①   98.3.1
b. anterodorsal pallidotomy   ②, ③
c. ventrolateral thalamotomy   ③, ④, ⑤
d. L-dopa   ⑥
e. transplantation   ⑦   98.3.2

4. **True or False. The following symptoms improve after anterodorsal pallidotomy:**
98.3.1
a. tremor ipsilateral   false
b. rigidity   true
c. bradykinesia   false
d. ataxia   false
e. tremor contralateral   false

5. **Ventrolateral thalamotomy can improve tremor; it cannot be performed bilaterally because bilateral thalamotomy causes**
98.3.1
a. d_____ and   dysarthria
b. g_____ d_____.   gait disturbance

6. **Complete the following about surgical treatment of Parkinson's disease:**
98.3.2
a. The target today is the _____ _____   anterodorsal pallidum
b. specifically the _____ which blocks the input from the _____ _____.   GPi–internal segment of the globus pallidus; STN–subthalamic nucleus

7. **How might pallidotomy work?**
98.3.2
a. direct destruction of the _____   GPi
b. interrupt _____ fibers   pallidofugal
c. diminish input from the _____ _____   subthalamic nucleus

8. **Answer the following about surgical treatment of Parkinson's disease:**
98.3.2
a. What was an early procedure for the treatment of Parkinson disease?   ligation of the anterior choroidal artery
b. What are the mechanisms by which pallidotomy may work?
  i. destroy _____   GPi
  ii. interrupt p_____ p_____   pallidofugal pathways
  iii. reduce input into m_____ p_____   medial pallidum
c. What is the target for the tremor treatment?   ventralis intermedius nucleus (VIM) of the thalamus
d. True or False. Pallidotomy is primarily focused on the treatment of motor symptoms.   true
e. What are the most common complications of pallidotomy? Hint: vhid
  i. v_____   visual field deficit
  ii. h_____   hemiparesis
  iii. i_____ h_____   intracerebral hemorrhage
  iv. d_____   dysarthria

98

98

9. **True or False. Indications for pallidotomy in parkinsonism include**   98.3.2
   a. refractory to drug therapy   true
   b. drug-induced dyskinesia   true
   c. rigidity   true
   d. tremor   false
   e. dementia   false

10. **Ipsilateral hemianopsia is a contraindication to ventral pallidotomy because one of the side effects of the procedure could be o_____ t_____ i_____ and would cause the patient to be _____.**   optic tract injury; blind (Visual field defects could occur in 2.5% of patients; blindness could result.)   98.3.2

11. **Bilateral pallidotomies carry an increased risk of**   98.3.2
    a. s_____ d_____ and   speech difficulties
    b. c_____ d_____.   cognitive decline

12. **True or False. What are the benefits for the patient from posteroventral pallidotomy as done currently?**   98.3.2
    a. motor symptoms   true
    b. dyskinesia   true
    c. rigidity   true
    d. bradykinesia   true
    e. tremor   true

13. **Characterize thalamic lesions.**   98.3.2
    a. Lesioning in the thalamic _____ nucleus   intermedius
    b. reduces parkinsonian _____,   tremor
    c. However, it does not improve _____   dyskinesia
    d. and may worsen
       i. g_____ s_____ and   gait symptoms
       ii. s_____ p_____.   speech problems

14. **Characterize subthalamatomy.**   98.3.2
    a. Lesions in the STN classically produced _____.   hemiballism
    b. Selective lesions may give relief on a par with _____.   pallidotomy

■ Dystonia

15. **Characterize dystonia.**   98.4
    a. Stimulation of the _____ is the primary surgical treatment for the dystonia.   pallidum
    b. Results are better for _____ dyskinesia.   tardive
    c. The most common target is _____.   GPi

98

16. True or False. Stimulation has attracted increasing interest in patients with Parkinson's disease who are refractory to medical drug treatment. The deep brain stimulator (the electrode) is placed in which of the following locations? (There are three true answers.)   98.4
    a. zona incerta   false
    b. posterior ventral pallidum (PV)   false
    c. substantia nigra (SN)   false
    d. Forel's field (H)   false
    e. subthalamic nucleus (STN)   true
    f. globus pallidus internus (GPi)   true
    g. pedunculopontine nucleus   true

■ Spasticity

17. True or False. A spastic bladder will   98.5.2
    a. have high capacity and empty spontaneously.   false
    b. have high capacity and empty with difficulty.   false
    c. have low capacity and empty spontaneously.   true (Low capacity and spontaneous emptying are the hallmarks of the spastic bladder.)
    d. have low capacity and empty with difficulty.   false

18. True or False. The onset of a spastic bladder after spinal cord injury is   98.5.2
    a. immediate   false
    b. delayed   true (Delayed onset is typical because the acute phase of spinal shock is hyporeflexic and hypotonic.)
    c. can occur at any time   false

19. True or False. The Ashworth score can grade severity of spasticity. The highest score in this system is given when there is   Table 98.2
    a. no increase in tone (full movement)   false
    b. rigidity in all flexors   false
    c. rigidity in all extensors   false
    d. rigidity in flexion and extension   true

20. The Ashworth score is the clinical grading of the _____ of_____.   severity of spasticity   98.5.2

98

21. **What are the medications used in the treatment of spasticity?**   98.5.3
    a. b_____   baclofen
    b. d_____   diazepam
    c. d_____   dantrolene
    d. p_____   progabide

22. **What are the nonablative procedures used for the treatment of spasticity?**   98.5.3
    a. i_____ b_____   intrathecal baclofen
    b. i_____ m_____   intrathecal morphine
    c. e_____ e_____ s_____ epidural electrical stimulation

23. **True or False. Fibers that are more sensitive to radiofrequency rhizotomy are**   98.5.3
    a. small unmyelinated sensory fibers.   true
    b. large myelinated alpha motor fibers. false

24. **What are the ablative procedures with preservation of ambulation used for the treatment of spasticity? Name one.**   motor point block; phenol nerve block; selective neurectomy; percutaneous radiofrequency foraminal rhizotomy; Bischof's myelotomy; selective dorsal rhizotomy; stereotactic thalamotomy; dentatotomy   98.5.3

25. **What are the ablative procedures with sacrifice of ambulation used for the treatment of spasticity? Name one.**   intrathecal injection of phenol; selective anterior rhizotomy; neurectomy; intramuscular neurolysis; cordectomy; cordotomy   98.5.3

26. **True or False. Spasticity can be treated with intrathecal baclofen pumps. Complications are mainly**   98.5.3
    a. pump under-infusion   false
    b. wound complications   false
    c. catheter complications   true (Catheter complications may have a frequency of up to 30% in baclofen pumps.)
    d. drug resistance   false

■ Torticollis

27. **What is another name for torticollis?**   wry neck   98.6.1

28. **What muscle is usually affected in spasmodic torticollis?**   sternocleidomastoid   98.6.2

29. **What are the surgical procedures used for the treatment of spasmodic torticollis?**   98.6.3
   a. stimulate _____ _____   dorsal cord
   b. inject _____ _____   botulinum toxin
   c. cut _____   rhizotomy Forel's H1
   d. coagulate _____ _____   vertebral artery

30. **What artery is most commonly implicated in the torticollis of the eleventh nerve origin?**   vertebral artery   98.6.6

■ Neurovascular Compression Syndromes

31. **Characterize root entry zone.**   98.7.1
   a. Syndromes due to compression of
      i.   _____ _____   cranial nerves
      ii. at the _____ _____   root entry zone
           _____.
   b. This site, also known as the _____-   Obersteiner-Redlich
      _____ zone,
   c. is the point where the central myelin   oligodendroglial
      from the _____ cells
   d. changes to the peripheral myelin of the   Schwann cells
      _____ cells.

32. **True or False. Hemifacial spasm (HFS) starts from the lower half of the face and spreads to the upper half of the face.**   false (starts with the orbicularis oculi)   98.7.2

33. **Complete the following about neurovascular compression syndromes:**   98.7.2
   a. On what side is HFS more common?   left
   b. What is the age and gender predilection? women, after the teen ages
   c. What is the most commonly involved   AICA
      artery?
   d. True or False. Carbamazepine and   false
      phenytoin are generally effective
      treatment.
   e. What is the material used as a cushion in Ivalon, polyvinyl formyl
      the microvascular decompression   alcohol foam
      (MVD)?

34. **What is the only other involuntary movement disorder besides HFS that persists during sleep?**   palatal myoclonus   98.7.2

98

98

35. What distinguishes HFS from facial myokymia (FM)?   98.7.2
   a. Hemifacial spasm (HFS) is _____.   unilateral
   b. Facial myokymia (FM) is _____.   bilateral

36. True or False. The vessel most commonly associated with hemifacial spasm is   98.7.2
   a. posterior inferior cerebellar artery (PICA)   false
   b. superior cerebellar artery (SCA)   false
   c. anterior inferior cerebellar artery (AICA)   true
   d. posterior cerebral artery (PCA)   false
   e. vertebral artery   false
   f. basilar artery   false

37. Hemifacial spasm   98.7.2
   a. is caused by compression at the   root entry zone
      _____ _____ _____
   b. of the _____ _____   facial nerve
   c. by the _____.   AICA
   d. This does not cause _____   ephaptic
      conduction but
   e. produces _____ and _____. kindling, synkinesis

38. Synkinesis is a phenomenon where   98.7.2
   a. stimulation of _____ _____ of   one branch
      the facial nerve
   b. results in _____ _____ through   delayed discharges;
      _____ _____.   another branch

39. True or False. Postoperatively after microvascular decompression for hemifacial spasm, the patient can expect   98.7.2
   a. immediate cessation of facial spasms.   false
   b. reduction starting 2 to 3 days later.   true
   c. better results the longer the patient has false
      had HFS.
   d. better results the older the patient is.   false
   e. complete resolution of spasms   true (in 81 to 93% of patients)
      eventually.
   f. possible relapse even if free of spasms   false (relapse after 2 years
      for a full 2 years.   only 1%)

40. Complications of hemifacial spasm (HFS) surgery include the following: 98.7.2
   Hint: hemifacial s
   a. h_____   hoarseness
   b. e_____   elderly do less well
   c. m_____   meningitis (aseptic)
   d. i_____ _____ _____   ipsilateral hearing loss
   e. f_____ _____   facial weakness
   f. a_____   ataxia
   g. c_____   CSF rhinorrhea
   h. i_____ _____   incomplete relief of
                                       symptoms

i.   a_____ _____   aseptic meningitis
j.   l_____ _____   lip (perioral) herpes
k.   s_____ _____   swallowing (dysphagia)

98

■ Hyperhidrosis

41. **Complete the following statements about hyperhidrosis:**
    a. It is due to overactivity of the _____ _____ glands.   eccrine sweat   98.8.1
    b. These glands are under control of the _____ _____ _____.   sympathetic nervous system
    c. The neurotransmitter is _____.   acetylcholine
    d. Most _____ end organs are _____.   sympathetic; adrenergic
    e. Some cases warrant _____ _____.   surgical sympathectomy   98.8.2

■ Sympathectomy

42. **Complete the following statements about sympathectomy:**
    a. What is the level for cardiac sympathectomy?   from stellate ganglion   98.10.1
    b. What is the level for UE sympathectomy?   second thoracic ganglia T2   98.10.2
    c. What is the level for lumbar sympathectomy?   L2 and L3 sympathetic ganglia   98.10.4
    d. What is the most commonly used approach for lumbar sympathectomy?   retroperitoneal

43. **Name five indications for upper extremity (UE) sympathectomy.**   Table 98.6
    Hint: "crash" the sympathetic ganglia
    a. c_____ _____ _____   causalgia major primary
    b. R_____ _____   Raynaud disease
    c. a_____ _____   intractable angina
    d. s_____-_____ _____   shoulder-hand syndrome
    e. h_____   hyperhidrosis

44. **What are the complications of UE sympathectomy?**   98.10.2
    a. p_____   pneumothorax
    b. i_____ n_____   intercostal neuralgia
    c. s_____ c_____ i_____   spinal cord injury
    d. H_____ s_____   Horner's syndrome

99

Pain Procedures

■ General Information

1. **Usual oral narcotic dose tolerated is M_____ c_____.**

    MS contin (up to 300 to 400 mg/day)

    99.1

■ Types of Pain Procedures

2. **Name intracranial ablative procedures to treat the following pains:**

    99.3

    a. cancer pain: m_____ t_____
    medial thalamotomy

    b. head, neck, face pain: s_____ m_____
    stereotactic mesencephalon

3. **Matching. Match the procedure and its application (some have more than one).**
    Applications for pain from:
    ① spinal cord injuries; ② post-laminectomy pain; ③ pelvic pain with incontinence; ④ at or below C5; ⑤ head, face, neck, upper extremity; ⑥ bilateral below the diaphragm; ⑦ causalgia; ⑧ bilateral below thoracic dermatomes; ⑨ avulsion injuries; ⑩ not for cancer pain
    Procedure: (a-h) below

    99.3

    a. stereotactic mesencephalotomy   ⑤
    b. cordotomy   ④
    c. spinal intrathecal   ⑥
    d. sacral cordotomy   ③
    e. sympathectomy   ⑦
    f. commissural myelotomy   ⑧
    g. dorsal entry zone (DREZ)   ①, ⑨, ⑩
    h. spinal cord stimulator   ②, ⑩

■ Cordotomy

4. **Complete the following concerning cordotomy:**

a. Your objective is to interrupt the fibers of the l_____ s_____ t_____ t_____ on the side thalamic tract c_____ to the pain.
   lateral spinal thalamic tract; contralateral
   99.4.1

b. Cordotomy is the procedure of choice for u_____ pain below the C_____ dermatome.
   unilateral; C5

c. Two ways to perform cordotomy:
   i. o_____
   ii. p_____
   open
   percutaneously

d. Loss of automatic breathing can occur after b_____ c_____ and is called O_____ c_____.
   bilateral cordotomy; Ondine's curse

e. What is the cutoff percentage on pulmonary function test before patients can undergo cordotomy?
   50%
   99.4.2

5. **Answer the following about pain procedures:**
   99.4.3

a. What kind of patients are candidates for cordotomy?
   terminally ill patients

b. On which side should the cordotomy be performed?
   contralateral to pain

c. What happens to impedance as the needle penetrates the cord?
   jumps from 300 to 500 ohms to 1200 to 1500 ohms

d. What response should stop cordotomy from being performed?
   muscle tetany upon stimulation

e. If you look at the patient's eyes, what will you learn?
   If an ipsilateral Horner's syndrome occurs, the procedure is satisfactory.

f. What percentage will have pain relief?
   94%

■ Commissural Myelotomy

6. **Answer the following concerning commissural myelotomy:**

a. What is the indication for commissural myelotomy?
   bilateral or midline pain
   99.5.2

b. What is the rate of complete pain relief after commissural?
   60%
   99.5.4

c. What is the special requirement for intrathecal morphine?
   preservative-free 0.9% saline
   99.7.1

99

99

■ CNS Narcotic Administration

7. **Answer the following regarding central nervous (CNS) narcotic administration:**   99.7.1

   a. Requirement for implantation of a morphine pump is p_____ t_____ d_____.   pre-operative testing dose

   b. B_____ i_____ can shorten the delay time for a morphine pump to function; otherwise the relief may not occur for d_____.   Bolus infusion; days

   c. Is meningitis common after pump placement?   no

   d. Is respiratory failure common after pump placement?   no

■ Spinal Cord Stimulation (SCS)

8. **Complete the following regarding spinal cord stimulation:**

   a. Site of spinal cord stimulation is the d_____ c_____.   dorsal columns   99.8.1

      i. The most common indication is p_____ p_____ s_____.   postlaminectomy pain syndrome   99.8.2

      ii. It is not usually indicated for c_____ p_____.   cancer pain

   b. Two kinds of electrodes:

      i. p_____-like   plate

      ii. w_____-like   wire

9. **Complete the following statements about complex regional pain syndrome (CRPS)?**   99.8.6

   a. It is a c_____ pain condition characterized by   chronic

   b. intense a_____ or b_____ pain.   aching; burning

10. **What is the difference between Type I and Type II chronic regional pain syndrome?**   Type I has no nerve injury and Type II follows a nerve injury.   99.8.6

11. **True or False. Regarding spinal cord stimulation:**   99.8.6

    a. Improves pain control over physical therapy or medical management alone in patients with failed back surgery.   true

    b. It helps with pain due to inoperable limb ischemia.   true

    c. Reduces angina pain and improves exercise capacity.   true

■ Deep Brain Stimulation (DBS)

12. **Complete the following regarding deep brain stimulation:**   99.9

    a. Deafferentiation pain syndromes may benefit from stimulation of the _____ _____ .   sensory thalamus

    b. DBS for chronic neuropathic pain produces a reduction of ___-___% in pain in about ___-___% of patients.   40-50%; 25-60%

    c. Nociceptive pain syndromes benefit from stimulation of _____ ____ _____ .   periaqueductal gray matter

    d. Cluster headaches may benefit from _____ _____ .   hypothalamic stimulation

■ Dorsal Root Entry Zone (DREZ) Lesions

13. **Complete the following about dorsal root entry zone (DREZ) lesions:**

    a. They are useful for d_____ pain.   deafferentiation   99.10.1

    b. They result from nerve root a_____ .   avulsion

    c. They most commonly occur from m_____ accidents.   motorcycle

    d. For such an injury, pain relief can be expected in _____%.   80 to 90%   99.10.5

99

100

Seizure Surgery

■ General Information, Indications

1. **What percent of patients are not controlled with medication?** — 20% — 100.1

2. **Characteristics of refractory seizures considered for surgery.** — 100.1
   a. Nature of seizures? — severe disabling
   b. Length of treatment? — at least 1 year

3. **Complete the following regarding medically refractory seizures.** — 100.1
   a. Medically refractory is usually considered _____ attempts of high dose monotherapy — two
   b. with _____ distinct AEDs, and — two
   c. _____ attempt at polytherapy. — one

■ Pre-surgical Evaluation

4. **True or False. Regarding pre-surgical evaluation.**
   a. All patients should undergo high resolution MRI as part of pre-surgical evaluation. — true — 100.2.1
   b. It is the best test to demonstrate hippocampal asymmetry. — true — 100.2.2

5. **Complete the following about noninvasive seizure evaluation techniques.** — 100.2.2
   a. Video-EEG monitoring is used to identify the s_____ f_____. — seizure focus
   b. In a CT with IV contrast the focus may e_____. — enhance
   c. Interictal PET scan shows h_____ in ____% of patients with refractory CPS. — hypometabolism; 70%
   d. During a seizure a SPECT will demonstrate b_____ f_____ during a s_____. — blood flow during a seizure

6. **Complete the following about the WADA test:**   100.2.3
   a. The purpose is to localize d_____ h_____.   dominant hemisphere
   b. You can be misled by
      i.   A_____   AVM
      ii. p_____ t_____ a_____   persistent trigeminal artery
      iii. h_____ s_____ by   hippocampus supplied by
      iv. p_____ c_____   posterior circulation

7. **When there is lack of lateralizing or localizing physiology in pre-operative evaluation, there are two surgical options for better definition of seizure focus:**   100.2.4
   a. d_____ e_____   depth electrode
   b. s_____ g_____ or s_____   surgical grids or strips

■ Surgical Techniques

8. **Surgical disconnection operations available are:**   100.3.1
   a. c_____   callosotomy
   b. h_____   hemispherectomy
   c. m_____ s_____ t_____   multiple subpial transections

■ Surgical Procedures

9. **Complete the following about corpus callosotomy (CC):**   100.4.1
   a. Indication for corpus callosotomy
      i. d____ a_____ – a_____ s_____   drop attacks – atonic seizures
      ii. i_____ h_____ s_____   infantile hemiplegia syndrome
   b. How much of the CC is resected?   anterior two-thirds
   c. Complication is a_____ m_____.   akinetic mutism (or reduced temporary verbalization)
   d. Must the anterior commissure also be sectioned?   no – less likely to get disconnection syndrome if spared
   e. Contraindication?   crossed dominance
   f. Exclude by W_____ t_____ on all l_____ h_____ persons.   Wada test on all left-handed persons

10. **Answer the following about**   100.4.1
    disconnection syndrome in a left-
    dominant person (i.e., right-handed):
    a. Usually lasts _____ months.   2 to 3 months
    b. Effect:
       i.   left hand t_____ a_____   tactile anomia
       ii. vision p_____   pseudohemianopsia
       iii. smell: a_____   anosmia
       iv. copying figures (i.e., spatial   poor with right hand
            synthesis): p_____ with r_____
            h_____
       v.   speech: r_____ s_____   reduced spontaneity
       vi. urinary i_____   incontinence
       vii. left-sided d_____   dyspraxia
    c. Occurs with l_____ l_____ of   large lesions of corpus
       c_____ c_____.   callosum
    d. Less likely to occur if a_____ c_____   anterior commissure is spared
       is s_____.

11. **Complete the following regarding**   100.4.2
    temporal lobectomy limits:
    a. On dominant side permitted
       i.   _____   4 to 5 cm
       ii. too much i_____ s_____   injures speech
    b. On nondominant side permitted
       i.   _____   6 to 7 cm
       ii. too much c_____p_____   contralateral partial upper
            u_____ h_____   hemianopsia
    c. Greater resection of
       i.   _____ will cause   8 to 9 cm
       ii. c_____ c_____ u_____   contralateral complete upper
            h_____   hemianopsia

■ MRI Guided Laser Interstitial Thermal Therapy (MRGLITT)

12. **Complete the following.**   100.6
    a. MRGLITT stands for M_____ g_____   MRI guided laser interstitial
       l_____ i_____ t_____ t_____.   thermal therapy
    b. It is performed with simultaneous MRI   stereotactic guidance
       s_____ g_____.
    c. It is considered l_____ invasive than   less
       microsurgery.
    d. What is the main advantage?   shorter post-op recovery
    e. Preliminary seizure control is ___ to   60 to 70%
       ___%.

■ Post-operative Management for Seizure Surgery (Epilepsy Surgery)

13. **True or False. Regarding post-operative management for epilepsy surgery.**   100.7

   a. Requires ICU observation for 24 hours.   true
   b. Not necessary to treat one brief generalized seizure.   true
   c. Administer 10 mg dexamethasone IV before surgery followed by q8 hours dosing as necessary.   true
   d. Anti-convulsants can be discontinued immediately after surgery.   false (need to be continued for 1-2 years even if no post-op seizures occur)
   e. Neuropsychiatric evaluation 6-12 months after surgery.   true

100

■ Outcome

14. **Describe seizure surgery outcome expectations.**   100.8.1

   a. The greatest effect of surgery is r____ of s____ f____.   reduction of seizure frequency
   b. Incidence of being seizure free is _____%.   50%
   c. Seizures reduced by at least 50% in _____%.   80%

15. **What is the main risk of surgery during vagus nerve stimulation?**   vocal cord paralysis   100.8.3

101

Radiation Therapy (XRT)

■ Conventional External Beam Radiation

1. Radiation injury to tissue is a function of:
a. d____   dose
b. e_____ ____   exposure time
c. a____   area

101.2.1

2. What are the four "R's" of radiobiology?
a. R_____   Repair of sublethal damage
b. R_____   Reoxygenation of previously hypoxic tumor cells
c. R_____   Repopulation of tumor cells following treatment
d. R_____   Redistribution of cells within the cell cycle

101.2.1

3. What is the linear-quadratic equation (LQ-model)?
Biologically effective dose $(Gy) = n \times d \times [1 + d / (\alpha/\beta)]$; where n = # of doses, d = dose per fraction, and α/β ratio = description of cell response to radiation with higher values corresponding to earlier-responding tissue such as tumor cells.

101.2.2

4. Complete the following about cranial radiation:
a. After surgery most surgeons wait __ to __ days before irradiating.   7 to 10
b. Tumors that are very responsive to XRT include:
    i. l_____   lymphomas
    ii. g__ c__ t_____   germ cell tumors

101.2.3

5. What are the two normal CNS cell types most vulnerable to radiation necrosis?
a. v_____ _____   vascular endothelium
b. o_____ ____   oligodendroglial cells

101.2.3

6. **Seven major side effects of radiation:**   101.2.3

a. d_____ c_____   decreased cognition

b. r_____ n_____   radiation necrosis

c. o___ p_____ injury   optic pathway injury

d. h_____   hypopituitarism

e. p_____ h_____   primary hypothyroidism

f. formation of new _____   formation of new tumors – gliomas, meningiomas, nerve sheath tumors

g. l_____   leukoencephalopathy

7. **Two major treatments of radiation necrosis are:**   101.2.3

a. s_____   steroids

b. s_____   surgery (if deterioration from mass effect)

8. **What is the estimated dose of XRT that can be tolerated by normal brain tissue?**   About 65-75 Gy given as 5 fractions/week over 6.5-8 wks. Radiation necrosis will occur in about 5% of patients after 60 Gy given as 5 fractions/week over wks.   101.2.3

9. **True or False. Regarding the following imaging studies to detect radiation necrosis:**   101.2.3

a. MR spectroscopy is useful if mass is pure tumor.   true

b. MR spectroscopy is useful if mass is pure necrosis.   true

c. MR spectroscopy is useful if mass is a mix of tumor and necrosis.   false

d. RN will lead to decreased radionuclide uptake on SPECT imaging.   true

e. RN will lead to increased regional glucose metabolism on PET imaging.   false (will be decreased)

10. **Has radiation of spinal metastases been shown to prolong survival?**   No definitive proof of prolonged survival. Often used for pain relief and preservation of function.   101.2.4

11. **Side effects of spinal radiation include:**   101.2.4

a. m_____ or n_____   myelopathy or neuropathy

b. n_____, v_____, d_____   nausea, vomiting, diarrhea

c. b_____ m_____ s_____   bone marrow suppression

d. g_____ r_____ in children   growth retardation in children

e. development of c_____ m_____   cavernous malformations

101

12. What are important factors relating to the occurrence of radiation myelopathy? 101.2.4

a. r_____   rate of application
b. t_____ r_____ d____   total radiation dose
c. extent of c_____ s_____   extent of cord shielding
d. i_____ s_____   individual susceptibility
e. amount of t_____ r_____   amount of tissue radiated
f. v_____ s_____ to the region radiated   vascular supply
g. s____ of r_____   source of radiation

13. Describe the 4 types of radiation myelopathy. Table 101.1

a. Type 1   Benign form, mild sensory symptoms/Lhermitte's sign, occurs several months following XRT but usually resolves within several months.

b. Type 2   Lower motor neuron signs in upper or lower extremities due to injury to anterior horn cells.

c. Type 3   Complete cord lesion within hours due to blood vessel injury.

d. Type 4   Most common, chronic progressive myelopathy with initial paresthesias/Lhermitte's sign and eventual spastic weakness with hyperreflexia.

14. What radiation doses are associated with negligible risk of radiation myelopathy?   Dependent on field size. Large field: negligible risk with ≤ 3.3 Gy over 6 weeks (0.55 Gy/wk). Small field: negligible risk with ≤ 4.3 Gy over 6 weeks (0.717 Gy/wk).   101.2.4

101

■ Stereotactic Radiosurgery and Radiotherapy

15. The three main categories for delivery of SRS/SRT are: 101.3.1

a. G_____ K_____   Gamma Knife (gamma ray)
b. l_____ a_____   linear accelerator (x-ray)
c. h_____ c_____ p_____   heavy charged particle
   r_____   radiosurgery

16. The main source of gamma decay used in Gamma Knife is _____.   Cobalt-60   101.3.1

17. **In general, lesions less than _____ in diameter are amenable to treatment with SRS.**

< 3 cm

101.3.2

18. **What is the maximum recommended radiation dose to the following organs?**
    a. eye lens: ___ Gy
    b. optic nerve: ___ Gy
    c. skin in beam: ___ Gy
    d. thyroid: ___ Gy

1 Gy
1 Gy
0.5 Gy
0.1 Gy

101.3.4

19. **Is SRS useful for**
    a. venous angiomas?
    b. an AVM with a compact nidus?
    c. dural AVF with cortical drainage?

no
yes
no – high risk of hemorrhage with cortical drainage

101.3.5

101

20. **The V_____ R_____ A____ scale and P_____-F_____ score are useful scales to predict favorable outcome with AVM radiosurgery.**

Virginia Radiosurgery AVM Scale; Pollock-Flickinger score

101.3.5

21. **The gold standard (Level 1) recommendation for a single brain metastasis in an accessible region is s_____ r_____ plus W_____.**

surgical resection; WBRT

101.3.5

22. **True or False. Based on prospective randomized study data involving patients with a single brain metastasis:**
    a. Survival between SRS vs. surgery + WBRT is equal.
    b. There was a higher incidence of distant recurrence in the SRS arm.

true

true

101.3.5

23. **In pituitary adenomas treated with SRS, is the percentage of tumor growth control rate or endocrine remission rate higher?**

Overall tumor control rate has been reported as 90% vs. endocrine remission rates ranging from 26 – 54% depending on the hormone being over-secreted. Typically a higher dose of radiation is required for secretory tumors.

101.3.5

24. **Immediate adverse reactions to SRS include:**
    a. p_____ h_____
    b. n_____ and v_____
    c. s_____
    d. Adverse events have been reduced by pre-medicating with m_____ and p_____.

post-procedural headaches
nausea and vomiting
seizures
methylprednisolone; phenobarbital

101.3.5

25. **Complications from SRS include:**   101.3.5
a. v_____   vasculopathy
b. c_____ n_____ deficits   cranial nerve deficits
c. radiation-induced t_____   radiation-induced tumors
d. radiation-induced i_____ c_____ radiation-induced imaging
                                          changes

■ Interstitial Brachytherapy

26. **What are three techniques for**   101.4.2
        brachytherapy?
a. insertion of i__-_____ p_____   Iodine-125 pellets
b. insertion of c_____ containing catheters
    radioactive source
c. administration of r_____   radioactive liquids
    l_____

102

Endovascular Neurosurgery

■ General Information

1. **Contraindications to catheter angiography:**   102.1.3
   a. uncorrected b_____ disorders   bleeding
   b. poor r_____ function due to i_____ dye load   renal; iodine

---

■ Pharmacologic Agents

2. **Pharmacologic agents:**
   a. Brand name of abciximab is R_____.   ReoPro;   102.2.2
   b. Mechanism of action is that it prevents binding of f_____ to p_____ GP IIb/IIIa r_____.   fibrinogen; platelet; receptors
   c. Aspirin works by irreversibly inactivating c_____.   cyclo-oxygenase   102.2.3
   d. Uncoated aspirin achieves peak plasma concentrations in ___ - ___ minutes, whereas enteric-coated aspirin reaches peak in _____ hours.   30-40 minutes; 6 hours
   e. Up to _____% of patients are resistant to aspirin 325 mg/day.   30%
   f. Brand name of clopidogrel is P_____.   Plavix   102.2.4
   g. It is a platelet A_____ receptor antagonist.   ADP
   h. Start _____ days before procedure because it takes ___ - ___ days to reach full therapeutic effect.   5 days; 3-7 days
   i. Use _____ mg loading dose it there is no time to reach therapeutic effect over a few days.   300 mg
   j. Brand name of eptifibatide is I_____.   Integrilin   102.2.5
   k. It is a r_____ inhibitor of p_____ aggregation.   reversible; platelet
   l. ACT goal for embolization of an aneurysm or AVM is ____ - ____ seconds.   300-350 seconds   102.2.6
   m. ACT goal for angioplasty with/without stenting is ____ - ____ seconds.   250-300 seconds

n. Agent used to reverse heparin is p_____ s_____.

protamine sulfate

o. Agent used during Wada test is s_____ a_____.

sodium amytal

102.2.9

p. _____ mg is injected through catheter for Wada test with additional boluses of _____ mg if needed.

100 mg; 25 mg

q. tPA converts p_____ to p_____.

plasminogen; plasmin

102.2.10

r. Can be administered i_____ or i_____.

intravenously; intraarterially

s. tPA can be reversed using F_____.

FFP

t. Verapamil is a c_____ c_____ blocker that enables v_____.

calcium channel; vasodilation

102.2.11

Neuroendovascular Procedure Basics

3. **Neuroendovascular procedure basics:**

a. Vascular access can be obtained via f_____ artery, r_____ artery, b_____ artery, or c_____ artery.

femoral; radial; brachial; carotid

102.3.1

b. Arteriotomy closure options include m_____ pressure or percutaneous c_____ devices.

manual; closure

102.3.3

Disease-Specific Intervention

4. **Endovascular treatment of aneurysms:**

102.5.1

a. Endovascular treatment has emerged as a f_____ l_____ therapy for most aneurysms, but surgery still remains a strong option for M_____ and P_____ aneurysms.

first line; MCA; PICA

b. Wide necked aneurysms were previously thought better suited for c_____ but the availability of s_____ increased the spectrum of aneurysms amenable to endovascular treatment.

clipping; stents

c. Small aneurysms ____ ____ ____ mm are less favorable for c_____.

less than 4 mm; coiling

d. Another endovascular option for wide necked aneurysms is b_____-assisted coiling.

balloon

e. Most coils are made from b_____ p_____.

bare platinum

f. The p_____ e_____ device prevents b_____ e_____ into aneurysm and therefore encourages s_____.

pipeline embolization; blood entry; stasis

g. _____ month follow-up angiogram   6 month;
    usually reveals complete o_____ of   obliteration
    aneurysm.
h. Treatment of aneurysm rupture during
    coiling:
    i.   lower b_____ p_____   blood pressure
    ii.   inflate b_____ if being used   balloon
    iii. reverse a_____   anticoagulation
    iv.   continue c_____   coiling
    v.   insert E_____   EVD

5. **Management of vasospasm:**   102.5.2
a. Endovascular options include c_____   chemical;
    spasmolysis and a_____.   angioplasty
b. Drug of first choice for spasmolysis is   verapamil
    v_____.
c. R_____ treatments may be   Repeat
    considered.

6. **AVM embolization:**   102.5.3
a. Indications:
    i.   Most common indication is   pre-operative
          p_____ embolization.
    ii.   Embolization of associated   feeders; nidus
          aneurysms located on f_____ or
          in n_____.
    iii. Curative AVM embolization is   rare;
          r_____ and limited to s_____   small;
          AVMs with s_____   simple
          angioarchitecture.
b. 2 most common embolic agents include   onyx;
    o_____ and N_____.   NBCA
c. Radiopaque component of Onyx is   tantalum
    t_____.
d. Onyx requires priming microcatheter   DMSO;
    with D_____ to prevent Onyx   solidification
    s_____ within microcatheter.
e. NBCA is an embolic agent that is a   glue
    g_____.

7. **Dural arteriovenous fistula (DAVF):**
a. DAVF with a_____ features are   aggressive   102.5.4
    always considered for treatment.
b. These features include c_____   cortical venous reflux,
    v_____ r_____, h_____,   hemorrhage, focal
    f_____ n_____ d_____,   neurological deficit,
    d_____, p_____, and   dementia, papilledema;
    i_____ i_____ p_____.   increased intraocular pressure
c. T_____ approach is preferred.   Transvenous
d. Embolic materials that can be used   coils, onyx;   102.5.3
    include c_____, o_____, and   NBCA
    N_____.

102

8. **Carotid cavernous fistula (CCF):**   102.5.5
   a. Direct fistula requires t_____   treatment;
      because they do not resolve s_____.   spontaneously
   b. Endovascular routes used to treat CCF   transarterial, transvenous;
      are t_____, t_____, and via   superior ophthalmic vein
      s_____ o_____ v_____.
   c. Route and technique of choice is   transarterial coil
      t_____ c_____ embolization.
   d. Detachable balloons are n_____   no longer available
      l_____ a_____ in the U.S.

9. **Vertebrojugular fistula:**   102.5.6
   a. 3 main etiologies are i_____,   iatrogenic, trauma;
      t_____, or v_____.   vasculitis
   b. 2 main endovascular treatments are   covered stent;
      c_____ s_____ or c_____   coil occlusion
      o_____ if there is adequate blood
      flow through contralateral vertebral
      artery.

10. **Carotid dissection:**   102.5.7
    a. The most common angiographic feature   luminal stenosis (65%)
       is l_____ s_____ (_____%).
    b. Indications for endovascular intervention   ischemic;
       are persistent i_____ symptoms   anticoagulation; flow-
       despite a_____ or f_____-limiting   limiting;
       lesion with h_____ compromise.   hemodynamic
    c. Endovascular treatment consists of   stenting;
       s_____ with either c_____ or   covered or uncovered
       u_____ stent.

11. **Subclavian artery stenosis:**   102.5.8
    a. Only _____% of patients with   2.5%;
       subclavian artery stenosis have flow   reversal
       r_____ in the vertebral artery.
    b. Indication for endovascular intervention   subclavian steal syndrome
       is stenosis resulting in s_____
       s_____ s_____.
    c. Intervention consists of a_____ and   angioplasty;
       s_____.   stenting

12. **Mechanical thrombectomy for**   102.5.9
    ischemic stroke:
    a. May be performed within _____   6 hours
       hours of symptom onset.
    b. May be performed for posterior   24 hours
       circulation strokes up to _____
       hours after symptom onset.
    c. Current device of choice is the   stent retriever
       s_____ r_____.
    d. Recanalization rate with this device is   88-100%
       ____ - ____ %.
    e. An older device used is p_____   penumbra aspiration
       a_____.

f. Has a recanalization rate of _____%.   80%

g. Recanalization with the older device takes l_____ to achieve.   longer

13. Tumor embolization: 102.5.11

a. Purpose is preoperative d_____ of v_____ tumors, such as m_____.   devascularization; vascular; meningiomas

b. Embolization with P_____ particles is not d_____ and so surgery should be performed within a f_____ days of embolization.   PVA; durable; few

14. The PVA particle size that is typically used to treat epistaxis is ____ - ____ mcgm.   250-300 mcgm   102.5.13